LABORATORY EXERCISES IN RESPIRATORY CARE

Laboratory Exercises in Respiratory Care

by

Daniel J. Grady, R.R.T.

Director of Clinical Education
Respiratory Therapy Technology
Sandhills Community College
Carthage, North Carolina

with contributions by

William A. Byrtus, B.A., R.R.T.
Respiratory Therapy Program Director
Sandhills Community College
Carthage, North Carolina

Mary S. Grady, R.R.T.
Technical Director
Respiratory Care Department
St. Joseph of the Pines Hospital
Southern Pines, North Carolina

Susan Rinaldo, M.Ed., R.R.T.
Education Coordinator
Duke University Medical Center
Durham, North Carolina

17 92

J. B. LIPPINCOTT COMPANY
Philadelphia

London New York São Paulo
Mexico City St. Louis Sydney

Acquisitions Editor: Lisa A. Biello
Sponsoring Editor: Delois Patterson
Manuscript Editor: Leslie E. Hoeltzel
Design Coordinator: Susan Hess Blaker
Designer: Jack Grady
Production Manager: Kathleen P. Dunn
Production Coordinator: Ken Neimeister
Compositor: Progressive Typographers
Printer/Binder: R. R. Donnelley & Sons Company

1 3 5 6 4 2

Library of Congress Cataloging-in-Publication Data

Grady, Daniel J.
Laboratory exercises in respiratory care.

Includes bibliographies.
1. Respiratory therapy—Laboratory manuals.
I. Title. [DNLM: 1. Respiratory Therapy—examination questions. 2. Respiratory Therapy—laboratory manuals. WF 25 G733L]
RC735.I5G73 1986 615.8'36 86-7398
ISBN 0-397-50767-4

The authors and publishers have exerted every effort to ensure that drug selection and dosage set forth in this text are in accord with current recommendations and practice at the time of publication. However, in view of ongoing research, changes in government regulations, and the constant flow of information relating to drug therapy and drug reactions, the reader is urged to check the package insert for each drug for any change in indications and dosage and for added warnings and precautions. This is particularly important when the recommended agent is a new or infrequently employed drug.

"What is most complete is still incomplete;
Yet it is as complete as it can be."

Lao Tzu

"There is just one way to treat a cold,
and that is with contempt."

Sir William Osler

To That Which Provides Our Breath

PREFACE

Within the past three decades, respiratory care has emerged as a new health profession. As the profession evolved, numerous textbooks addressing respiratory care theory and equipment have been published. To date, very few introductory laboratory manuals have been available. *Laboratory Exercises in Respiratory Care* was written to introduce students to respiratory care procedures and equipment in the laboratory setting. Because laboratory courses frequently precede clinical application, it is hoped that this book may bridge the gap between introductory laboratory work and the clinical practice of respiratory care. The purpose of this book is to develop the cognitive and psychomotor skills of respiratory care students through laboratory practice.

Laboratory Exercises in Respiratory Care contains a number of unique features. The book has been designed specifically for students who may have had no previous exposure to respiratory care laboratory practices. Contained within the book are 48 different topics and more than 250 exercises. Each exercise is described in a detailed, step-by-step approach. The following elements are an integral part of each chapter: an introduction, behavioral objectives, requisite equipment, individual exercises, laboratory reports, recommended reading, and performance evaluation checklists. A concerted effort has been made to provide illustrations of critical performance elements and the technical apparatus needed to perform the exercises. The book also contains sections on laboratory safety and recommended laboratory techniques. In addition, the outline format moves the beginning student smoothly from the fundamental to the advanced procedures.

The individual exercises contained within each chapter were designed to be both flexible and clinically relevant. Many different brands of equipment may be used in completing the exercises. In several exercises, illustrations of "generic" equipment have been provided to allow fundamental component identification by the student. This design provides the instructor with the flexibility to select either available brands of equipment or the brands that the student is most likely to encounter in regional clinical settings.

Many of the exercises in *Laboratory Exercises in Respiratory Care* are clinically relevant because they involve the performance of respiratory care procedures, physiologic measurements, or the determination of "unknown" samples. As an example of an exercise requiring the determination of an "unknown," a student may be asked to analyze the oxygen concentration in a high flow system that had been previously set up and analyzed by the laboratory instructor. Exercises of this type provide both the student and the instructor with valuable feedback concerning the student's accuracy in laboratory practice. In addition, with creativity and careful planning, the laboratory instructor may develop an infinite number of exercises requiring individual determinations of an "unknown."

Because of the great variance in the clinical practice of respiratory care, it has been difficult to identify topics and procedural performance elements that are universally acceptable to most instructors. For these reasons, many of the topics relate to the competencies expected of entry-level respiratory care practitioners that have been identified by the National Board for Respiratory Care (NBRC). Since an actual patient care environment does not exist in the laboratory, only the performance elements relevant to the laboratory setting are emphasized.

Laboratory Exercises in Respiratory Care describes one way (not necessarily the only way) to perform procedures. Although I have tried to synthesize an enormous amount of technical information from widely dispersed sources, additional research is needed to establish firmly the scientific basis of respiratory care procedures.

DANIEL J. GRADY, R.R.T

ACKNOWLEDGMENTS

*LABORATORY EXERCISES IN RESPIRATORY CARE has been possible because of the dedication, commitment, and hard work of many people. The authors would like to express their sincere thanks to **Mary S. Grady, R.R.T.**, for the original illustrations and excellent visual art; **Carolyn Mitchell** for manuscript preparation; **Carole Browning** for secretarial services; **Kathleen Butz** for graphic design and preparation; **Arletta Gardner, R.T.(R.)**, and **Barbara McCullough, R.N.**, for technical research; **John Winks, C.R.T.T.**, for manuscript review and advice; **Dr. Vaud Travis** for motivation and support; **Dr. F. Farrell Collins** for inspiration; the authors who have kindly granted permission for reproduction of their work; the entire professional staff at **J. B. Lippincott Company** for advice, assistance, and support; **Jack Grady** for book design; and finally to our families, friends, and colleagues who sacrificed much while this book was being written.*

CONTENTS

LABORATORY EXERCISES IN RESPIRATORY CARE

INTRODUCTION

Laboratory Exercises in Respiratory Care has been written for the purpose of reinforcing respiratory care concepts and theory through laboratory practice. The exercises contained within this book are intended to supplement the material taught in didactic courses, and the book is not intended to be used exclusively as a textbook. For additional information on a specific topic, a recommended reading list is included at the end of each chapter.

The topics presented in the table of contents are not necessarily the sequence that may be selected by the laboratory instructor. I have noted, however, a consistently positive student response to laboratory work by beginning with the topics related to basic life support and cardiopulmonary resuscitation (CPR). As noted by the University of Hawaii Medical School faculty, an early introduction to CPR provides a practical foundation upon which to build concepts of cardiopulmonary anatomy, physiology, and pathology. In addition, students may recertify in CPR the following year and become eligible to meet the requirements for instructor certification.

The exercises in *Laboratory Exercises in Respiratory Care* should be set up before the scheduled laboratory session. Equipment function should be checked before demonstrations. Laboratory instructors may find it desirable to set up stations identified by letters (''A,'' ''B,'' ''C,'' and so forth) that correspond to individual exercises. In general, the laboratory functions best when supervised by an instructor.

Laboratory Safety

The following guidelines must be observed during all laboratory sessions.

GENERAL

1. Smoking, eating, and drinking are not allowed in the laboratory.
2. Instructor permission must be obtained before removing any equipment from the laboratory.
3. Instructor supervision is required if invasive procedures are practiced on classmates.
4. The administration of all medications and gases other than air or oxygen must be supervised by an instructor.
5. "No-smoking" signs must be posted during oxygen administration.

GAS CYLINDERS

1. Protective valve caps must be used whenever cylinders are transported or are not in use.
2. Gas cylinders must never violently strike another object.
3. Gas cylinders must be stabilized in a cart by a restraining chain or strap.
4. Small gas cylinders must be stabilized by a cart or stand.
5. Gas cylinder valves must never be opened or "cracked" while facing another person.
6. Equipment designed for a single gas type must not be modified or used for another gas type.
7. Oil and grease must never be allowed to come into contact with cylinder valve outlets or oxygen administration equipment.
8. The gas cylinder label should always match the color code. If the label does not match, do *not* use the cylinder.
9. Gas cylinders without a label should never be used.

Laboratory Techniques

PLANNING • NOTEBOOKS • REPORTS • INSTRUCTION • EVALUATION • EQUIPMENT

1. PLANNING

Efficient use of laboratory time is dependent upon adequate preparation by the student. Assigned topics should be reviewed before the scheduled laboratory session.

Students are highly encouraged to practice the performance of laboratory procedures. Extensive practice may be required in order to master invasive procedures.

2. LABORATORY NOTEBOOK

A loose-leaf notebook should be maintained. The laboratory notebook should contain all laboratory procedures, experiments, results, and reports.

3. LABORATORY REPORTS

Completed laboratory reports must be turned in no later than 1 week after the assigned topic. Late reports will be penalized. Incomplete laboratory reports are not acceptable.

4. METHOD OF INSTRUCTION

A lecture and demonstration of the assigned procedure will precede each laboratory session. After the lecture and demonstration, the student may complete the assigned procedure during the remaining time period or at any time that the laboratory is open. Available laboratory time will be posted.

5. METHODS OF EVALUATION

The student is evaluated by written reports and laboratory performance. Completion of individual procedure performance evaluations is required. The student should schedule an appointment or see the laboratory instructor for procedure performance evaluation.

6. EQUIPMENT CLEANING AND STORAGE

All equipment used by the student is to be completely disassembled, cleaned, and properly stored after use.

chapter 1

Single-rescuer cardiopulmonary resuscitation

INTRODUCTION

No skill is more fundamental in the practice of respiratory care than the ability to detect the presence (or absence) of adequate ventilation and circulation. Clinical death, consisting of absent breathing and circulation, may progress to irreversible biological death if basic resuscitative measures are not immediately instituted. The technique of cardiopulmonary resuscitation (CPR) consists of artificial ventilation combined with artificial circulation. The purpose of this chapter is to introduce you to the procedure of CPR performed by a single rescuer.

OBJECTIVES

After completing this chapter, you should be able to do the following:

1. *Position a victim for effective chest compression.*
2. *Identify three techniques for relieving acute airway obstruction caused by soft tissue (the tongue).*
3. *Establish the presence or absence of effective ventilation.*
4. *Establish the presence or absence of effective circulation.*
5. *Perform single-rescuer CPR.*

EQUIPMENT NEEDED

- ☐ CPR mannequin (recording mannequin or torso)
- ☐ Alcohol
- ☐ 4″ by 4″ gauze pads
- ☐ Size "D" batteries and paper for recording mannequin
- ☐ Watch with a second hand
- ☐ Sodium hypochlorite solution

ACTIVITIES

Exercise A: Establishing Unresponsiveness and Positioning

1. Upon encountering an apparently unconscious person or one with suspected cardiac, respiratory, or cardiopulmonary arrest, establish unresponsiveness by gently shaking the shoulder and loudly asking, "Are you all right?"
2. If the victim is unresponsive, request help from other people nearby.
3. Place the victim in the supine position. If the victim is lying face down, gently roll him as a unit by supporting the head, neck, and hips (Fig. 1-1). If positioning is required, grasp the head and neck with one hand to prevent twisting and possible cervical damage.
4. For chest compressions to be effective, it is necessary to place the back of the victim against a firm surface. If the victim is discovered in bed, insert a board or other rigid structure beneath his back.

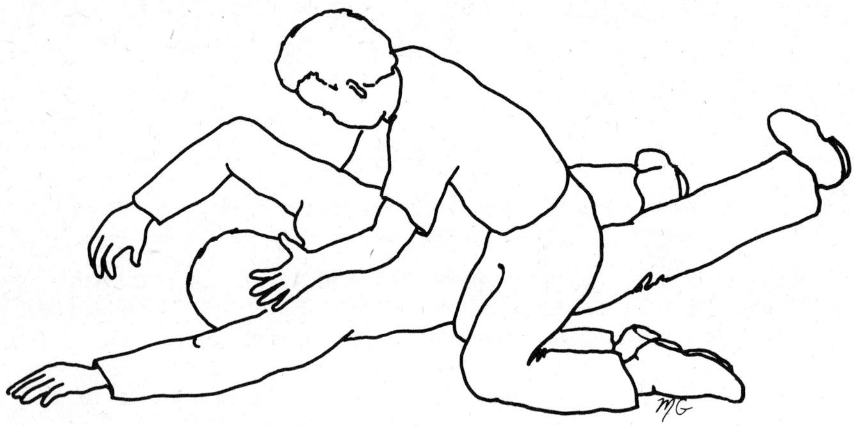

Fig. 1-1. Positioning the victim.

Exercise B: Opening the Airway

1. During unconsciousness or anoxia, the tongue may block the flow of gas between the upper and lower airway by falling against the posterior wall of the pharynx. Since the tongue is attached to the jaw, the manipulation of the jaw may lift the base of the tongue from the pharynx and create a clear path for gas flow between upper and lower airway (Fig. 1-2).
2. Three maneuvers may be used to open the airway and relieve soft tissue obstruction, including the head tilt–neck lift, the head tilt–chin lift, and the jaw thrust maneuvers.
3. Perform the head tilt–neck lift by positioning yourself at the victim's side. Place one hand on the victim's forehead. Place your other hand under his neck near the base of the skull. *Gently* lift the neck with one hand while tilting the forehead backward (Fig. 1-3).

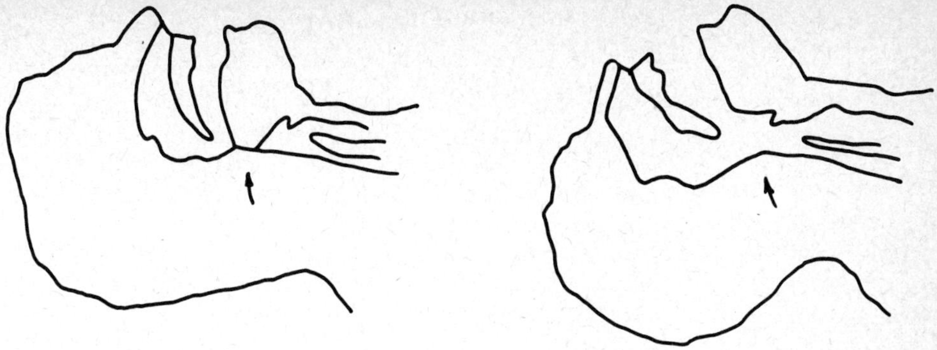

Fig. 1-2. Opening the airway. *(Reproduced with permission from Shapiro BA et al: Clinical Application of Respiratory Care, 3rd ed. Copyright © 1985 by Year Book Medical Publishers, Inc., Chicago).*

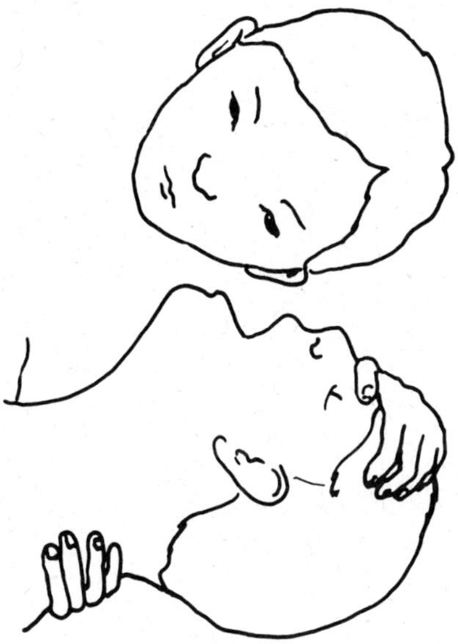

Fig. 1-3. Head tilt–neck lift.

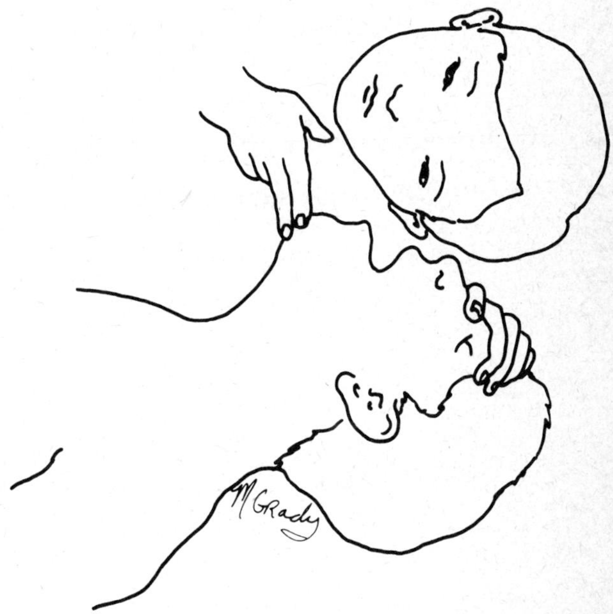

Fig. 1-4. Head tilt–chin lift.

4. Perform the head tilt–chin lift by positioning yourself at the victim's side. Place one hand on the victim's forehead. Place the other hand on the bony portion (not soft tissue) of the chin. Gently push the forehead backward while lifting the chin (Fig. 1-4). The head tilt–chin lift is the most effective way to open the airway manually.
5. Perform the jaw thrust maneuver by positioning yourself at the top of the patient's head. The jaw thrust maneuver is usually reserved for situations in which neck hyperextension is *not* desirable, as in suspected cervical injuries. During the maneuver, the head and neck are stabilized by placing the heels of your hands on the victim's cheek bones. Grasp the short portion of the jaw beneath the victim's ear lobes. Lift the jaw with your fingers (Fig. 1-5).

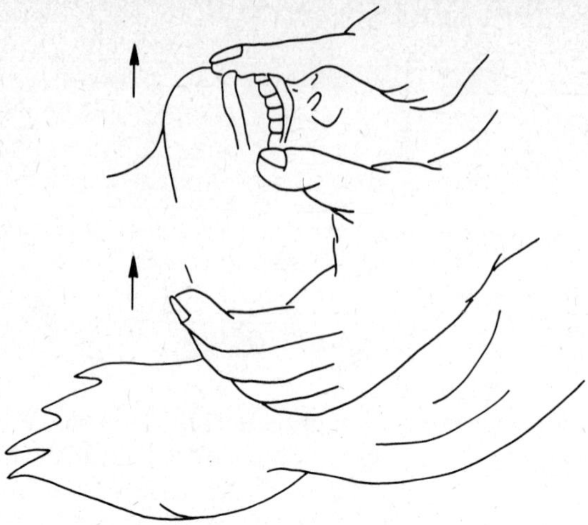

Fig. 1-5. Jaw thrust.

Exercise C: Establishing Breathlessness and Artificial Ventilation

1. After opening the airway, determine the presence (or absence) of adequate breathing by placing your ear directly over the victim's mouth and nose (Fig. 1-6).
2. While listening and feeling for exhaled air, observe the chest for movement. The presence of chest movement without hearing and feeling airflow does *not* guarantee adequate ventilation.
3. If breathing is absent, initiate a signal for advanced life support. To administer artificial ventilation, occlude the victim's external nares with your fingers and cover the victim's mouth with your mouth. Give two, deep breaths to reinflate the victim's lungs (Fig. 1-7). The two initial ventilations are given at 1.0 to 1.5 seconds per breath.

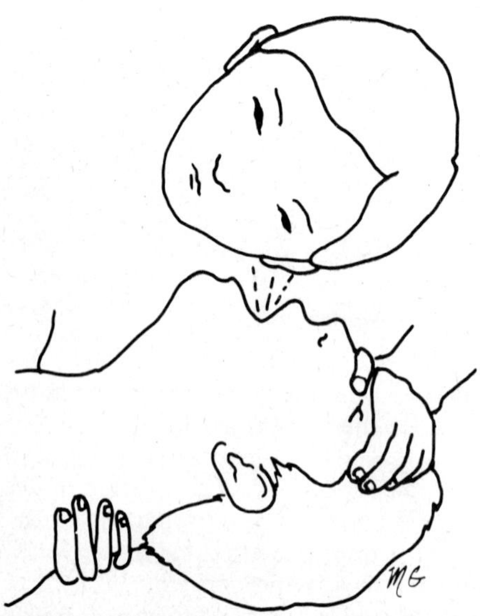

Fig. 1-6. Establishing breathlessness by looking, listening, and feeling for air flow.

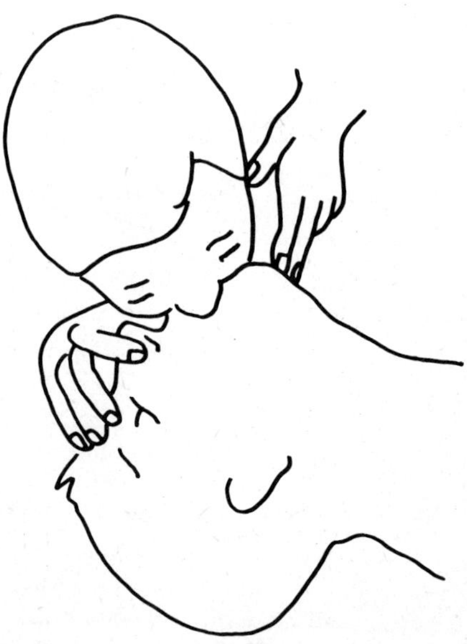

Fig. 1-7. Artificial ventilation by mouth-to-mouth breathing.

4. Variations in mouth-to-mouth breathing for artificial ventilation may include mouth-to-nose breathing, mouth-to-tracheostomy stoma breathing, and mouth-to-tube breathing. Practice as many of the variations in artificial ventilation as required by your laboratory instructor.

Exercise D: Establishing Pulselessness and Chest Compressions

1. After opening the airway and giving artificial ventilation, evaluate the presence (or absence) of circulation by palpating the carotid pulse.
2. To locate the carotid pulse, palpate the thyroid cartilage (Adam's apple) in the neck. After locating the thyroid cartilage, slide your fingers into the first large groove to the side of the cartilage (Fig. 1-8).
3. To avoid the accidental administration of chest compressions when a palpable pulse exists, be sure to palpate the carotid pulse for 5 to 10 seconds.
4. When the pulse is absent, chest compressions must be administered. To give effective chest compressions, proper hand location is essential. Using two fingers, locate the notch between the ribs and the xiphoid process. While maintaining two fingers in the notch, place the heel of your other hand midline and on the lower half of the sternum (Fig. 1-9).
5. Both of your shoulders should be directly over the victim's sternum. Only the heel of your hand should contact the victim's sternum. Your fingers may be interlaced. Your elbows should be "locked." Compress the sternum with smooth, even compressions to a depth of 1 ½ to 2 inches. Compress the chest at a rate of 80 to 100 compressions/minute (Fig. 1-10).
6. After 15 compressions, move to the victim's head and open the airway. Give two quick, full breaths.
7. After two ventilations, return to the chest and check for proper hand placement. Continue to administer 15 compressions alternating with two breaths as directed by your laboratory instructor.

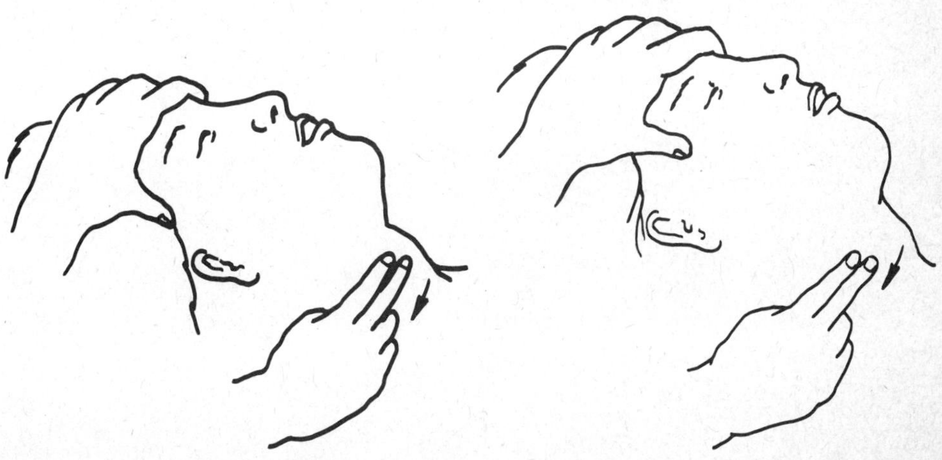

Fig. 1-8. Establishing pulselessness by carotid artery palpation. *(Modified from American Heart Association: Standards and guidelines for cardiopulmonary resuscitation (CPR) and emergency cardiac care (ECC). JAMA 255:2919, 1986)*

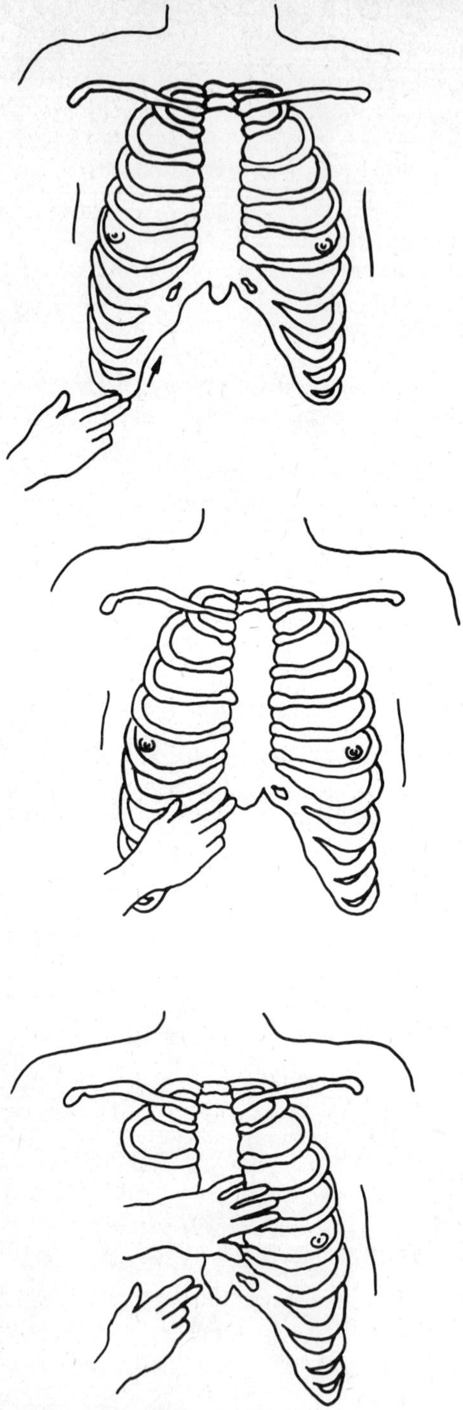

Fig. 1-9. Location of xiphoid process for external chest compression.

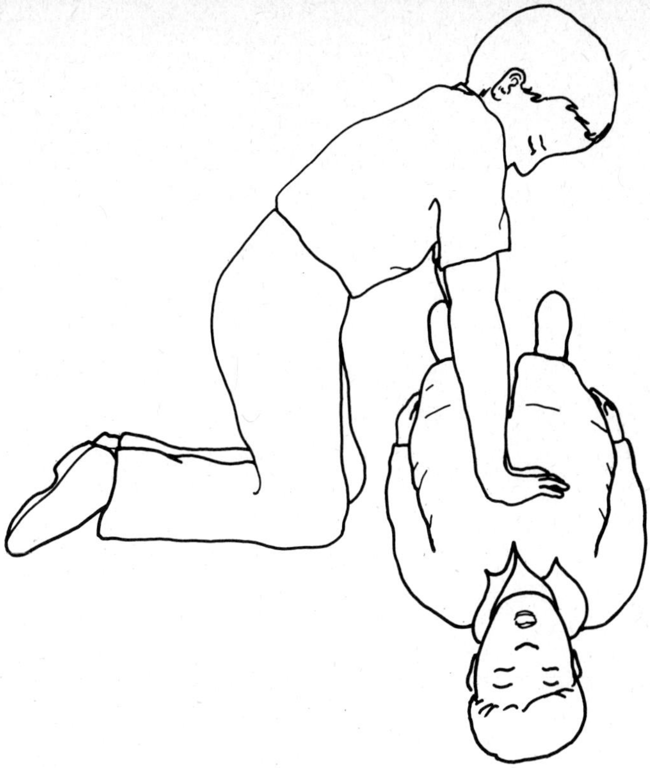

Fig. 1-10. Adult chest compression technique.

Exercise E: Evaluating the Effectiveness of CPR

1. After the first minute of CPR, and after every few minutes, stop CPR and check for the return of spontaneous breathing and a palpable pulse.
2. If breathing is absent but a pulse is palpable, provide artificial breathing about 12 times/ minute.
3. If neither breathing nor a pulse is present, continue to administer artificial ventilation and artificial circulation for 1 minute.
4. It is optional to check for constriction of the pupil when the pupil is exposed to light.

RECOMMENDED READING

Burton GG, Hodgkin JE: Respiratory Care. A Guide to Clinical Practice, 2nd ed. Philadelphia, JB Lippincott, 1984

Lewis AJ, Montgomery WH, Guildner CW et al: A Manual for Instructors of Basic Cardiac Life Support. Dallas, Ameican Heart Association, 1981

Montgomery WH, Herrin TJ (eds): Student Manual for Basic Life Support. Dallas, American Heart Association, 1981

Safar P: Cardiopulmonary Cerebral Resuscitation. Philadelphia, WB Saunders, 1981

Standards and Guidelines for Cardiopulmonary Resuscitation (CPR) and Emergency Cardiac Care (EEC). JAMA 255;21, 1986

Laboratory Performance Evaluation (#1)

Topic: Single-Rescuer Cardiopulmonary Resuscitation

Student ______________________ Course ______________________

Date ______________________ Section ______________________

Performance Elements	Acceptable	Unacceptable	Not Applicable	Comments
1. Establishes unresponsiveness				
2. Calls for help				
3. Positions victim				
4. Opens airway				
5. Establishes breathlessness				
6. Initiates signal for advanced life support				
7. Administers two ventilations				
8. Establishes pulselessness (5–10 seconds)				
9. Determines proper hand placement				
10. Administers chest compressions				
11. Administers combination of 2 ventilations and 15 compressions for 8 cycles				
12. Evaluates victim for return of pulse and spontaneous breathing after 1 minute				

Knowledge of Procedure

- ☐ Good; student is knowledgeable about rationale and theory related to procedure
- ☐ Fair; student has adequate understanding of rationale and theory related to procedure
- ☐ Poor; student has inadequate understanding of rationale and theory related to procedure

Performance Deficiencies (check those that apply)

- ☐ Excessive time needed to complete procedure
- ☐ Broke aseptic or sterile technique
- ☐ Gross inaccuracy noted
- ☐ Technique may be harmful to patient
- ☐ Incorrect dosage or gas concentration
- ☐ Incorrect equipment assembly/use
- ☐ Unable to answer questions correctly about rationale and/or theory related to procedure
- ☐ Other ______________________________

Evaluation Summary

- ☐ Satisfactory performance
- ☐ Unsatisfactory performance

Recommendations of Evaluator

- ☐ Skills may be applied/observed in clinical setting
- ☐ Specific evaluation deficiencies require correction
- ☐ Complete re-evaluation required
- ☐ Additional laboratory practice required

Signatures:

Evaluator ______________________ Date ______________________

Student ______________________ Date ______________________

Laboratory Report

Student ______________________ Acceptable ______________________

Date ______________________ Unacceptable ______________________

Course ______________________

Topic: Single-Rescuer Cardiopulmonary Resuscitation

Scenario: As you enter the emergency room, you happen to glance into one of the medical rooms in time to hear the audible alarm on the patient's ECG monitor sound. As you approach the patient, you notice that he does not seem to be breathing. His eyes stare blankly at the ceiling, and his pupils are fixed and dilated. Please answer the following questions:

1. How should the airway be opened for this victim who presents in the emergency room with a suspected neck injury?

2. What are three ways to detect the presence of adequate spontaneous breathing?

3. Why must a victim of a cardiac arrest be placed in the supine position against a firm surface?

4. After attempting the head tilt–neck lift maneuver for an unconscious victim, what should be suspected if the victim has chest movement but airflow is neither felt nor heard while checking for adequate breathing?

5. Why is it important to palpate the pulse for a period of 5 to 10 seconds?

6. Describe briefly how you would proceed if a victim

A. is *not* breathing and has no pulse.

B. is not breathing and has a palpable pulse.

C. resumes spontaneous breathing and has a pulse after 10 minutes of CPR.

chapter 2

Two-rescuer cardiopulmonary resuscitation

INTRODUCTION

Prolonged basic life support frequently is performed by two (or more) members of the health care team. When properly performed, two-rescuer CPR may be more efficient than single-rescuer CPR since momentary pauses between compressions and breaths are avoided. Although differences exist, the fundamental ABC's (airway, breathing, and circulation) of two rescuer CPR are similar to those of single-rescuer CPR. The purpose of this chapter is to introduce you to the technique of two-rescuer CPR.

OBJECTIVES

After completing this chapter you should be able to do the following:

1. *Perform two-rescuer CPR.*
2. *Compare and contrast the technique of two-rescuer CPR with single-rescuer CPR.*
3. *Efficiently change positions during two-rescuer CPR.*
4. *Evaluate the effectiveness of chest compressions by another rescuer.*

EQUIPMENT NEEDED

- ☐ CPR mannequin (recording mannequin or torso)
- ☐ Alcohol pads
- ☐ 4″ by 4″ gauze pads
- ☐ Size "D" batteries and paper for recording mannequin.
- ☐ Watch with a second hand
- ☐ Replacement lungs
- ☐ Disinfectant solution (sodium hypochlorite solution: household bleach)

ACTIVITIES

Exercise A: Evaluating CPR in Progress

1. Initiate CPR using the single-rescuer technique for a minimum of four complete cycles.
2. Upon arrival of a second rescuer, the second rescuer indicates that assistance will be given.
3. The second rescuer should obtain a position beside the victim's head and across from the first rescuer.
4. While chest compressions are delivered by the first rescuer, the newly arrived rescuer palpates the carotid artery to check for effective compressions (Fig. 2-1).
5. In reality, when compressions are adequate, a pulse may be palpated with each compression.
6. The second rescuer maintains an open airway and places an ear directly over the victim's mouth and nose to assess ventilation.
7. The second rescuer informs the first rescuer to "stop compressions" in order to check for the return of spontaneous breathing and pulse. Both breathing and circulation are simultaneously checked for about 5 seconds.

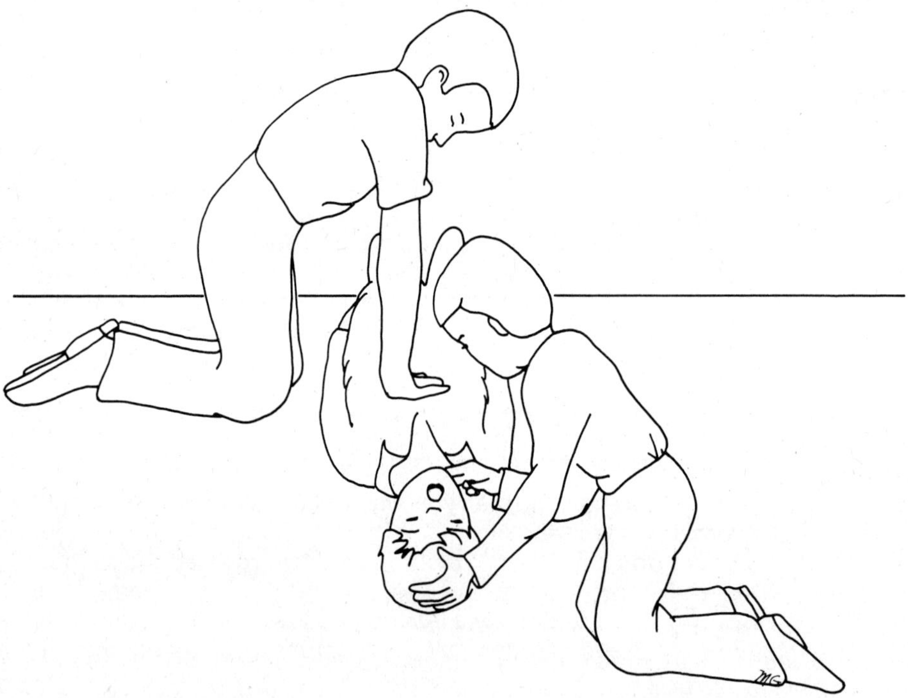

Fig. 2-1. Evaluation of chest compressions by checking the pulse during compressions.

Exercise B: Initiating Two-Rescuer CPR

1. If neither spontaneous breathing nor a pulse is present, two-rescuer CPR is initiated.
2. The second rescuer opens the airway and delivers a single ventilation (Fig. 2-2).
3. After the delivery of a single ventilation, the second rescuer informs the first rescuer to "continue compressions" (if a pulse was not palpable).

4. The rescuer compressing the chest provides about 80 to 100 compressions per minute.
5. Breaths are administered at a minimum rate of 12–16/minute during two-rescuer CPR, yielding a ratio of compressions to breaths of about 5:1.
6. The rescuer delivering compressions may elect to use a mnemonic to set the pace for the two-rescuer technique. The mnemonic recommended by the American Heart Association is "one-and, two-and, three-and, four-and, five-and, one and, . . ." and so on.
7. The rescuer providing compressions should pause 1.0 to 1.5 seconds to allow a breath to be given.

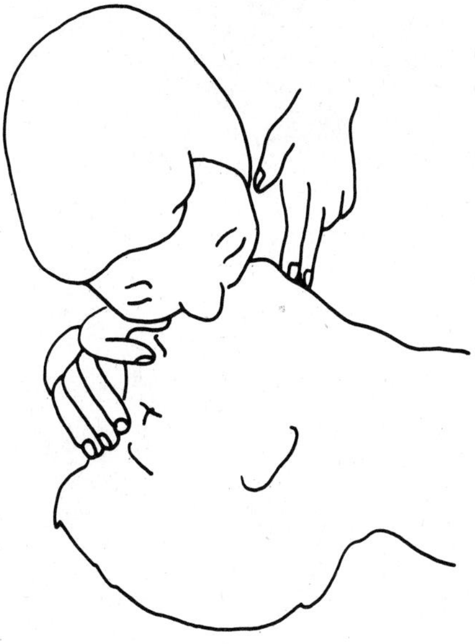

Fig. 2-2. Opening the airway and delivery of ventilation by second rescuer.

Exercise C: Maintaining Airway Patency and Ventilation

1. During two-rescuer CPR, a ventilation is given after every fifth compression.
2. The airway is completely opened after the fourth compression, and a mouth-to-mouth seal with slight pressurization of the airway is made during the downstroke of the fifth compression.
3. The breath is given during the upstroke of the fifth compression. The rescuer giving ventilations may attempt to blow the compressor's hands up from the victim's chest during the upstroke of the fifth compression (Fig. 2-3).
4. Should vomiting occur during CPR, the victim's body is turned to the side, the mouth and oropharynx are swept clear, and the airway is reopened for resumption of CPR.

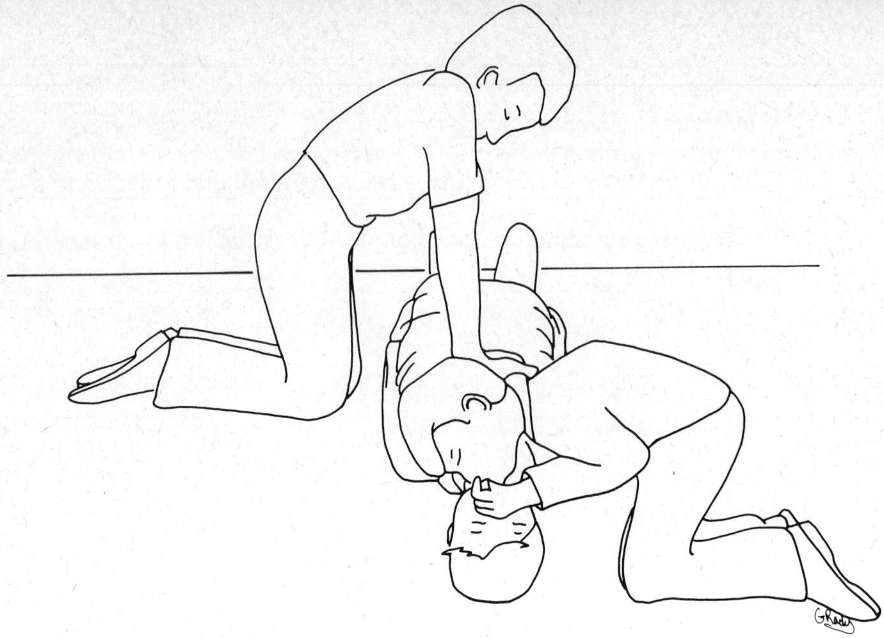

Fig. 2-3. Technique of two-rescuer CPR.

Exercise D: Changing Position During Two-Rescuer CPR

1. Initiate two-rescuer CPR for about 2 minutes.
2. After 2 minutes of CPR, the rescuer performing compressions may call for a change in positions by using the following mnemonic: "one-and, two-and, three-and, four-and, five-and, next-time-change-on-five, one-and, two-and, three-and, four-and five."
3. The rescuer at the head gives a breath, moves adjacent to the chest, and finds proper hand location and placement in preparation for compressions (Fig. 2-4).
4. The rescuer at the chest moves to the victim's head, opens the airway, and simultaneously checks for the return of spontaneous breathing and a pulse.
5. If neither spontaneous breathing nor a pulse is present, the rescuer at the head gives a breath and states "continue CPR" (Fig. 2-5).

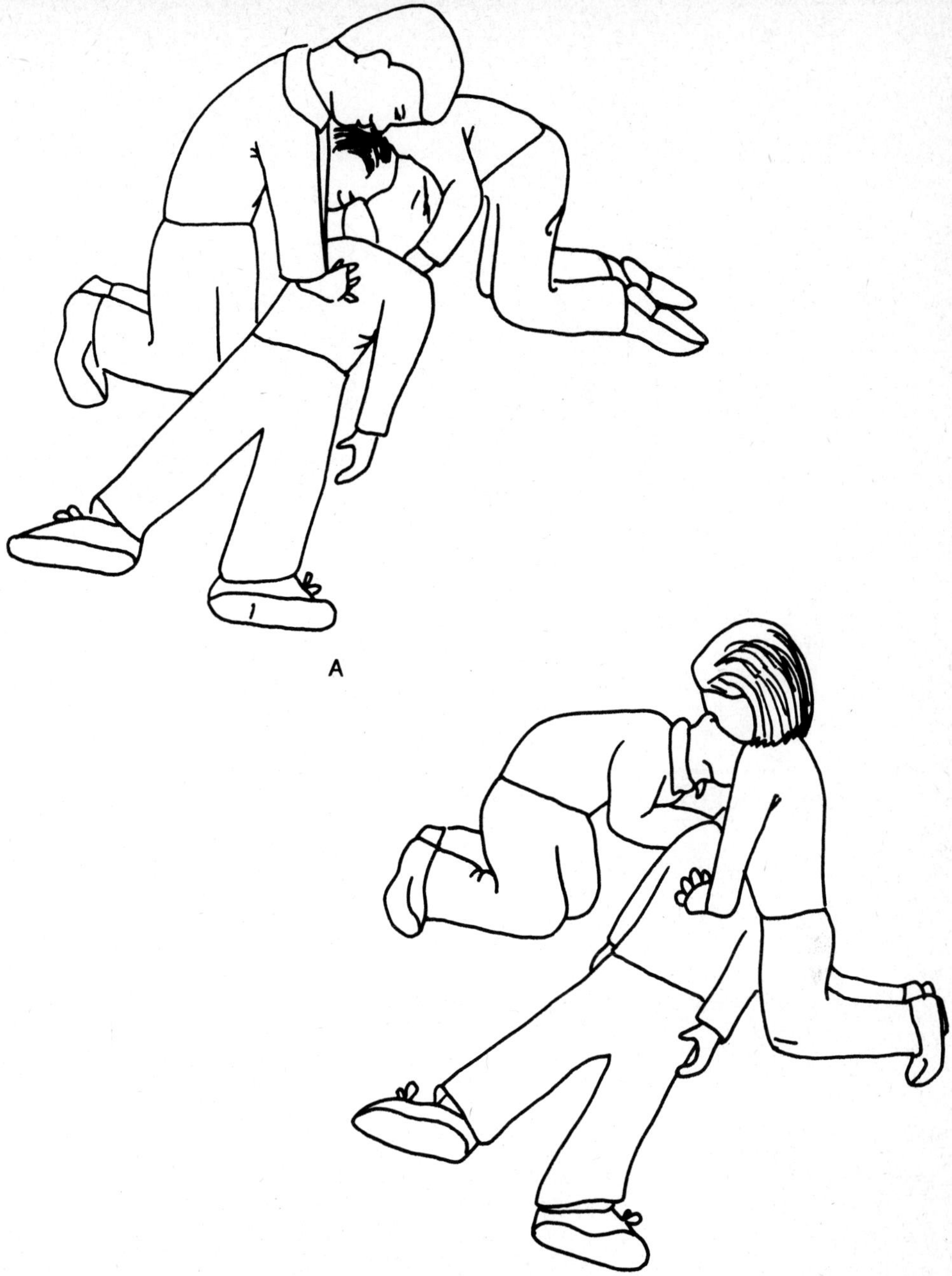

A

B

Fig. 2-4. Delivery of a breath immediately before position change during two-rescuer CPR.

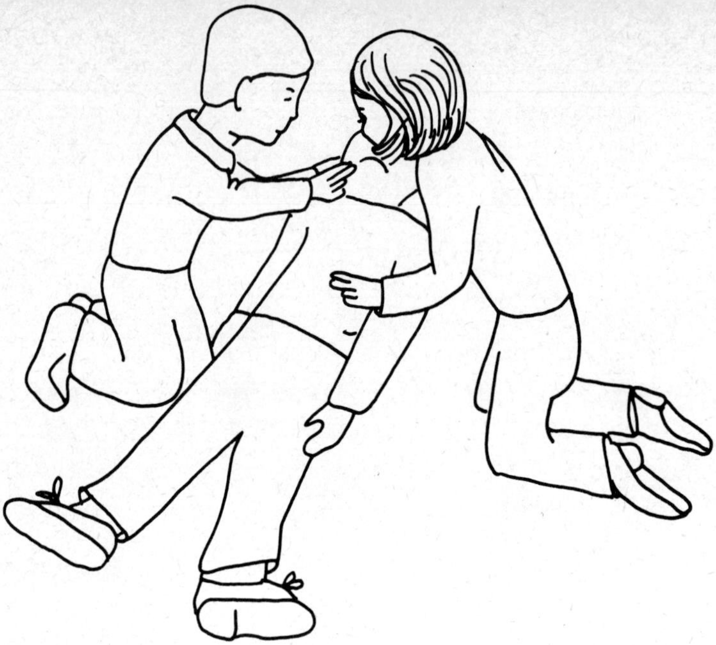

Fig. 2-5. Palpation of pulse and assessment of ventilation by second-rescuer after position change.

RECOMMENDED READING

Burton GG, Hodgkin JE: Respiratory Care. A Guide to Clinical Practice, 2nd ed. Philadelphia, JB Lippincott, 1984

Lewis AJ, Montgomery WH, Guildner CW et al: A Manual for Instructors of Basic Cardiac Life Support. Dallas, American Heart Association, 1981

Montgomery WH, Herrin TJ (eds): Student Manual for Basic Life Support. Dallas, American Heart Association, 1981

Safar P: Cardiopulmonary Cerebral Resuscitation. Philadelphia, WB Saunders, 1981

Standards and Guidelines for Cardiopulmonary Resuscitation (CPR) and Emergency Cardiac Care (EEC). JAMA 255:21, 1986

Laboratory Performance Evaluation (#2)

Topic: Two-Rescuer Cardiopulmonary Resuscitation

Student ______________________ Course ______________________

Date ______________________ Section ______________________

Performance Elements	Acceptable	Unacceptable	Not Applicable	Comments
1. Single-rescuer CPR initiated				
2. Second rescuer arrives and monitors carotid pulse				
3. Second rescuer requests that compressions be stopped				
4. Second rescuer simultaneously checks for spontaneous breathing and pulse (5 seconds)				
5. Activates "code" signal for advanced life support				
6. Second rescuer gives a ventilation				
7. Second rescuer states "continue CPR"				
8. Two-rescuer CPR technique includes A. Compression rate: 80/minutes B. One ventilation follows every fifth compression				
9. Ratio of compression to breaths is 5:1				
10. Two-rescuer technique continues for 2 minutes				
11. Rescuers switch positions to instructor's satisfaction				

Knowledge of Procedure

- ☐ Good; student is knowledgeable about rationale and theory related to procedure
- ☐ Fair; student has adequate understanding of rationale and theory related to procedure
- ☐ Poor; student has inadequate understanding of rationale and theory related to procedure

Performance Deficiencies (check those that apply)

- ☐ Excessive time needed to complete procedure
- ☐ Broke aseptic or sterile technique
- ☐ Gross inaccuracy noted
- ☐ Technique may be harmful to patient
- ☐ Incorrect dosage or gas concentration
- ☐ Incorrect equipment assembly/use
- ☐ Unable to answer questions correctly about rationale and/or theory related to procedure
- ☐ Other ______________________________

Evaluation Summary

- ☐ Satisfactory performance
- ☐ Unsatisfactory performance

Recommendations of Evaluator

- ☐ Skills may be applied/observed in clinical setting
- ☐ Specific evaluation deficiencies require correction
- ☐ Complete re-evaluation required
- ☐ Additional laboratory practice required

Signatures:

Evaluator ______________________ Date ______________________

Student ______________________ Date ______________________

Laboratory Report

Student ______________________ Acceptable ______________________

Date ______________________ Unacceptable ______________________

Course ______________________

Topic: Two-Rescuer Cardiopulmonary Resuscitation

Scenario: You are about to leave the emergency room on your way back to the surgery crash room when a medical patient suffers a cardiac arrest. You don't know how long you have been performing single-rescuer CPR, but just when you think that help will never arrive, a nurse's aide happens by. Please answer the following questions:

1. When monitoring the pulse during compressions by another rescuer, briefly describe what you would do if you were unable to palpate a pulse.

2. Briefly state the difference in technique between two- and one-rescuer CPR for
   A. rate of compressions

   B. rate of ventilations

   C. ratio of compressions to breaths

3. Under most circumstances (other than transporting patients, intubation, and calling for help), what is the maximum length of time allowable for interruptions in CPR?

4. Describe what you would do if the victim vomits during CPR.

5. During two-rescuer CPR, why is the proper rate of compressions important for allowing effective ventilations to be administered?

chapter 3

Infant and child cardiopulmonary resuscitation

INTRODUCTION

Regardless of the age or size of a person experiencing a respiratory arrest (absence of effective breathing) or a cardiac arrest (absence of effective circulation), the fundamental principles of resuscitation are similar. The essence of basic life support and CPR is that when breathing is absent, ventilation is given through an open airway. When the pulse is absent, chest compressions are given. Although the fundamental principles of CPR for adults are similar to those used for infants and children, major differences exist between the techniques. The purpose of this chapter is to introduce you to the techniques of CPR for infants and children.

OBJECTIVES

After completing this chapter, you should be able to do the following:

1. *Perform infant and child CPR.*
2. *Identify differences in airway management, artificial ventilation, and chest compression that exist among infant, child, and adult CPR.*
3. *Cite the American Heart Association specifications for both one and two rescuer cardiopulmonary resuscitation techniques applied to an adult, child, or infant victim.*

EQUIPMENT NEEDED

- ☐ CPR mannequins (infant and child)
- ☐ 70% isopropyl alcohol
- ☐ 4″ by 4″ gauze pads
- ☐ Watch with a second hand
- ☐ Replacement lungs
- ☐ Disinfectant solution (sodium hypochlorite: bleach solution)

ACTIVITIES

Exercise A: Establishing Unresponsiveness and Positioning an Infant

1. Your instructor will provide you with an infant mannequin.
2. Establish unresponsiveness by *gently* tapping or shaking the infant and saying, "Wake up!" An alternative physical stimulus such as flicking the infant's toes with your finger is acceptable (Fig. 3-1).
3. If the infant is unresponsive, call for help.
4. While supporting the head and neck, turn, if necessary, and place the infant in a supine, horizontal position.

Exercise B: Opening the Infant Airway and Establishing Breathlessness

1. Open the infant's airway by moderately lifting the neck (or chin) while gently tipping back the forehead. It is essential to avoid extreme hyperextension of the head and neck because airway obstruction may be paradoxically produced owing to compression of the soft, developing trachea (Fig. 3-2).
2. The airway may be opened by using the head tilt–chin lift or the head tilt–neck lift maneuvers.
3. After opening the infant's airway, evaluate the presence (or absence) of breathing by looking at the chest and by listening and feeling for gas flow. To listen and feel for gas flow, place your ear directly over the infant's nose and mouth while looking at the chest (Fig. 3-3).
4. If breathing is present, you should see the chest (or abdomen) rise upward and outward during inspiration, and you should hear and feel exhaled air.

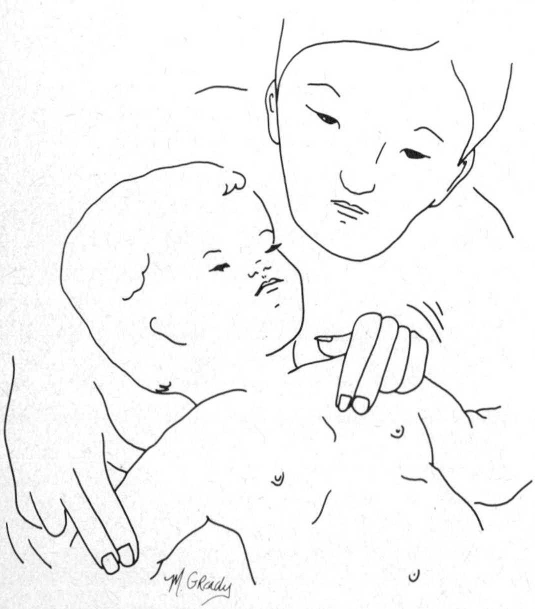

Fig. 3-1. Establishment of unresponsiveness in an infant.

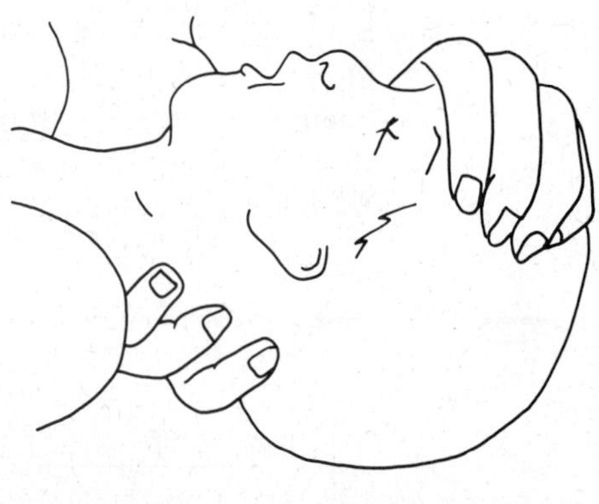

Fig. 3-2. Opening the airway of an infant. *(Modified from American Heart Association: Standards and guidelines for CPR and ECC. JAMA 255:2956, 1986)*

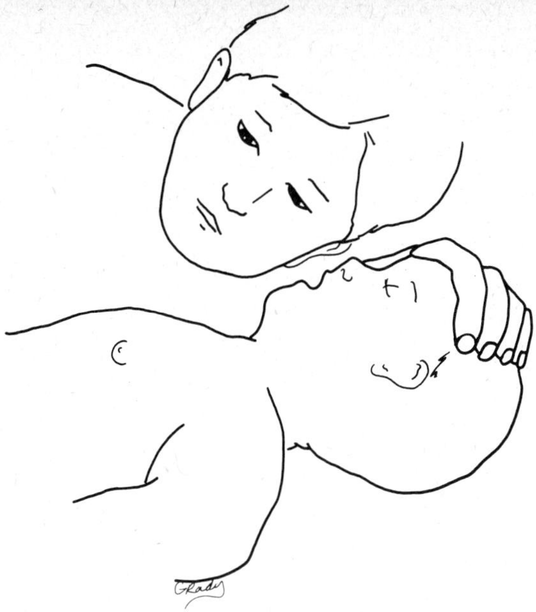

Fig. 3-3. Detection of breathlessness by looking, listening, and feeling for airflow.

Exercise C: Artificially Ventilating an Infant

1. If breathing is absent, maintain an open airway and give artificial ventilation. Simulate the initiation of a "code" signal for advanced life support.
2. While maintaining an open airway, cover both the nose and mouth of the infant with your mouth. Give two puffs of air to reinflate the infant's lungs (Fig. 3-4). Allow a slight pause between breaths.
3. When giving breaths to an infant, attempt to use the smallest volume of air that causes effective chest movement. Because of the risks of gastric inflation or pneumothorax, it is essential to limit the volume of ventilation to that which moves the chest.

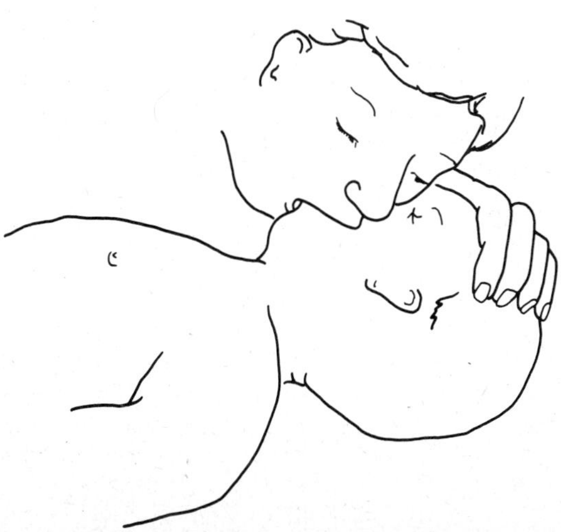

Fig. 3-4. Artificial ventilation of a neonate. *(Modified from American Heart Association: Standards and guidelines for CPR and ECC. JAMA 255:2956, 1986)*

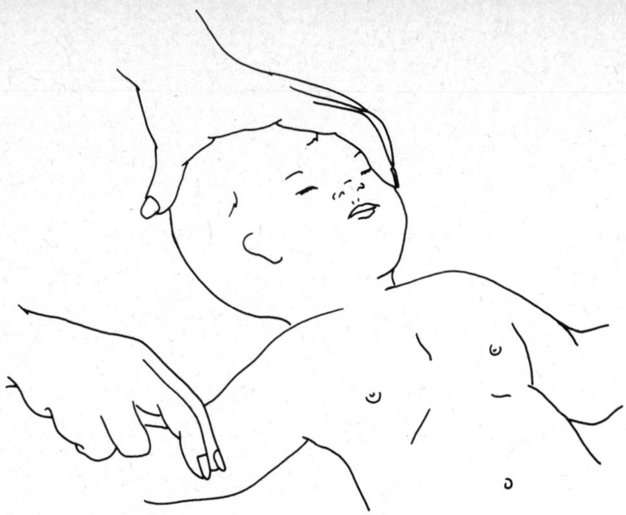

Fig. 3-5. Establishing pulselessness in a neonate by brachial artery palpation.

Exercise D: Establishing Pulselessness and Infant Chest Compressions

1. After delivering two ventilations, evaluate the pulse.
2. In an infant, palpate the brachial pulse for about 5 seconds. (The brachial pulse is checked because the short neck of an infant makes it difficult to palpate the carotid pulse.) The brachial pulse is located near the medial side of the elbow (Fig. 3-5).
3. When no pulse is present, give chest compressions.
4. Using two fingers, the index and middle fingers, locate the middle of the sternum, about one fingerbreadth below the intermammary line. Place two fingers midline on the sternum and compress straight down to a depth of 0.5 to 1.0 inch. The chest is compressed at the rate of 100 compressions/minute. A breath is given after every fifth compression, regardless of the number of rescuers involved (Fig. 3-6).
5. An alternative method of infant chest compression is to encircle the chest with both your hands and to compress the midsternum with both thumbs. This technique is useful when a firm surface is unavailable for compression or during two-rescuer CPR (Fig. 3-7).

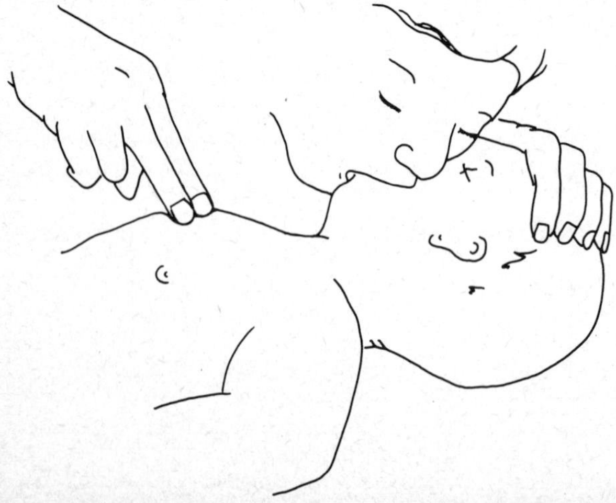

Fig. 3-6. Techniques of artificial ventilation and chest compressions of a neonate.

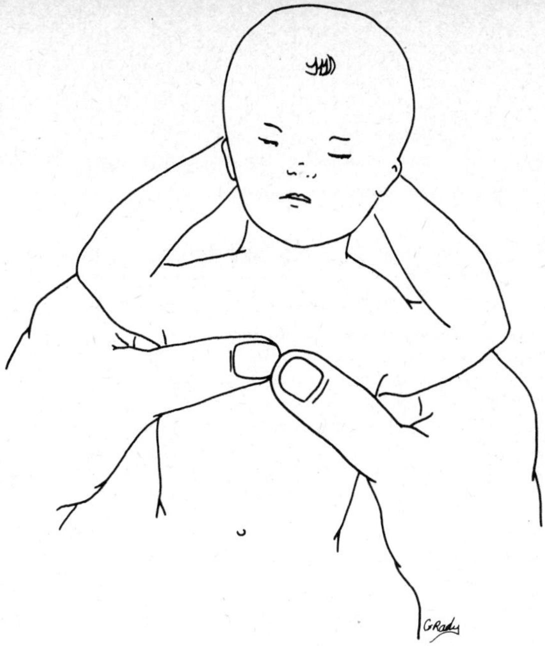

Fig. 3-7. Alternative method of chest compression of a neonate.

Exercise E: CPR of a Child

1. Your instructor may provide you with a child mannequin, which may be used for practicing resuscitation for individuals between 1 and 8 years of age. The age and the size of the individual determine the resuscitative technique used.
2. Establish responsiveness by gently shaking the shoulder and asking, "Are you all right?"
3. If unresponsive, call for help.
4. Open the airway using the head tilt–chin lift method.
5. After opening the airway, evaluate breathing adequacy by looking at the chest and by listening and feeling for exhaled gas flow.
6. If breathing is absent, maintain an open airway, pinch the nose, and give two quick breaths. Watch the chest to be certain that the breaths provide adequate lung inflation.

Table 3-1. CPR Specifications

	Approximate Breath Rate per Minute	Compression Rate per Minute	Compression Depth (inches)	Ratio Compressions/ Breath
One Rescuer				
Infant	20	100	0.5–1.0	5:1
Child	16	80	1.0–1.5	5:1
Adult	12	80	1.5–2.0	15:2
Two Rescuer				
Infant	20	100	Same as one rescuer	5:1
Child	16	80	Same as one rescuer	5:1
Adult	16	80	1.5–2.0	5:1

7. After giving two breaths, check the carotid pulse for about 5 seconds.
8. If no pulse is present, compress the chest.
9. Give chest compressions to a child by positioning the heel of one hand at the middle of the sternum.
10. Compress the chest with the heel of one hand to a depth of 1 to 1.5 inches.
11. Give chest compressions at a rate of 80 compressions/minute.
12. A breath is given after every fifth compression regardless of the number of rescuers involved.
13. Review the summary of American Heart Association specifications for CPR in Table 3-1.

RECOMMENDED READING

Burgess WR, Chernick V: Respiratory Therapy in Newborn Infants and Children. New York, Thieme-Stratton, 1982

Burton GG, Hodgkin JE: Respiratory Care. A Guide to Clinical Practice, 2nd ed. Philadelphia, JB Lippincott, 1984

Goldsmith JP, Karotkin EH: Assisted Ventilation of the Neonate. Philadelphia, WB Saunders, 1981

Klaus MH, Fanaroff AA: Care of the High Risk Neonate. Philadelphia, WB Saunders, 1973

Lough MD, Williams TJ, Rawson JE: Newborn Respiratory Care. Chicago, Year Book Medical Publishers, 1979

Standards and Guidelines for Cardiopulmonary Resuscitation (CPR) and Emergency Cardiac Care (ECC). JAMA 255:21, 1986

Laboratory Performance Evaluation (#3)

Topic: Infant and Child Cardiopulmonary Resuscitation

Student ______________________ Course ______________________

Date ______________________ Section ______________________

Performance Elements	Acceptable	Unacceptable	Not Applicable	Comments
1. Establishes unresponsiveness				
2. Calls for help				
3. Positions infant				
4. Opens the airway				
5. Looks, listens, and feels for breathing				
6. Activates signal for advanced life support				
7. Gives two breaths				
8. Checks the brachial pulse for 5 seconds to determine pulselessness				
9. Compresses midsternum at a rate of 100/minute				
10. Compresses chest to a depth of ½ to 1 inch				
11. Maintains a ratio of compressions to breaths of 5:1				
12. Continues infant CPR for 1 minute				

Performance Elements	Acceptable	Unacceptable	Not Applicable	Comments
13. Rechecks for spontaneous breathing and pulse				
14. Continues sequence to satisfaction of the instructor				

Knowledge of Procedure

☐ Good; student is knowledgeable about rationale and theory related to procedure

☐ Fair; student has adequate understanding of rationale and theory related to procedure

☐ Poor; student has inadequate understanding of rationale and theory related to procedure

Performance Deficiencies (check those that apply)

☐ Excessive time needed to complete procedure

☐ Broke aseptic or sterile technique

☐ Gross inaccuracy noted

☐ Technique may be harmful to patient

☐ Incorrect dosage or gas concentration

☐ Incorrect equipment assembly/use

☐ Unable to answer questions correctly about rationale and/or theory related to procedure

☐ Other ____________________

Evaluation Summary

☐ Satisfactory performance

☐ Unsatisfactory performance

Recommendations of Evaluator

- ☐ Skills may be applied/observed in clinical setting
- ☐ Specific evaluation deficiencies require correction
- ☐ Complete re-evaluation required
- ☐ Additional laboratory practice required

Signatures:

Evaluator ______________________ Date ______________________

Student ______________________ Date ______________________

Laboratory Report

Student ______________________ Acceptable ______________________

Date ______________________ Unacceptable ______________________

Course ______________________

Topic: Infant and Child Cardiopulmonary Resuscitation

Scenario: You and several other members of the staff have been invited to the tenth annual reunion party of intensive care nursery graduates. Suddenly, the party atmosphere is interrupted by the hysterical screams of a young woman standing over her child. The child is a small 4-year-old boy who has apparently stopped breathing.

It is assumed that you are the only person in the group who is certified in CPR. Please answer the following questions:

1. How would you establish the level of consciousness of the child?

2. Would you place the child in the horizontal position? Why?

3. With regard to the airway, why is hyperextension of the neck not indicated?

4. How do you establish breathlessness in the toddler?

5. Initially, how many ventilations should the child receive?

6. In this situation, which of the arteries listed below is palpated to establish pulselessness?
   - ☐ **A.** Femoral artery
   - ☐ **B.** Brachial artery
   - ☐ **C.** Radial artery
   - ☐ **D.** Temporal artery
   - ☐ **E.** Carotid artery

7. Mouth-to-mouth, mouth-to-nose, or mouth-to-mouth and -nose is the method used to ventilate infants and very small children. (Circle the most appropriate.)

chapter 4

Management of complete airway obstruction

INTRODUCTION

The maintenance of a clear path for gas flow between the upper and lower airway is essential for both spontaneous breathing and effective artificial ventilation. During unconsciousness, the tongue frequently produces blockage or acute obstruction of the airway. In conscious individuals with intact airway reflexes, acute airway obstruction may be caused by large pieces of food, dentures, or foreign bodies such as small toys. Unrelieved, total, or complete airway obstruction may cause irreversible central nervous system damage or progress to death within a matter of minutes. Both rapid recognition and prompt treatment of complete airway obstruction are essential. In this chapter you will be introduced to the assessment and management of airway obstruction in the adult, child, and infant.

OBJECTIVES

After completion of this chapter you should be able to do the following:

1. *Recognize the signs and universal distress signal for choking and complete airway obstruction.*
2. *Differentiate between partial and complete airway obstruction.*
3. *Perform the techniques recommended by the American Heart Association for relieving complete airway obstruction in an adult, infant, or child.*
4. *Modify the treatment of complete airway obstruction for pregnant or obese individuals.*
5. *Evaluate and manage unwitnessed airway obstruction.*

EQUIPMENT NEEDED

- ☐ CPR mannequin or choking simulator mannequin
- ☐ 70% isopropyl alcohol
- ☐ Sodium hypochlorite solution
- ☐ Gauze pads or paper towels

ACTIVITIES

Caution: Do *not* forcefully practice the techniques for relieving airway obstruction on students.

Exercise A: Airway Obstruction in a Conscious Adult or Child

1. Choking or airway obstruction frequently occurs during eating. Upon encountering an apparent victim of airway obstruction, determine whether the airway is partially or completely obstructed.
2. If a victim is obviously choking but is able to speak or forcefully cough, do *not* interfere with his attempts to clear the obstruction.
3. A person with complete airway obstruction cannot breathe, speak, or cough. He usually appears to be in obvious respiratory distress and may exhibit cyanosis of the tongue and lips. In addition, a victim of complete airway obstruction may demonstrate the "universal" distress signal for choking by placing a hand around the throat (Fig. 4-1).
4. Establish complete airway obstruction by asking the victim, "Can you speak?"
5. If the victim cannot speak or cough forcefully, assume that complete airway obstruction exists. Inform the victim that you will help him breathe.
6. Deliver abdominal thrusts.
7. To deliver an abdominal thrust, or Heimlich maneuver, stand behind the victim. Encircle the victim's abdomen with your arms. Place the thumb side of your fist midline in the area between the navel and xiphoid process. Grasp the fist with your other hand to encircle the victim. Thrust upward and inward using enough force to dislodge the object (Fig. 4-2).
8. Repeat the abdominal thrusts until the object is expelled or until unconsciousness occurs.

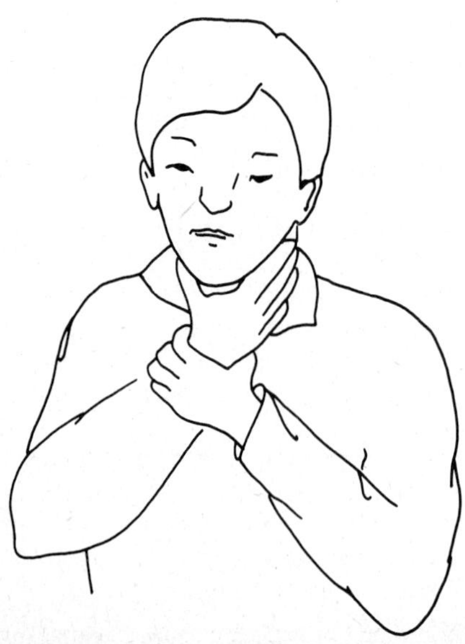

Fig. 4-1. Universal distress signal of choking: hand encircling the throat.

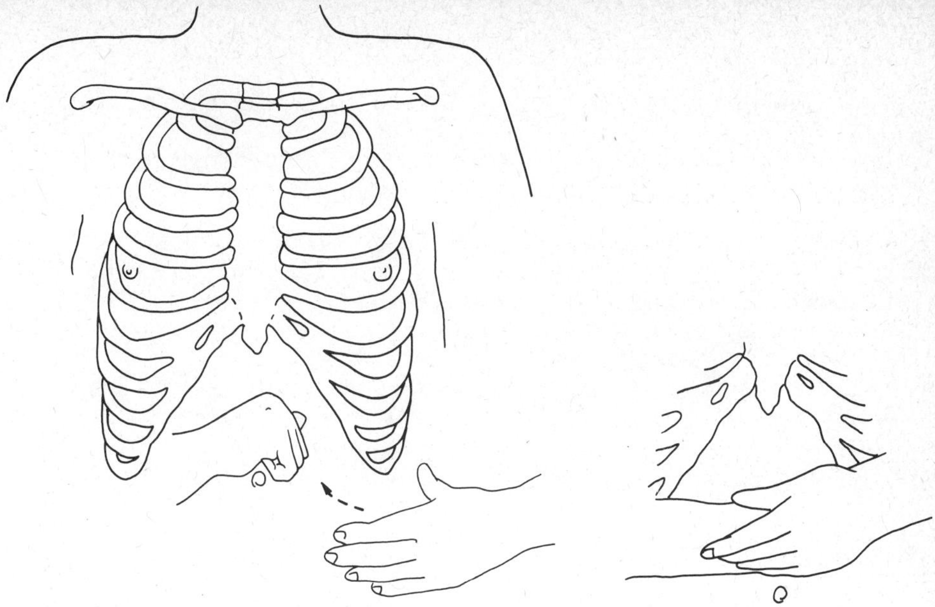

Fig. 4-2. Hand positions for abdominal thrust to an adult. *(Modified from Standards and Guidelines for Cardiopulmonary Resuscitation [CPR] and Emergency Cardiac Care [ECC]. JAMA 244:453, 1980)*

Exercise B: Airway Obstruction in an Adult or Child Becoming Unconscious

1. The conscious victim with complete airway obstruction will usually become unconscious within a short period of time owing to brain hypoxia.
2. When an adult experiencing complete airway obstruction becomes unconscious, place him in the supine position (Fig. 4-3).
3. Call for advanced life support.
4. Open the airway using the head tilt–chin lift technique. Quickly inspect the oropharynx.
5. Attempt to ventilate the victim (Fig. 4-4).
6. If ventilation around the obstruction is possible, continue to ventilate using very slow, deep breaths. The rationale for attempting ventilation is that some air flow may prevent death even at the risk of forcing an object deeper into the airway.
7. If ventilation is ineffective, kneel astride the victim.
8. Administer six to ten abdominal thrusts. Position yourself straddling the victim.
9. To administer abdominal thrusts, place the heel of one hand midline in the area between the navel and xiphoid process. Place your other hand on top of the hand in contact with the epigastrum. Give quick inward and upward thrusts (Fig. 4-5)
10. If abdominal thrusts are ineffective, perform a jaw lift and finger sweep.
11. To perform a jaw lift and finger sweep, position the victim in the supine position with the victim's face up. Be certain that the head and neck are in a midline position. Open the victim's mouth. Using your fingers and thumb of one hand, lift the victim's jaw upward. While entering the side of the mouth with a finger, deeply sweep across the oropharynx using a hooking motion (Fig. 4-6). *Note:* Do *not* perform blind finger sweeps on a child.

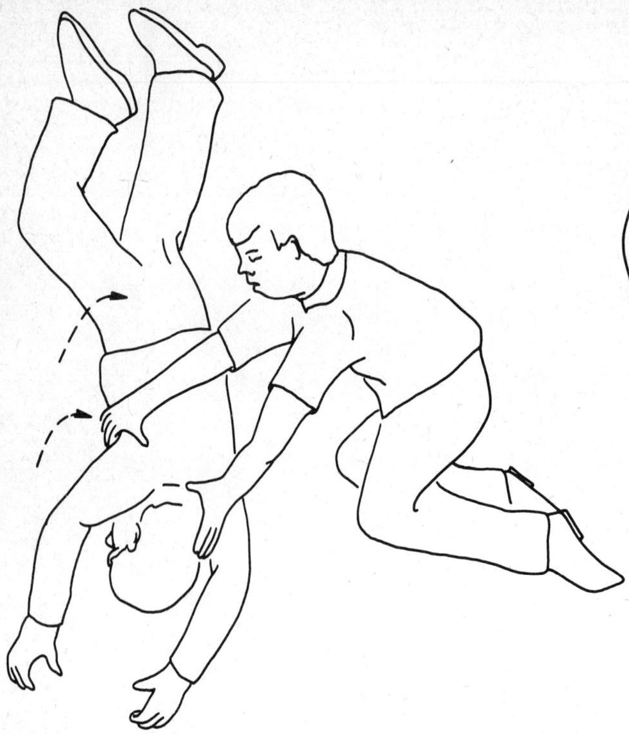

Fig. 4-3. Positioning the unconscious choking victim.

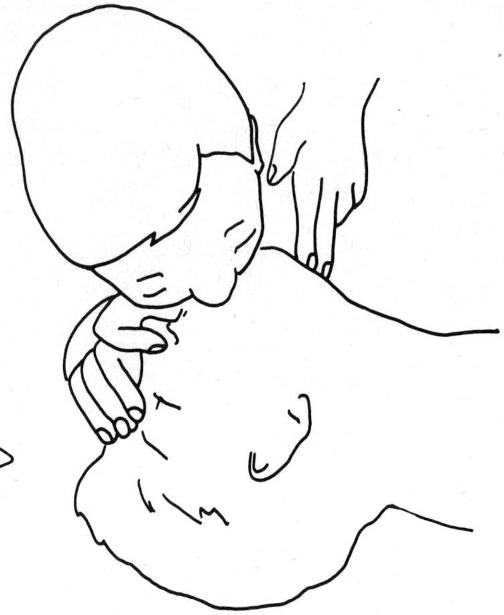

Fig. 4-4. Opening the airway and attempting ventilation before abdominal thrusts.

12. If the preceding actions are ineffective, repeat the entire sequence of steps until the obstruction is removed:
    Open airway and attempt ventilation
    Give six to ten abdominal thrusts
    Perform jaw lift and finger sweep
13. Although initial attempts to relieve an obstruction may be unsuccessful, it is extremely important to continue the effort because prolonged hypoxia during choking may cause muscular relaxation in the throat. As the musculature in the throat relaxes, it may become easier to remove the object.
14. The obstruction has been adequately treated when the victim can effectively ventilate.
15. Practice these techniques to the satisfaction of your laboratory instructor.

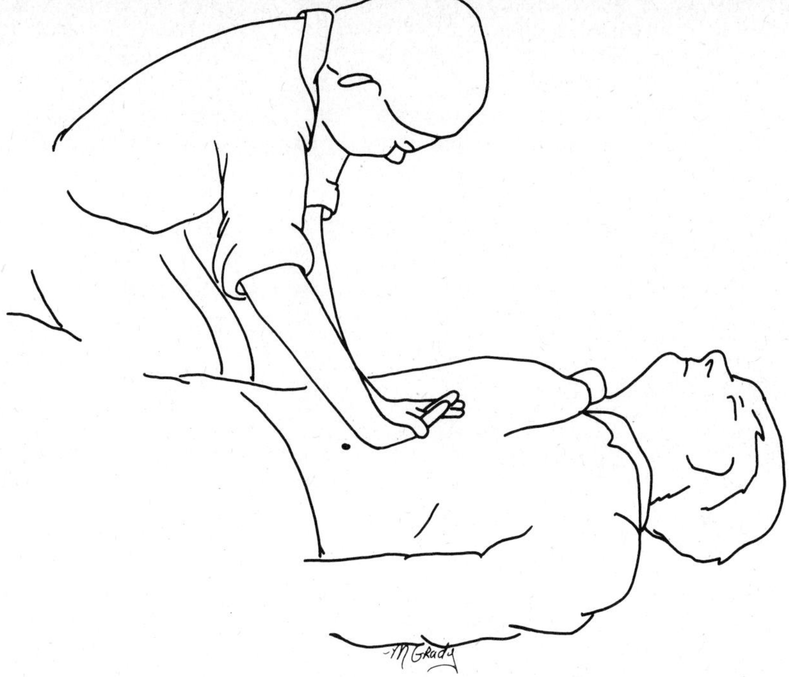

Fig. 4-5. Abdominal thrust to an unconscious victim.

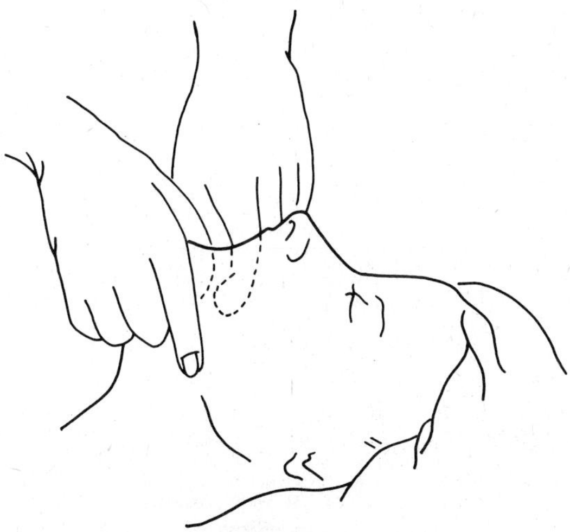

Fig. 4-6. Jaw lift and finger sweep in an unconscious adult choking victim. *(Modified from Montgomery WH, Herrin TJ [eds.]: Student Manual for Basic Life Support. Dallas, American Heart Association, 1981)*

Exercise C: Modification of the Abdominal Thrust

1. In very obese or pregnant individuals, it may be impossible to encircle the abdomen adequately to provide abdominal thrusts or the Heimlich maneuver. In these situations, chest thrusts are an acceptable alternative to abdominal thrusts.
2. To perform chest thrusts, stand behind the victim.
3. Place the thumb side of your fist midline near the center of the sternum. Be certain that your fist is *not* near the xiphoid process.
4. Encircle the victim's chest with your other arm and grasp the fist that was placed against the victim's sternum.

5. Administer four chest thrusts by compressing the chest inward (Fig. 4-7).
6. Use the minimum amount of force necessary to cause displacement of the object.
7. Another modification to the abdominal thrust may be applied to yourself if choking occurs while you are alone.
8. To apply abdominal thrusts to yourself, compress the area between your navel and xiphoid process by gently pushing against an object such as the arm of a chair or a chair railing.

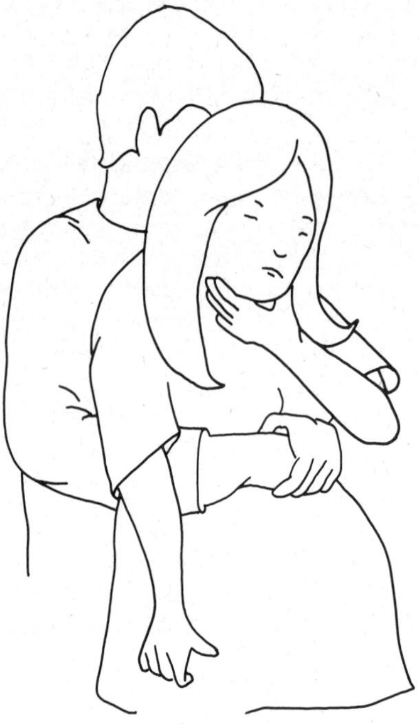

Fig. 4-7. Delivery of a chest thrust.

Exercise D: Unwitnessed Airway Obstruction

1. When encountering an unresponsive person who may have experienced a respiratory or cardiac arrest, attempt to open the airway and ventilate.
2. If ventilation is ineffective because of airway obstruction, you may experience difficulty inflating the lungs, the chest may not move adequately during inspiration, and you may be unable to feel or hear air flow during exhalation. Airway obstruction should be suspected.
3. Because the tongue is a common cause of airway obstruction, the airway once again should be opened manually. The oropharynx may be quickly examined for the presence of a foreign body.
4. If ventilation remains ineffective after attempting to open the airway again, proceed through the steps for relieving acute airway obstruction in an unconscious person. These steps are as follows:
   Open airway and attempt ventilation
   Give six to ten abdominal thrusts
   Perform jaw lift and finger sweep
   Open airway again and reattempt ventilation
5. Frequently evaluate the airway for the expelled foreign object in the oropharynx.
6. Practice the management of unwitnessed airway obstruction to the satisfaction of your instructor.

Exercise E: Complete Airway Obstruction in Infants

1. Airway obstruction may be suspected in infants (younger than 12 months old) and small children who suddenly exhibit respiratory distress, chest retractions, cyanosis, and an inability to cough, speak, or cry. In addition, infants and small children may demonstrate stridor or a high-pitched whistling or crowing noise during breathing.
2. When encountering an infant with suspected airway obstruction, determine whether the victim can clear the obstruction by coughing. If the victim has an adequate cough, do *not* interfere with the victim's efforts. Closely monitor the victim's progress.
3. When complete airway obstruction exists, place the infant in a face-down position with the head lower than the chest.
4. Administer four back blows by striking the infant between the shoulder blades. Use the minimum force necessary to dislodge the object (Fig. 4-8).
5. If back blows are unsuccessful, turn the infant over while supporting the infant's head, neck, and spine.
6. Administer four chest compressions by placing two fingers midline in the center of the sternum. Compress the chest four times using the minimum force required to displace the obstruction. The chest compressions are similar to those given during CPR.
7. Because of potential damage to internal organs and especially the liver, abdominal thrusts are *not* administered to infants.
8. Continue the sequence of four back blows followed by four chest thrusts until the obstruction is expelled.

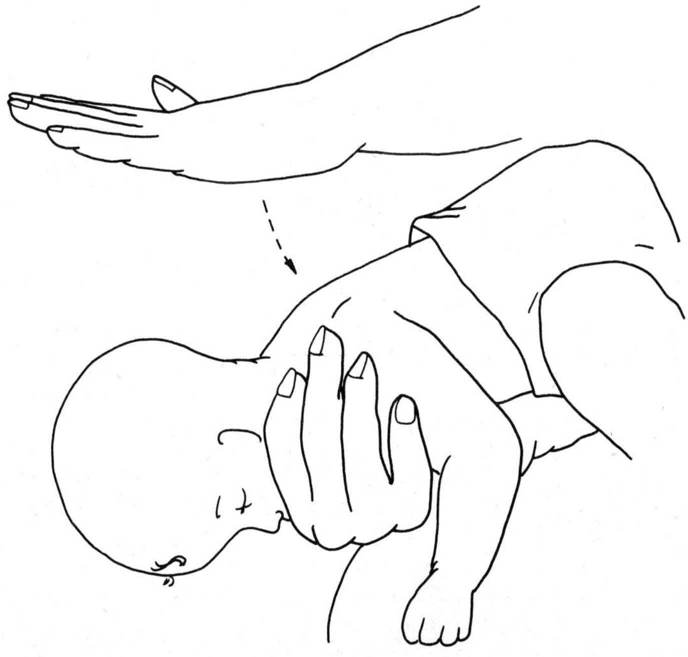

Fig. 4-8. Back blows to a choking infant victim. *(Modified from American Heart Association: Standards and guidelines for CPR and ECC. JAMA 244:2959, 1986)*

9. Because of the relatively large size of an adult's finger compared to the size of an infant's oropharynx, blind finger sweeps are *not* performed on an infant or child with airway obstruction. A finger sweep is performed on a neonate only if the object is visualized in the oropharynx.
10. If unwitnessed airway obstruction is suspected in an infant, as with an adult, open the airway a second time and attempt to ventilate again before treatment for airway obstruction.

RECOMMENDED READING

Burton GG, Hodgkin JE: Respiratory Care. A Guide to Clinical Practice, 2nd ed. Philadelphia, JB Lippincott, 1984

Lewis AJ, Montgomery WH, Guidner CW et al: A Manual for Instructors of Basic Cardiac Life Support. Dallas, American Heart Association, 1981

Montgomery WH, Herrin TJ (eds): Student Manual for Basic Life Support. Dallas, American Heart Association, 1981

Safar P: Cardiopulmonary Cerebral Resuscitation. Philadelphia, WB Saunders, 1981

Standards and Guidelines for Cardiopulmonary Resuscitation (CPR) and Emergency Cardiac Care (EEC). JAMA 255:21, 1986

Laboratory Performance Evaluation (#4a)

Topic: Complete Airway Obstruction: Conscious Adult or Child

Student ______________________ Course ______________________

Date ______________________ Section ______________________

Performance Elements	Acceptable	Unacceptable	Not Applicable	Comments
1. Determines complete obstruction by asking, "Can you speak?"				
2. Informs victim that assistance will be given				
3. Administers abdominal thrusts				
4. Reassesses the obstruction				
5. Repeats the above sequence until the airway becomes patent or to satisfaction of instructor				

Knowledge of Procedure

☐ Good; student is knowledgeable about rationale and theory related to procedure

☐ Fair; student has adequate understanding of rationale and theory related to procedure

☐ Poor; student has inadequate understanding of rationale and theory related to procedure

Performance Deficiencies (check those that apply)

- ☐ Excessive time needed to complete procedure
- ☐ Broke aseptic or sterile technique
- ☐ Gross inaccuracy noted
- ☐ Technique may be harmful to patient
- ☐ Incorrect dosage or gas concentration
- ☐ Incorrect equipment assembly/use
- ☐ Unable to answer questions correctly about rationale and/or theory related to procedure
- ☐ Other ______________________

Evaluation Summary

- ☐ Satisfactory performance
- ☐ Unsatisfactory performance

Recommendations of Evaluator

- ☐ Skills may be applied/observed in clinical setting
- ☐ Specific evaluation deficiencies require correction
- ☐ Complete re-evaluation required
- ☐ Additional laboratory practice required

Signatures:

Evaluator ______________________ Date ______________________

Student ______________________ Date ______________________

Laboratory Performance Evaluation (#4b)

Topic: Complete Airway Obstruction: Adult or Child Becomes Unconscious

Student ______________________ Course ______________________

Date ______________________ Section ______________________

Performance Elements	Acceptable	Unacceptable	Not Applicable	Comments
1. Positions victim in a supine position				
2. Calls for help				
3. Signals for advanced life support				
4. Opens airway and checks for foreign body				
5. Attempts ventilation				
6. Administers six to ten abdominal thrusts				
7. Performs jaw lift and finger sweep *Note:* A blind finger sweep is *not* performed on a child.				
8. Re-evaluates obstruction				
9. Opens airway and repeats ventilation attempt				
10. Repeats above sequence until the airway becomes patent or to satisfaction of instructor				

Knowledge of Procedure

- ☐ Good; student is knowledgeable about rationale and theory related to procedure
- ☐ Fair; student has adequate understanding of rationale and theory related to procedure
- ☐ Poor; student has inadequate understanding of rationale and theory related to procedure

Performance Deficiencies (check those that apply)

- ☐ Excessive time needed to complete procedure
- ☐ Broke aseptic or sterile technique
- ☐ Gross inaccuracy noted
- ☐ Technique may be harmful to patient
- ☐ Incorrect dosage or gas concentration
- ☐ Incorrect equipment assembly/use
- ☐ Unable to answer questions correctly about rationale and/or theory related to procedure
- ☐ Other ______________________________

Evaluation Summary

- ☐ Satisfactory performance
- ☐ Unsatisfactory performance

Recommendations of Evaluator

- ☐ Skills may be applied/observed in clinical setting
- ☐ Specific evaluation deficiencies require correction
- ☐ Complete re-evaluation required
- ☐ Additional laboratory practice required

Signatures:

Evaluator ______________________ Date ______________________

Student ______________________ Date ______________________

Laboratory Performance Evaluation (#4c)

Topic: Complete Airway Obstruction: Unconscious Adult or Child

Student ______________________ Course ______________________

Date ______________________ Section ______________________

Performance Elements	Acceptable	Unacceptable	Not Applicable	Comments
1. Establishes unresponsiveness				
2. Calls for help				
3. Places victim in a supine position and face up				
4. Opens the airway				
5. Determines breathlessness by looking, listening, and feeling for breathing.				
6. Activates signal for advanced life support				
7. Attempts ventilation				
8. Reopens airway				
9. Attempts again to ventilate				
10. Gives six to ten abdominal thrusts				
11. Performs jaw lift and finger sweep*				
12. Reopens airway and attempts to ventilate				
13. Repeats the above sequence until the airway becomes patent or to satisfaction of instructor				

* A blind finger sweep is *not* performed on a child.

Knowledge of Procedure

- ☐ Good; student is knowledgeable about rationale and theory related to procedure
- ☐ Fair; student has adequate understanding of rationale and theory related to procedure
- ☐ Poor; student has inadequate understanding of rationale and theory related to procedure

Performance Deficiencies (check those that apply)

- ☐ Excessive time needed to complete procedure
- ☐ Broke aseptic or sterile technique
- ☐ Gross inaccuracy noted
- ☐ Technique may be harmful to patient
- ☐ Incorrect dosage or gas concentration
- ☐ Incorrect equipment assembly/use
- ☐ Unable to answer questions correctly about rationale and/or theory related to procedure
- ☐ Other ______________________________

Evaluation Summary

- ☐ Satisfactory performance
- ☐ Unsatisfactory performance

Recommendations of Evaluator

- ☐ Skills may be applied/observed in clinical setting
- ☐ Specific evaluation deficiencies require correction
- ☐ Complete re-evaluation required
- ☐ Additional laboratory practice required

Signatures:

Evaluator ______________________ Date ______________________

Student ______________________ Date ______________________

Laboratory Performance Evaluation (#4d)

Topic: Complete Airway Obstruction: Infant

Student ______________________ Course ______________________

Date ______________________ Section ______________________

Performance Elements	Acceptable	Unacceptable	Not Applicable	Comments
1. Determines presence of complete airway obstruction				
2. Positions infant with head lower than chest and supports head and neck				
3. Gives four back blows				
4. Gives four chest thrusts				
5. Repeats above sequence until airway becomes patent or to satisfaction of instructor				

Knowledge of Procedure

- ☐ Good; student is knowledgeable about rationale and theory related to procedure
- ☐ Fair; student has adequate understanding of rationale and theory related to procedure
- ☐ Poor; student has inadequate understanding of rationale and theory related to procedure

Performance Deficiencies (check those that apply)

- ☐ Excessive time needed to complete procedure
- ☐ Broke aseptic or sterile technique
- ☐ Gross inaccuracy noted
- ☐ Technique may be harmful to patient
- ☐ Incorrect dosage or gas concentration
- ☐ Incorrect equipment assembly/use
- ☐ Unable to answer questions correctly about rationale and/or theory related to procedure
- ☐ Other ______________________________

Evaluation Summary

- ☐ Satisfactory performance
- ☐ Unsatisfactory performance

Recommendations of Evaluator

- ☐ Skills may be applied/observed in clinical setting
- ☐ Specific evaluation deficiencies require correction
- ☐ Complete re-evaluation required
- ☐ Additional laboratory practice required

Signatures:

Evaluator ______________________ Date ______________________

Student ______________________ Date ______________________

Laboratory Report

Student ______________________ Acceptable ______________________

Date ______________________ Unacceptable ______________________

Course ______________________

Topic: Management of Complete Airway Obstruction

Scenario: Today, you have been assigned to the pediatric area. Upon your arrival to monitor an oxygen tent, a 9-month-old boy is having marked chest and abdominal retractions. His lips are very blue and his eyes have rolled back so that only the white areas are visible. As you approach the bed, the blueness is replaced by paleness, and the child demonstrates a very high-pitched, crowing noise during inspiration. Please answer the following questions:

1. How would you establish partial or complete airway obstruction in this situation?

2. If your initial attempt to ventilate is unsuccessful, would you make another attempt to ventilate? Yes __________ No __________ Why? __________

3. How many back blows are delivered (circle best choice)?
   1 — 2 — 3 — 4 — 8
4. To where, anatomically, are the "chest thrusts" delivered? Be specific.

5. How many chest thrusts are administered (circle best choice)?
   1 — 2 — 3 — 4 — 6

6. Why are "blind" finger sweeps avoided in infants and small children?

7. Having gone through the appropriate sequence for relieving an obstruction one time and not being successful in accomplishing ventilation, would you repeat the procedure? Yes ________ No ________ Why?

chapter 5

Gas administration systems

INTRODUCTION

In many clinical environments, the respiratory care department is responsible for utilizing and monitoring a variety of gas administration systems. These systems may include a liquid oxygen storage vessel, gas bank or manifold, gas cylinders, oxygen concentrators, and air compressors.

Large quantities or reserves of oxygen may be stored using a liquid storage vessel or cylinder manifold. A liquid storage vessel is designed to maintain oxygen in the liquid state, thereby conserving storage space. A gas bank or manifold consists of a series of cylinders that, depending on the number and size of cylinders, can store large gaseous reserves. With both the liquid and manifold storage systems, oxygen may be distributed from the storage system throughout a facility by means of a piping distribution system. The piping distribution system usually includes pressure reducing valves, zone valves, and gas outlets.

Portable gas administration systems include gas cylinders, oxygen concentrators, and air compressors. Gas cylinders are available in a variety of sizes and may readily be transported throughout a facility. Oxygen concentrators are portable units that can produce high concentrations of oxygen when relatively low flowrates are required. An air compressor may be used as a portable source of compressed air for operating various respiratory care equipment or for titrating inspired gas mixtures. The purpose of this chapter is to familiarize you with several types of gas administration systems.

OBJECTIVES

After completing this chapter, you should be able to do the following:

1. *Discuss the types and advantages of bulk oxygen storage systems.*
2. *Describe and diagram a gas piping system.*
3. *Demonstrate the proper methods of preparing, transporting, and stabilizing gas cylinders.*
4. *Identify cylinder gases according to the label and color code.*

5. *Interpret gas cylinder markings.*
6. *Identify the components of an air compressor and oxygen concentrator.*
7. *Operate an air compressor and oxygen concentrator.*
8. *Understand the function of a zone valve and wall outlet.*

EQUIPMENT NEEDED

- ☐ Laboratory gas storage and piping system
- ☐ Large gas cylinders ("H" or "K")
- ☐ Small gas cylinders ("E" or "D")
- ☐ Cylinder stand or cart
- ☐ Wall outlet manometer
- ☐ Air compressor
- ☐ Oxygen concentrator
- ☐ Cylinder wrenches for large and small cylinders

ACTIVITIES

Exercise A: Examination of Bulk Gas Storage and Piping Systems

1. Using the diagram provided, examine a liquid oxygen storage system. (Fig. 5-1).
2. Identify the following components of a liquid oxygen storage system:
   - A. Liquid container
   - B. Pressure regulators
   - C. Vaporizer
   - D. Auxiliary gas supply cylinder manifold
   - E. Piping system
3. Using the diagram provided, examine a gas manifold bulk storage system (Fig. 5-2).

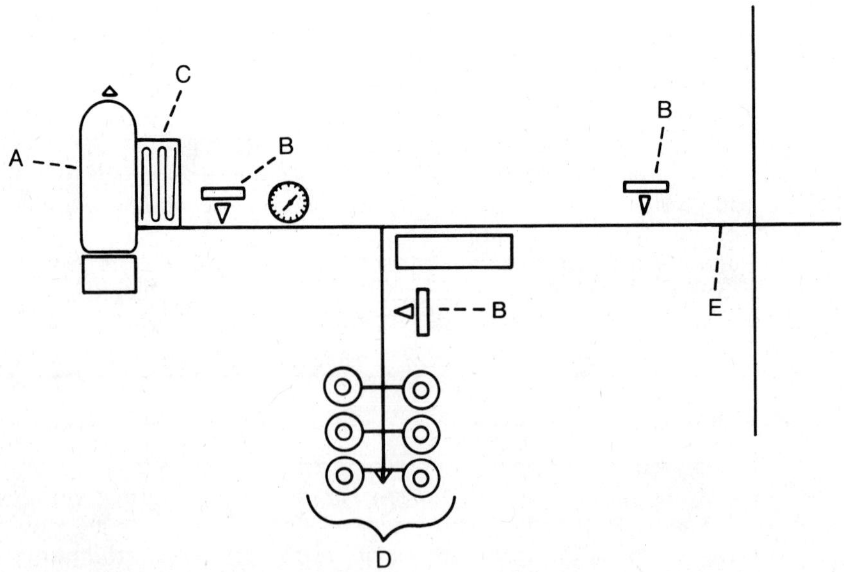

Fig. 5-1. Liquid oxygen storage system.

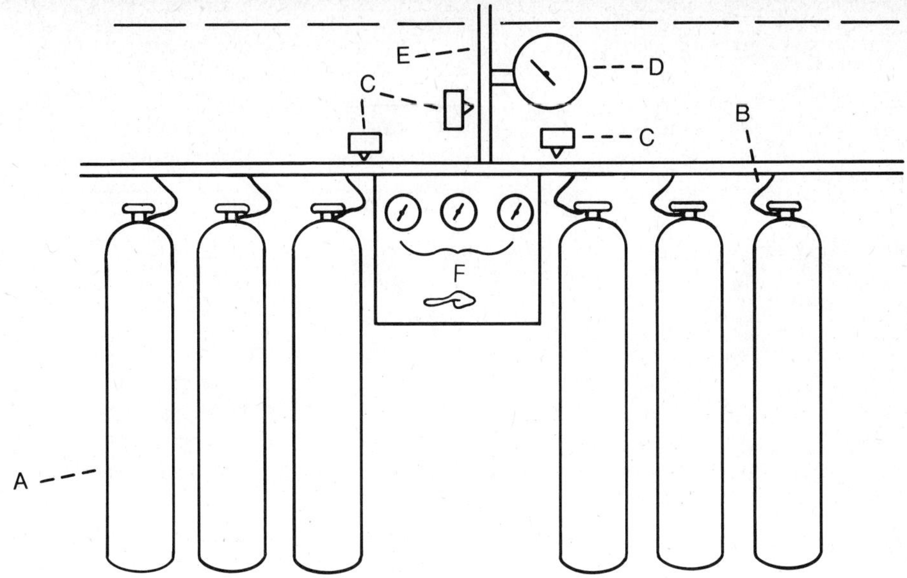

Fig. 5-2. Cylinder manifold storage system.

4. Identify the following components of a manifold:
   A. Gas cylinders
   B. Copper connection tubing
   C. Reducing valves
   D. Piping line manometers

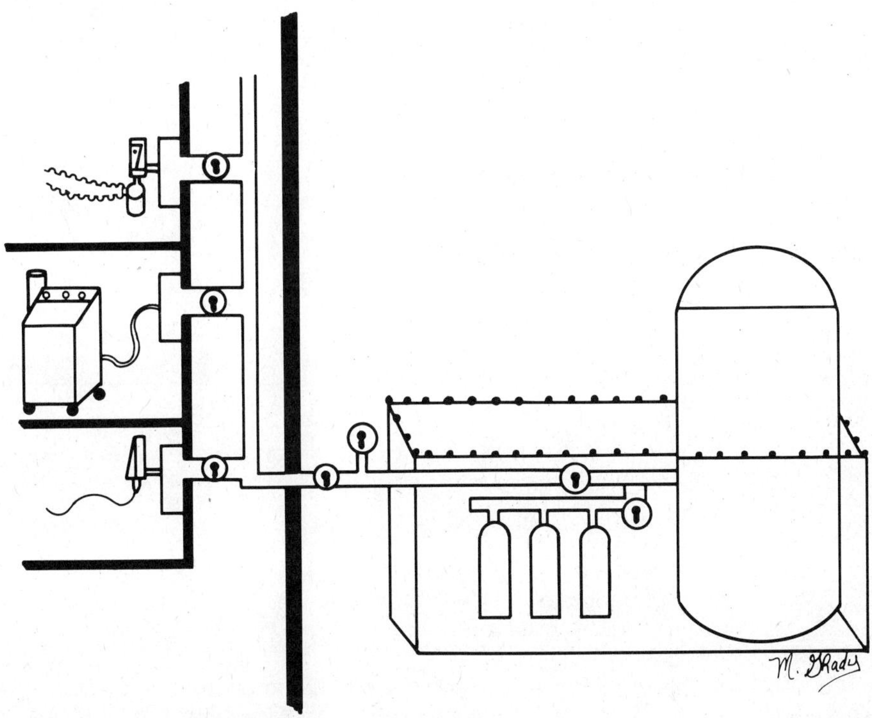

Fig. 5-3. Piping system.

E. Piping line
F. System manometers
5. Using the provided diagram, examine the laboratory gas piping system (Fig. 5-3).
6. The force that causes gas to flow through the piping system from the gas storage system to the wall outlet is gas pressure. For gas flow to occur, a pressure gradient or difference in pressure must exist between the storage system and the wall outlet. Trace the path or gas flow from the bulk storage system to the wall outlet. Note the pressure of gas at the storage system, in the piping system, and at the wall outlet.

Exercise B: Identification of a Zone Valve and Measurement of Wall Outlet Pressure

1. If applicable, locate a zone valve incorporated in the gas piping system (Fig. 5-4).
2. Familiarize yourself with the operation of the zone valve.
3. Identify various types of wall outlets such as air, oxygen, and suction (Fig. 5-5).
4. Using a manometer provided by your instructor, measure the wall outlet pressure for oxygen. Record your results on the laboratory report.
5. Compare the pressure of the wall outlet with the manifold pressures. Record your findings on the laboratory report.

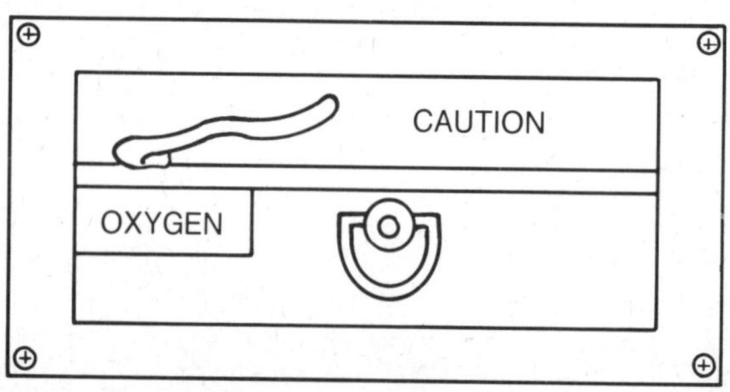

Fig. 5-4. Zone valve.

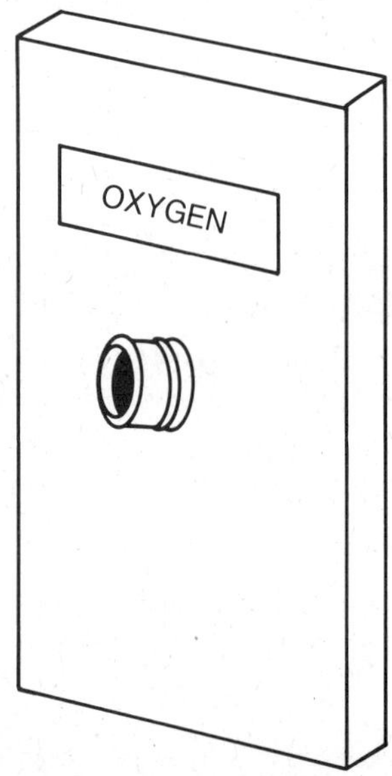

Fig. 5-5. Wall outlet.

Exercise C: Identification and Operation of an Air Compressor

1. Using the provided diagram, observe a portable air compressor (Fig. 5-6)
2. Identify the following components:
   A. Electrical cord
   B. Filter
   C. On/off switch
   D. Pressure manometer
   E. Pressure-regulating mechanism
   F. Gas outlet
3. Activate the air compressor. Adjust the outlet pressure to provide 50 pounds per square inch (50 psi). A working pressure of 50 psi frequently is used to power additional equipment such as flowmeters and mechanical ventilators.

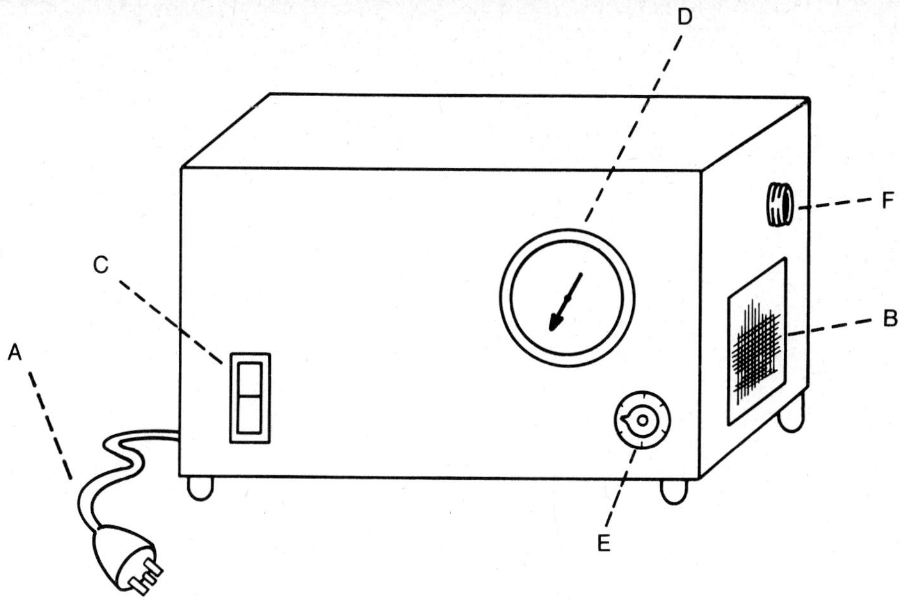

Fig. 5-6. Assembled air compressor.

Exercise D: Identification and Operation of an Oxygen Concentrator

1. Using the provided illustration, examine an oxygen concentrator (Fig. 5-7).
2. Identify the following components:
   - **A.** Power source
   - **B.** Filter
   - **C.** On/off switch
   - **D.** Gas flowmeter
   - **E.** Gas outlet
   - **F.** Alarm and battery
   - **G.** Chronometer (time use indicator)
   - **H.** Auxiliary connection to cylinder reserve (if applicable)
3. Activate the oxygen concentrator. Obtain a gas flowrate of 3 liters/min. The precise flowrate is obtained by reading the center of the float.
4. Record the maximum attainable gas flowrate on the laboratory report.
5. Verify the function of the power-loss alarm by disconnecting the power source while the concentrator is turned on.
6. Check the filter. Clean the filter according to manufacturer's recommendations.

Exercise E: Examination and Preparation of a Large Gas Cylinder

1. Using the diagram provided, identify the available sizes of gas cylinders (Fig. 5-8).
2. Select a size "H" cylinder.
3. Stabilize the gas cylinder by placing it in a cart or stand. Secure the cylinder with a chain or appropriate restraining device (Fig 5-9).
4. Remove the cylinder valve cover. Visually inspect the gas outlet for debris. Identify the main valve.
5. Direct the gas outlet away from everyone, including yourself.

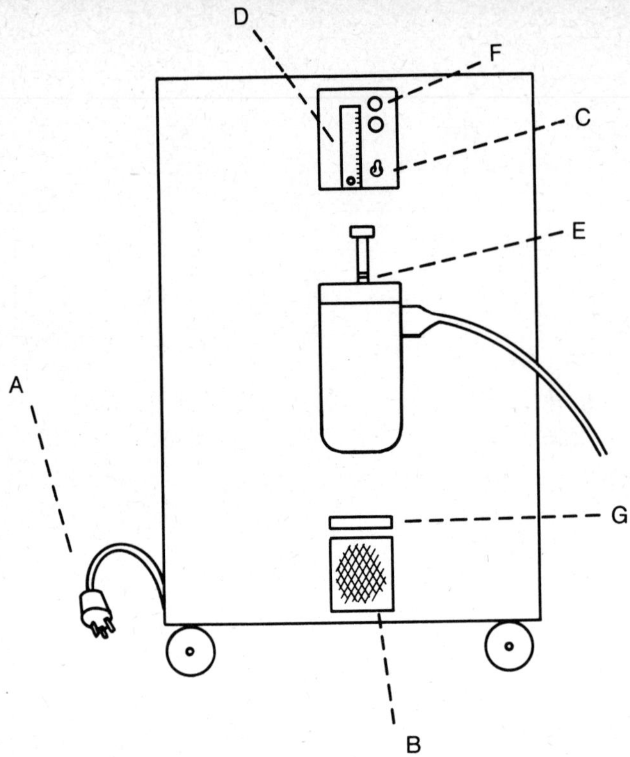

Fig. 5-7. Oxygen concentrator.

6. *Slowly* open the cylinder valve by turning it counterclockwise. Close the valve by turning it clockwise. (*Remember*: Clockwise closes the valve.) The term for this procedure of clearing the valve outlet is "cracking" the cylinder (Fig. 5-10)
7. Repeat your inspection of the valve outlet for debris.
8. Using the following diagram, examine the cylinder markings on both sides of the cylinder shoulder (Fig. 5-11).
9. Identify the following markings:
   - **A.** ICC/DOT
   - **B.** Serial number
   - **C.** Ownership
   - **D.** Inspector's mark
   - **E.** Service pressure
   - **F.** Hydrostatic test date
   - **G.** Elastic expansion results
   - **H.** Hydrostatic retest dates
10. Read the cylinder label. *Note:* If a label is not present, *do not* use the cylinder.
11. Observe the color of the cylinder.
12. Confirm the agreement between the labeled contents and color code.
13. On the laboratory report, record the cylinder contents, color code, and cylinder markings.
14. Refer to Table 5-1 for information on cylinder gases. Using the gas cylinder provided by your instructor, identify the gas contained in the cylinder, its primary use, flammability, color code, physical state, and volume in cubic feet.

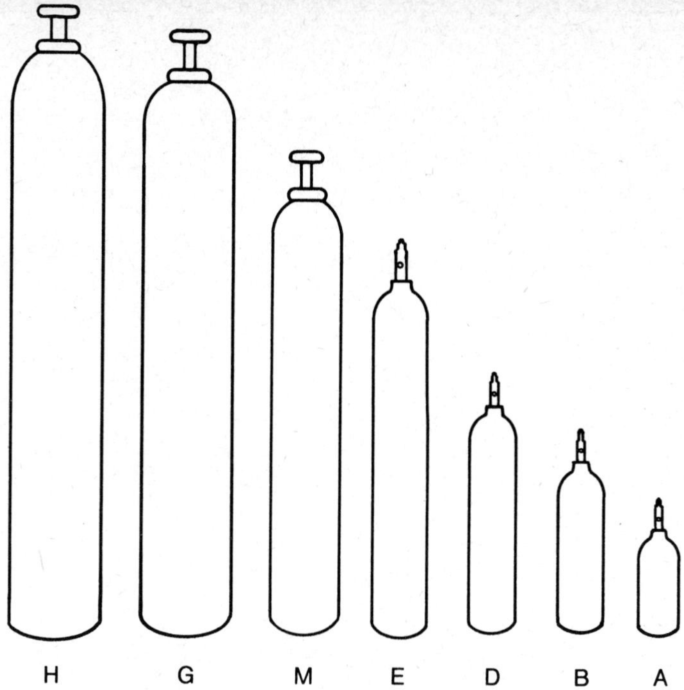

Fig. 5-8. Gas cylinder sizes for oxygen. *(Modified from Puritan Bennett Corporation, Los Angeles, CA)*

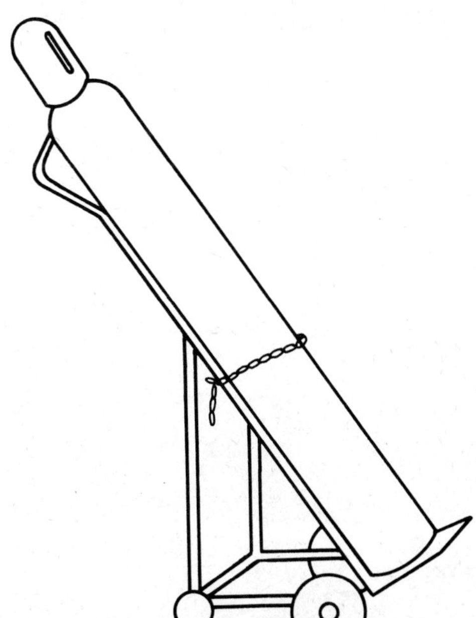

Fig. 5-9. Large cylinder stabilized by a cart or stand.

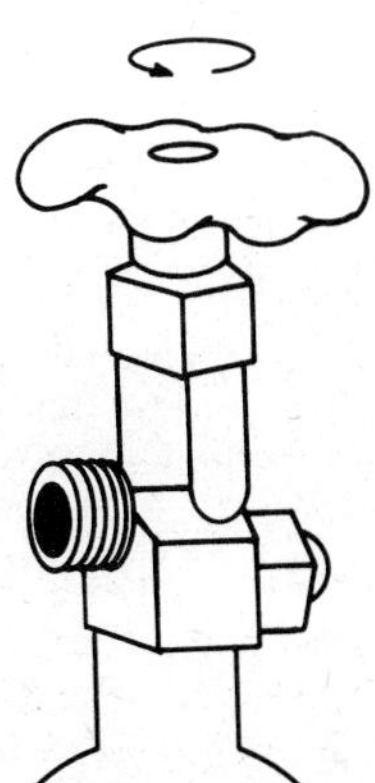

Fig. 5-10. "Cracking" a cylinder to clear the valve outlet.

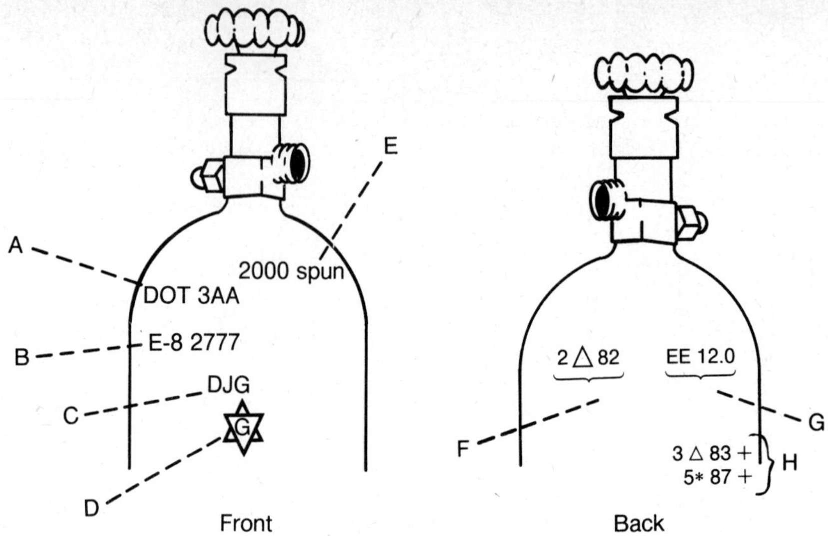

Fig. 5-11. Typical markings found on a cylinder shoulder.

Table 5-1. Information on Cylinder Gases

Gas	Primary Use	Flammability	(U.S.) Color Code	70°F Pressure and Physical Nature	Volume in Cubic Feet			
					D	E	G	H
Oxygen (O_2)	Therapy	Supports combustion	Green	2200 PSIG Gas	12.7	22.0	187	244
Air (O_2 and N_2)	Therapy	Supports combustion	Green/silver or black	1800–2000 PSIG Gas	12.7	22.0	187	220–244
Carbon dioxide (CO_2)	Laboratory	Nonflammable prevents combustion	Gray	825 PSIG Liquid/gas	34.7	56.1	427	Not supplied in this size cylinder
CO_2–O_2 mixtures	Therapy	Supports combustion	Gray/green	1600–2200 PSIG Gas	12.7	22.0	187	244
Nitrogen (N_2)	Laboratory	Nonflammable prevents combustion	Silver or yellow	1800–2200 PSIG Gas	12.7	22.0	187	244
Helium (He)	Laboratory	Nonflammable prevents combustion	Brown	1600–2000 PSIG Gas	10.6	17.5	147	191
He–O_2 mixture	Therapy	Supports combustion	Brown/green	1600–2000 PSIG Gas	10.8	17.7	150	194
Nitrous Oxide (N_2O)	Anesthesia	Supports combustion	Blue	745–900 PSIG Liquid/gas	—	57.6	488.6	—
Cyclopropane $(CH_2)_3$	Anesthesia	Flammable	Orange or orange/chrome	75.0 PSIG Liquid/gas	—	33.2	—	—

(Reproduced with permission from Grenard S et al: Introduction to Respiratory Therapy, 3rd ed. Copyright © 1981 by Year Book Medical Publishers, Inc., Chicago)

Exercise F: Examination and Preparation of a Small Gas Cylinder

1. Select a size "E" or "D" gas cylinder.
2. Stabilize the cylinder by placing it in a stand or cart (Fig. 5-12).
3. On the laboratory report, identify and record the contents of the gas cylinder by label and color code.
4. Identify the cylinder markings. Record the cylinder markings on the laboratory report.
5. If present, remove the valve wrapper and plastic washer. Save the plastic washer for use with pressure and flow-regulating equipment.
6. Check the cylinder valve outlet for debris (Fig. 5-13).
7. Practice "cracking" the small cylinder. Note that the main cylinder valve requires the use of a wrench for opening and closing the valve.

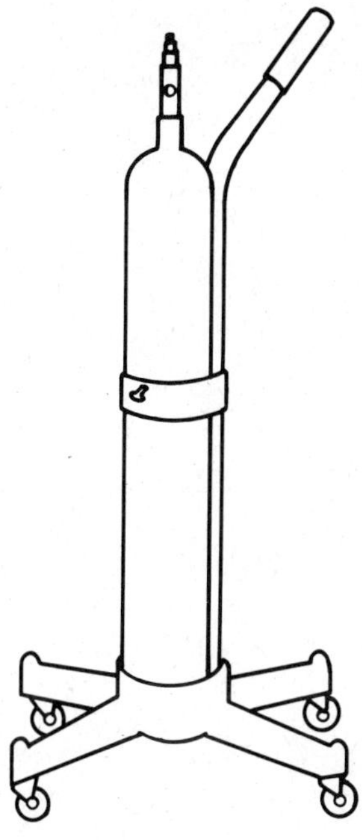

Fig. 5-12. Small cylinder stabilized by a cart or stand.

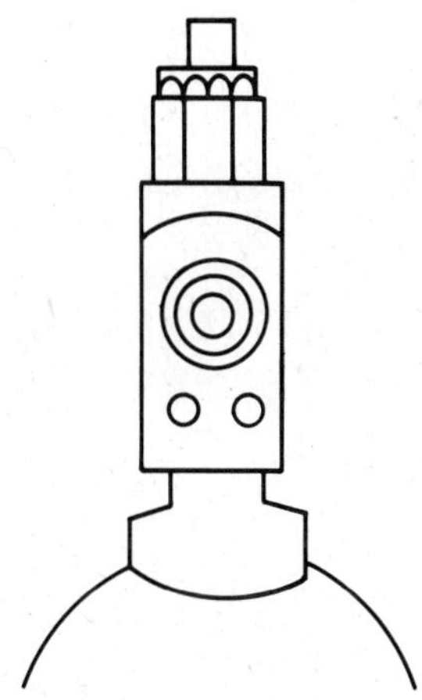

Fig. 5-13. Small cylinder valve.

Exercise G: Determination of "Unknown"

1. Your laboratory instructor will provide you with two cylinders of medical gases. Identify the contents of the medical gases, and record the results on the laboratory report.

RECOMMENDED READING

Burton GG, Hodgkin JE: Respiratory Care. A Guide to Clinical Practice, 2nd ed. Philadelphia, JB Lippincott, 1984

Grenard S, Beck GJ, Rich GW, Shapira M: Introduction to Respiratory Therapy, 3rd ed. Chicago, Year Book Medical Publishers, 1981

Kacmarek RM, Dimas S, Mack C: Essentials of Respiratory Therapy, 2nd ed. Chicago, Year Book Medical Publishers, 1985

McPherson SP, Spearman CB: Respiratory Therapy Equipment, 3rd ed. St Louis, CV Mosby, 1985

Rau J, Rau M: Fundamental Respiratory Therapy Equipment: Principles of Use and Operation. Sarasota, Glenn Educational Medical Services, 1977

Spearman CB, Sheldon RL: Egan's Fundamentals of Respiratory Therapy, 4th ed. St Louis, CV Mosby, 1982

Laboratory Performance Evaluation (#5)

Topic: Gas Administration Systems

Student ______________________ Course ______________________

Date ______________________ Section ______________________

Performance Elements	Acceptable	Unacceptable	Not Applicable	Comments
1. Selects a gas cylinder				
2. Demonstrates proper stabilization and transportation of cylinders: **A.** Applies valve cover **B.** Uses cart **C.** Secures cylinder with strap or chain **D.** Stabilizes cylinder with stand				
3. Identifies cylinder size				
4. Identifies cylinder contents by label and color code				
5. Identifies two cylinder markings				
6. Prepares the cylinder for use: **A.** Removes valve cover **B.** "Cracks" cylinder **C.** Checks for debris				
7. Turns main cylinder valve on, then off				
8. Locates, then operates zone valve				
9. Measures wall outlet pressure with appropriate manometer				

Knowledge of Procedure

- ☐ Good; student is knowledgeable about rationale and theory related to procedure
- ☐ Fair; student has adequate understanding of rationale and theory related to procedure
- ☐ Poor; student has inadequate understanding of rationale and theory related to procedure

Performance Deficiencies (check those that apply)

- ☐ Excessive time needed to complete procedure
- ☐ Broke aseptic or sterile technique
- ☐ Gross inaccuracy noted
- ☐ Technique may be harmful to patient
- ☐ Incorrect dosage or gas concentration
- ☐ Incorrect equipment assembly/use
- ☐ Unable to answer questions correctly about rationale and/or theory related to procedure
- ☐ Other ______________________________

Evaluation Summary

- ☐ Satisfactory performance
- ☐ Unsatisfactory performance

Recommendations of Evaluator

- ☐ Skills may be applied/observed in clinical setting
- ☐ Specific evaluation deficiencies require correction
- ☐ Complete re-evaluation required
- ☐ Additional laboratory practice required

Signatures:

Evaluator ______________________ Date ______________________

Student ______________________ Date ______________________

Laboratory Report

Student ______________________ Acceptable ______________________

Date ______________________ Unacceptable ______________________

Course ______________________

Topic: Gas Administration Systems

Data and Measurements:

1. Wall outlet pressure (PSI) ______________________
2. Manifold pressure ______________________
3. Difference between wall outlet pressure and manifold pressure ______________________
4. Oxygen concentrator maximum flow obtained ______________________
5. Diagram of laboratory gas storage and piping system:

6. "Unknown" contents of gas cylinders:

   Cylinder #1: ______________________

   Cylinder #2: ______________________

7. Gas cylinder information:

	Size "H" Cylinder	Size "E" Cylinder
Cylinder contents		
Color Code		
Cylinder Markings:		
Manufacturer's mark		
Serial number		
DOT/ICC specifications		
Service/filling/pressure		
Hydrostatic test		

Retest date ____________________ ____________________

Gas volume (cubic feet) ____________________ ____________________

Scenario: You have been notified by the shift supervisor that the bulk liquid oxygen supply system and the reserve bank will be "shut off" at 2:00 a.m. The systems will be down for about 1 hour.

The supervisor has assigned each staff member to a specific area within the hospital. It is his responsibility to (a) provide all patients in the area who are receiving oxygen with an appropriate portable delivery system and (b) to shut off the area (zone) valve.

Using clear and concise sentences, diagrams, or drawings, please answer the following questions:

1. What is the purpose of the zone shut-off valve?

2. Describe the safety precautions you would take while obtaining and transporting cylinders from the storage area to the patients's bedside.

3. How do you know what gas is contained in the cylinders you plan to transport to your assigned area?

4. Describe the method you would use to check the function of an oxygen concentrator.

5. Describe any differences between the valve of an "E" cylinder and that of an "H" cylinder.

6. What is the color code of the below gases, and which are flammable, which nonflammable, and which support combustion?

	Color Code	Flammability
A. Nitrous oxide	__________	__________
B. Carbon dioxide	__________	__________
C. Oxygen	__________	__________
D. 80% helium/20% oxygen	__________	__________
E. Ethylene oxide	__________	__________
F. Cyclopropane	__________	__________

chapter 6

Gas pressure and flow regulation

INTRODUCTION

Before administering medical gases from storage systems, it is necessary to regulate the gas pressure and flowrate. A device that reduces gas pressure is called a reducing valve. A flowmeter measures and controls gas flow, and a regulator will both reduce gas pressure and control gas flow.

When administering medical gases in the clinical setting, mistakes and accidents may be harmful or *fatal* to patients. For these reasons, safety systems have been devised to help prevent accidents when using gas pressure and flow-regulating equipment. These safety systems include the American Standard Valve Outlet Connection System, The Pin Index Safety System, and the Diameter Index Safety System. The Pin Index Safety System applies to size "E" cylinders and smaller; the American Standard Valve Outlet Connection System applies to cylinders larger than size "E"; and the Diameter Index Safety System applies to equipment connections that require an operational gas pressure of 200 psi or less.

To help ensure both precision and accuracy, specific types of pressure and flow-regulating equipment are intended to be used with specific gas mixtures. An oxygen flowmeter should be used only to regulate the flow of 100% oxygen. An oxygen flowmeter will not be accurate, for example, if used to deliver a gas mixture containing both helium and oxygen. In addition, gas pressure or flow-regulating equipment that is damaged or broken should never be used. The purpose of this chapter is to introduce you to equipment that will regulate gas pressure and flow.

OBJECTIVES

After completing this chapter, you should be able to do the following:

1. *Explain the purposes of reducing valves, regulators, and flowmeters.*
2. *Select, identify, and assemble a gas regulator, Bourdon gauge regulator, and a gas flowmeter.*
3. *Identify the primary components of reducing valves, regulators, and flowmeters.*

4. *Examine the American Standard Valve Outlet Connection (ASVOC) Safety System, Pin Index Safety System (PISS), and Diameter Index Safety System (DISS).*
5. *Measure and record the gas pressure, and regulate the gas flowrate from a cylinder.*
6. *Determine the duration of gas flow from a cylinder.*

EQUIPMENT NEEDED

- ☐ Large gas cylinder ("H" or "K")
- ☐ Small gas cylinder ("E" or "D")
- ☐ Preset, adjustable, and multistage reducing valves
- ☐ PISS Bourdon gauge
- ☐ DISS flowmeter (air and oxygen)

ACTIVITIES

Exercise A: Identification of Single and Multistage Reducing Valves

1. Your instructor will provide you with an adjustable, multistage reducing valve.
2. Using the diagram provided, examine the primary components of an adjustable, multistage reducing valve. (Fig. 6-1).
3. Identify the following components:
   A. High-pressure gas inlet
   B. Gas outlet
   C. Manometer indicating cylinder pressure

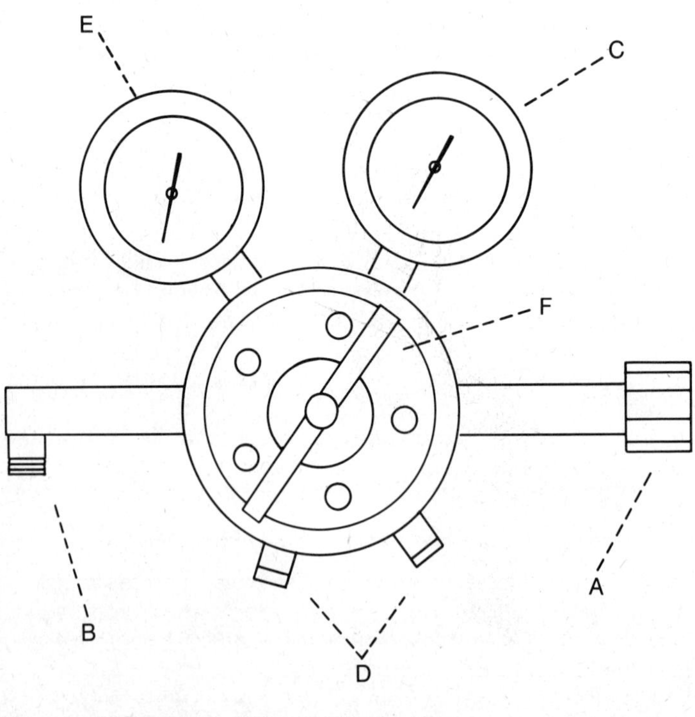

Fig. 6-1. Adjustable, multistage reducing valve.

D. Pressure relief valves indicating the number of stages of pressure reduction
E. Manometer indicating pressure of gas at outlet
F. Adjustable valve for outlet pressure regulation
4. An adjustable regulator or reducing valve frequently is used to reduce cylinder pressure to 50 psi (working pressure) in order to operate a variety of equipment.
5. Do not connect a reducing valve to a gas cylinder unless the 50 psi outlet pressure is diverted. See your laboratory instructor for assistance.

Exercise B: Identification and Assembly of a Gas Regulator

1. Select an oxygen regulator (reducing valve combined with a flowmeter) for use with a large gas cylinder.
2. Using the following diagram, examine the primary components (Fig. 6-2).
3. Identify the following components:
   A. High-pressure gas inlet
   B. Gas outlet from reducing valve
   C. Manometer (indicating cylinder pressure)
   D. Flowmeter
   E. Pressure chamber
   F. Pressure release valve(s)
   G. Flowmeter needle valve
4. Practice the assembly and disassembly of a regulator to a large gas cylinder. Observing the following steps, connect the regulator to a gas cylinder.
   A. Secure the cylinder in the proper stablizing device.
   B. Match the cylinder gas with the proper regulator.
   C. Move the cylinder away from everyone (especially patients) for connections.
   D. "Crack" the cylinder to avoid blowing debris into the regulator.
   E. Connect the regulator inlet to the cylinder outlet.
   F. Tighten the nut by hand, then with a wrench (Fig. 6-3).
   G. Turn the main cylinder valve on *slowly* for about a ¼ turn.

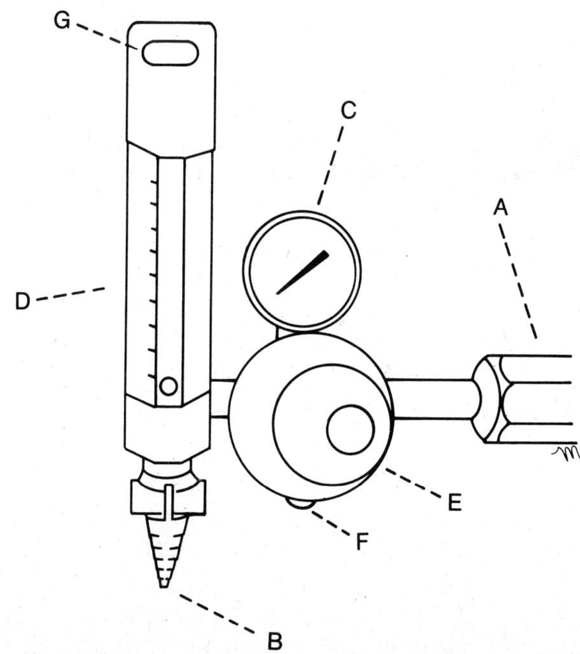

Fig. 6-2. Preset, single-stage gas regulator.

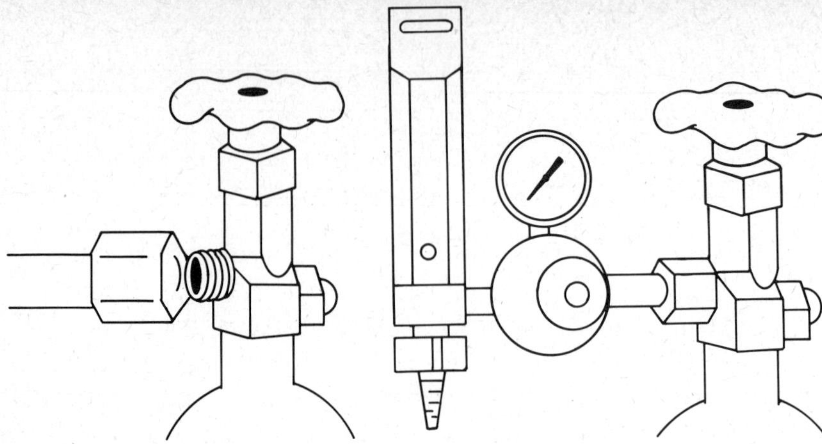

Fig. 6-3. American Standard Valve Outlet Connection: assembled regulator to a large gas cylinder.

H. After the regulator has been charged with gas pressure as indicated on the manometer, open the cylinder's main valve completely.
I. Adjust the flowmeter.

5. Observe and record cylinder pressure on the laboratory report.
Note: If oxygen cylinder pressure is 500 psi or less, the cylinder is almost empty and should be replaced.
6. Disassemble the regulator from the large cylinder.
Note: When removing a regulator from a cylinder, do the following:
A. Relieve the "trapped" pressure in the regulator by first turning the main cylinder valve off and the flowmeter on.
B. Using a wrench, loosen the connector.
C. Disassemble the regulator.

Exercise C: Identification and Assembly of a Bourdon Gauge

1. Select a Bourdon gauge regulator for use with a small cylinder (size "E").
2. Using the diagram provided, examine the components of a Bourdon gauge (Fig. 6-4).
3. Identify the following components:
A. Gas inlet
B. PISS connector pins
C. Gas outlet
D. Manometer (cylinder pressure)
E. Bourdon flow gauge
F. Flow needle valve
G. Pressure-release valve
H. Sealing washer (not shown)
I. Wing bolt (not shown)
4. Practice the assembly and disassembly of a Bourdon gauge to a size "E" cylinder containing oxygen. To attach a Bourdon gauge, do the following:
A. Secure the cylinder to a stabilizing device.
B. Verify that the Bourdon gauge regulator is to be used with oxygen and that the cylinder contains oxygen.

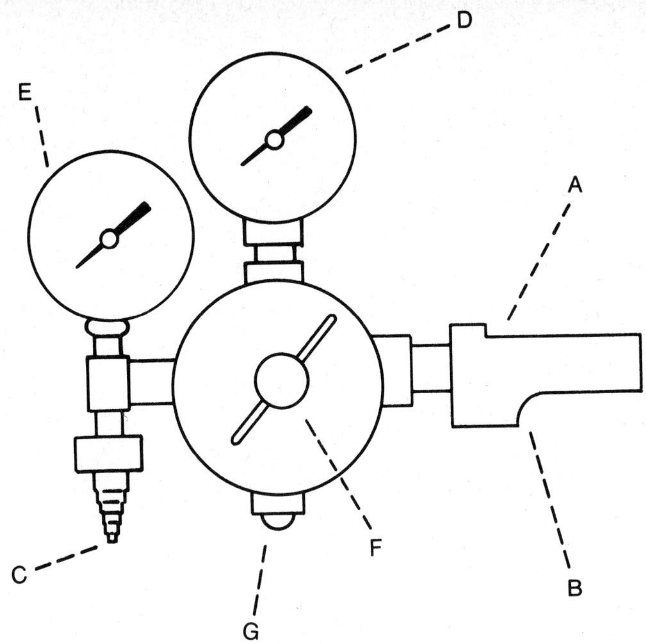

Fig. 6-4. Components of a Bourdon gauge regulator.

C. Remove the wrapper from the cylinder (if applicable) and save the enclosed sealing washer.
D. Be sure that a sealing washer is placed on the Bourdon gauge inlet yoke to prevent a gas leak and to ensure a seal.
E. Place the Bourdon gauge over the cylinder valve. Be certain that the Bourdon gauge inlet yoke mates with the cylinder gas outlet. Also, the pins on the Bourdon gauge should mate with the pins bored into the cylinder valve.
F. Tighten the wing nut by hand and then with a wrench (Fig. 6-5).
G. Using a wrench, slowly open the main cylinder valve. After the regulator has been charged with gas pressure, as indicated on the manometer, open the cylinder's main valve completely.
H. Listen for a hissing sound, which usually indicates a gas leak. If a gas leak is present, examine the sealing washer and repeat the procedure.
I. To regulate gas flow from the Bourdon gauge, adjust the needle valve.

5. Observe and record cylinder pressure on the laboratory report.
Note: An oxygen cylinder pressure of 500 psi or less usually indicates that replacement of the cylinder is needed because the cylinder is nearly empty.
6. Adjust the flow-regulating needle valve to sample flows of 3, 5, and 7 liters/minute.
Note: Connection of a wing nut may be necessary to generate adequate flowrates.
7. While a set flowrate is operational (such as 5 liters/minute), completely occlude the gas outlet with your finger. Is the indicated flowrate accurate when the gas outlet is occluded? Record your results on the laboratory report.
8. Disassemble the Bourdon gauge using the following steps:
A. Using a wrench, turn the main cylinder valve off.
B. While observing the manometer, "bleed" out the pressure trapped within the Bourdon gauge by adjusting the needle valve.
C. Using a wrench, loosen the wing bolt and store the Bourdon gauge.

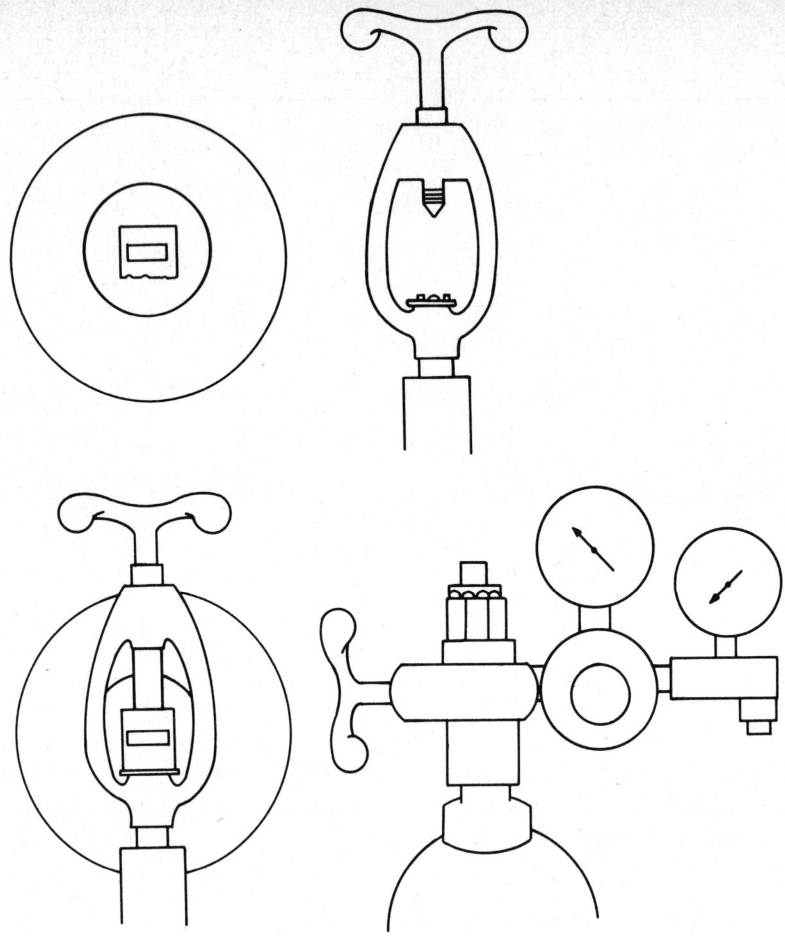

Fig. 6-5. Pin index safety system: assembled Bourdon gauge regulator to small cylinder valve.

Exercise D: Identification and Assembly of a Flowmeter

1. Select a flowmeter using the DISS.
2. Determine the type of gas with which the flowmeter should be used. (The flowmeter should be labeled and may be color coded.)
3. If the flowmeter is labeled, determine whether it is back-pressure compensated or nonback-pressure compensated. (Indicated flow is accurate when back pressure is applied to the gas outlet in a back-pressure compensated flowmeter.)
4. Using the diagram provided, examine the primary components of a DISS flowmeter (Fig. 6-6).
5. Identify the following components:
   - **A.** DISS connector
   - **B.** Gas inlet
   - **C.** Thorpe tube
   - **D.** Float or plunger
   - **E.** Gas outlet
   - **F.** Needle valve
   - **G.** 50 psi connector (if applicable)

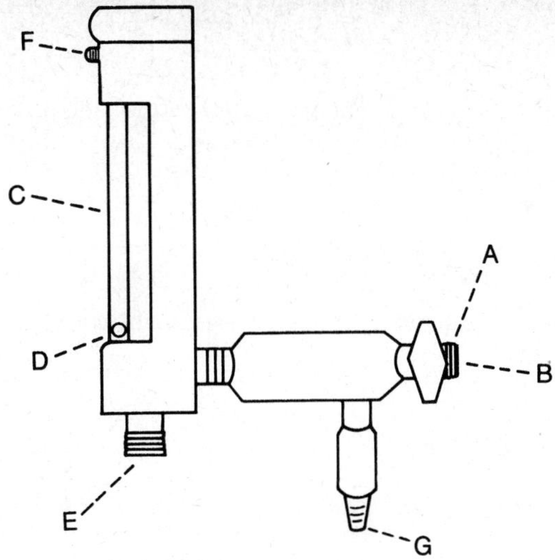

Fig. 6-6. Diameter index safety system: gas flowmeter.

6. Practice the assembly and disassembly of a DISS flowmeter. To connect the flowmeter to a wall outlet, do the following:
   A. Verify that the correct flowmeter is used for the desired gas.
   B. Push the flowmeter gas inlet into the wall outlet connection. If a back-pressure compensated flowmeter is used, observe the "popping" of the float as the flowmeter is pressurized.
   C. Engage the flowmeter nut with the wall outlet threads. Tighten by hand until the threads are completely engaged (Fig. 6-7). Do not use a wrench to tighten.
   D. Verify that no significant gas leak exists at the DISS connection.
7. Adjust the flow to 3, 5, and 7 liters/minute.
   Note: When adjusting flowrates, center the ball float on the calibrated line. For a flowrate of 3 liters/minute, for example, the middle of the ball should float on the calibration line indicating 3.

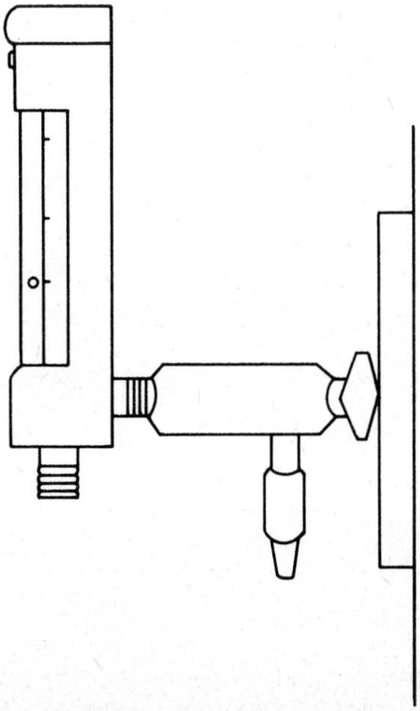

Fig. 6-7. Assembled gas flowmeter connected to a wall outlet.

8. Disconnect the flowmeter by loosening the nut while pushing the flowmeter toward the gas outlet.
9. Compare and contrast the DISS connection between an air and oxygen flowmeter. What happens if an attempt is made to connect an air flowmeter to an oxygen wall outlet? Record your results on the laboratory report.

Exercise E: Determination of "Unknown"

1. After connecting the regulator to a gas cylinder, determine the duration of gas flow using the following formula:

$$X = \frac{P \times C}{V}$$

X = Duration of gas flow in minutes
P = Cylinder pressure in psig (from manometer on regulator)
C = Cylinder factor (constant for different-sized cylinders)
V = Gas flowrate in liters/minute (from regulator flowmeter)

2. The following cylinder factors apply to sizes D, E, G, and H cylinders.

Cylinder Size	Factor
D	0.16
E	0.28
G	2.41
H or K	3.14

Example #1: An "E" cylinder of oxygen contains a pressure of 2000 psi and the flowmeter is operating at a flowrate of 5 liters/minute. What is the duration of gas flow in minutes?

$$X = \frac{P \times C}{V}$$

$$X = \frac{2000 \text{ psi} \times 0.28}{5 \text{ liters/minute}}$$

$$X = \frac{560}{5}$$

$$X = 112 \text{ minutes}$$

Example #2: A size "H" cylinder of oxygen indicates a cylinder pressure of 1000 psi and is used to provide a flowrate of 10 liters/minute to an oxygen mask. What is the duration of gas flow in hours?

$$X = \frac{P \times C}{V}$$

$$X = \frac{1000 \text{ psi} \times 3.14}{10 \text{ liters/minute}}$$

$$X = \frac{3140}{10}$$

$$X = 314 \text{ minutes}$$

$$314 \text{ minutes} \times \frac{1 \text{ hour}}{60 \text{ minutes}} = \frac{314 \times 1 \text{ (minute) (hours)}}{60 \text{ minutes}}$$

$$= \frac{314 \text{ hours}}{60}$$

$$= 5.23 \text{ hours}$$

3. Your laboratory instructor will provide you with a cylinder of oxygen. Using the appropriate wrench, connect a regulator to the cylinder. Adjust the gas flowrate to 5 liters/minute, and monitor the cylinder pressure. Determine the duration of gas flow and record your results on the laboratory report.

RECOMMENDED READING

Burton GG, Hodgkin JE: Respiratory Care. A Guide to Clinical Practice, 2nd ed. Philadelphia, JB Lippincott, 1984

Grenard S, Beck GJ, Rich GW, Shapira M: Introduction to Respiratory Therapy, 3rd ed. Chicago, Year Book Medical Publishers, 1981

Kacmarek RM, Dimas S, Mack C: Essentials of Respiratory Therapy, 2nd ed. Chicago, Year Book Medical Publishers, 1985

McPherson SP, Spearman CB: Respiratory Therapy Equipment, 3rd ed. St Louis, CV Mosby, 1985

Rau J, Rau M: Fundamental Respiratory Therapy Equipment: Principles of Use and Operation. Sarasota, Glenn Educational Medical Services, 1977

Spearman CB, Sheldon RL: Egan's Fundamentals of Respiratory Therapy, 4th ed. St Louis, CV Mosby, 1982

Laboratory Performance Evaluation (#6)

Topic: Gas Pressure and Flow Regulation

Student ______________________ Course ______________________

Date ______________________ Section ______________________

Performance Elements	Acceptable	Unacceptable	Not Applicable	Comments
1. Identifies various cylinder regulators/reducing valves				
2. Attaches regulator/ reducing valve to cylinder				
3. Stabilizes cylinder				
4. "Cracks" cylinder valve				
5. Turns cylinder valve on				
6. Checks regulator/ reducing valve for gas leaks				
7. Monitors cylinder pressure				
8. Records cylinder pressure				
9. Adjusts flow to prescribed flowrate				
10. Turns cylinder gas flow off				
11. "Bleeds" pressure from regulator				
12. Removes regulator/ reducing valve from cylinder				
13. Applies flowmeter to wall outlet				
14. Identifies ASVOC, PISS, and DISS systems				

Knowledge of Procedure

- ☐ Good; student is knowledgeable about rationale and theory related to procedure
- ☐ Fair; student has adequate understanding of rationale and theory related to procedure
- ☐ Poor; student has inadequate understanding of rationale and theory related to procedure

Performance Deficiencies (check those that apply)

- ☐ Excessive time needed to complete procedure
- ☐ Broke aseptic or sterile technique
- ☐ Gross inaccuracy noted
- ☐ Technique may be harmful to patient
- ☐ Incorrect dosage or gas concentration
- ☐ Incorrect equipment assembly/use
- ☐ Unable to answer questions correctly about rationale and/or theory related to procedure
- ☐ Other ______________________________

Evaluation Summary

- ☐ Satisfactory performance
- ☐ Unsatisfactory performance

Recommendations of Evaluator

- ☐ Skills may be applied/observed in clinical setting
- ☐ Specific evaluation deficiencies require correction
- ☐ Complete re-evaluation required
- ☐ Additional laboratory practice required

Signatures:

Evaluator ______________________ Date ______________________

Student ______________________ Date ______________________

Laboratory Report

Student ____________________ Acceptable ____________________

Date ____________________ Unacceptable ____________________

Course ____________________

Topic: Gas Pressure and Flow Regulation

Data or Measurements:

Large cylinder pressure __________ psi

Small cylinder pressure __________ psi

Determination of Unknown:

Cylinder size ____________________

Cylinder pressure ____________________

Cylinder flow ____________________

Duration of flow ____________________

Scenario. A premature infant requires oxygen during transportation to a medical center about 3 hours away. A size "E" cylinder of oxygen contains 2000 psig and is operating at a flow of 5 liters/minute.

1. How long will the cylinder last? (Show your calculations.)

   Answer = __________ minutes = __________ hours

   Will the "E" cylinder be adequate for the trip?

2. Perform the same calculation for an "H" cylinder containing 2200 psig and operating at a flowrate of 10 liters/minute.

   Answer = __________ minutes

3. (T or F) The glass Thorpe tube on a flowmeter is obviously shattered. The device may be used for gas delivery if low oxygen concentrations are needed.
4. The actual flow leaving a Bourdon gauge regulator is __________ than the indicated reading when the gas outlet is partially occluded.

5. The ________ ________ safety system applies to size "E" cylinders and smaller.
6. The ________ ________ safety system applies to cylinders larger than size "E."
7. The ________ ________ safety system applies to flowmeters and wall outlets as well as to equipment using less than 200 psi.
8. What is the purpose of gas safety systems?

9. Briefly describe the connections used for the
   A. American Standard Safety System.

   B. Pin Index Safety System.

   C. Diameter Index Safety System.

10. Preset reducing valves usually produce an outlet pressure of ________.

chapter 7

Oxygen therapy delivery devices

INTRODUCTION

Numerous devices are used to deliver oxygen, including nasal catheters, nasal cannulas, and simple, partial, nonrebreathing, and air entrainment (Venturi) masks. Depending on the delivery device, the gas flowrate, and the patient's ventilatory pattern, the fractional inspired oxygen concentration (FI_{O_2}) may vary from approximately that of room air ($FI_{O_2} = 21\%$) to that of pure oxygen ($FI_{O_2} = 100\%$).

Oxygen delivery devices may be classified as components of a high- or low-flow system, depending on the total gas flowrate delivered. A delivery device that provides supplemental oxygen to the volume of gas spontaneously breathed by a patient is a low-flow system. In contrast, a device that meets or exceeds all of the inspiratory requirements of a patient (tidal volume, minute volume, and peak inspiratory flowrate) may be classified as a high-flow system. A nonrebreathing mask is an example of a high-flow system. This chapter will introduce you to several types of oxygen delivery devices.

OBJECTIVES

After completing this chapter, you should be able to do the following:

1. *Classify an oxygen delivery device as a high- or low-flow system.*
2. *Assemble and identify the primary components of a nasal cannula, nasal catheter, and simple, partial, nonrebreathing, and air entrainment masks.*
3. *Given the operating flowrate, predict the delivered oxygen concentration from an oxygen delivery device.*
4. *Explain the function of a reservoir bag in partial and nonrebreathing devices.*
5. *Explain the functions of valves in a nonrebreathing mask.*
6. *Discuss the principles of gas mixing applied to air entrainment masks.*

EQUIPMENT NEEDED

- ☐ Gas supply system (cylinder or wall outlet)
- ☐ Regulator (for cylinder)
- ☐ Flowmeter (for wall outlet)
- ☐ Humidifier (bubble)
- ☐ Nasal catheter
- ☐ Nasal cannula
- ☐ Simple mask
- ☐ Partial rebreathing mask
- ☐ Nonrebreathing mask
- ☐ Air-entrainment mask

ACTIVITIES

Exercise A: Identification and Assembly of a Nasal Cannula

1. Select a nasal cannula.
2. Examine the primary components of a nasal cannula using the following diagram (Fig. 7-1).
3. Identify the following components:
   - **A.** Gas inlet connection
   - **B.** Nasal prongs
   - **C.** Elastic strap
4. Connect a flowmeter to a wall outlet, or connect a regulator to a gas cylinder.
5. Wash your hands.
6. Connect the humidifier to the flowmeter.
7. Connect small-bore oxygen tubing to the humidifier outlet.
8. Connect the cannula to the tubing. Verify that a tight connection exists.
9. Adjust the flowrate to sample flows of 3 and 6 liters/minute.
10. Check the system for proper function.
11. Apply to a mannequin or simulated patient (Fig. 7-2).

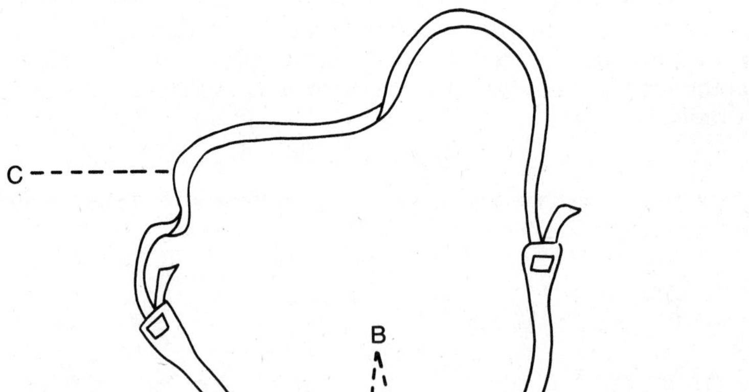

Fig. 7-1. Nasal cannula components.

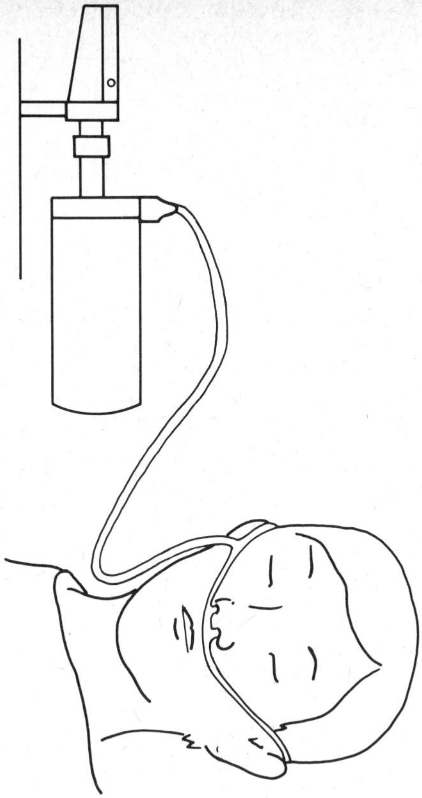

Fig. 7-2. Assembled nasal cannula, tubing, humidifier, and flowmeter.

12. Explain the fire hazards of oxygen and that the cannula should be worn continuously during oxygen therapy.
13. Post a no-smoking sign.
14. Disassemble all equipment.
    Note: A modified version of a nasal cannula currently is used to provide long-term oxygen therapy to neonates. Since neonates are obligate nasal breathers, a pediatric cannula may be modified by cutting away the nasal prongs, which allows low flowrates of oxygen to be delivered atraumatically to the nose.

Exercise B: Identification and Assembly of a Nasal Catheter

1. Select a nasal catheter. Using the following diagram, examine the components of a nasal catheter (Fig. 7-3).
2. Identify the following components:
   A. Gas inlet connector
   B. Gas outlet perforations
3. Using a mannequin, briefly explain the procedure and its purpose. Wash your hands.
4. Connect an oxygen flowmeter to a wall outlet or to a gas cylinder.
5. Attach a humidifier to the flowmeter.
6. Connect small-bore oxygen tubing to the nasal catheter and to the humidifier.
7. Turn on the gas flow and verify the patency of the catheter.
8. Estimate the depth of catheter insertion by placing the catheter tip near the lobe of the ear and marking the distance with tape.

9. Lubricate the catheter with a sterile water-soluble lubricant.
10. Place the catheter in the nose and gently advance it.
11. Advance the catheter until it is proximal to the uvula.
12. Verify the position of the catheter tip. If gagging occurs, the catheter probably is inserted too deeply.
13. Stabilize the catheter with tape. Refer to the following diagram for proper placement of a nasal catheter (Fig. 7-4).
14. Post a no-smoking sign, and reassure the patient.

Special Considerations

1. Nasal catheters are rarely used in the clinical setting.
2. A nasal catheter may be useful in severe facial trauma or burn cases.
3. Before insertion in the clinical setting, check patency of the nares by alternately occluding each external nare and requesting exhalation. Insert the catheter into the most patent side of the nose.

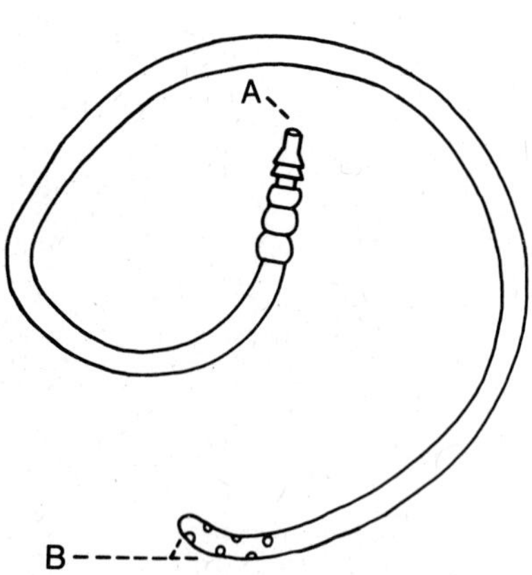

Fig. 7-3. Nasal catheter components.

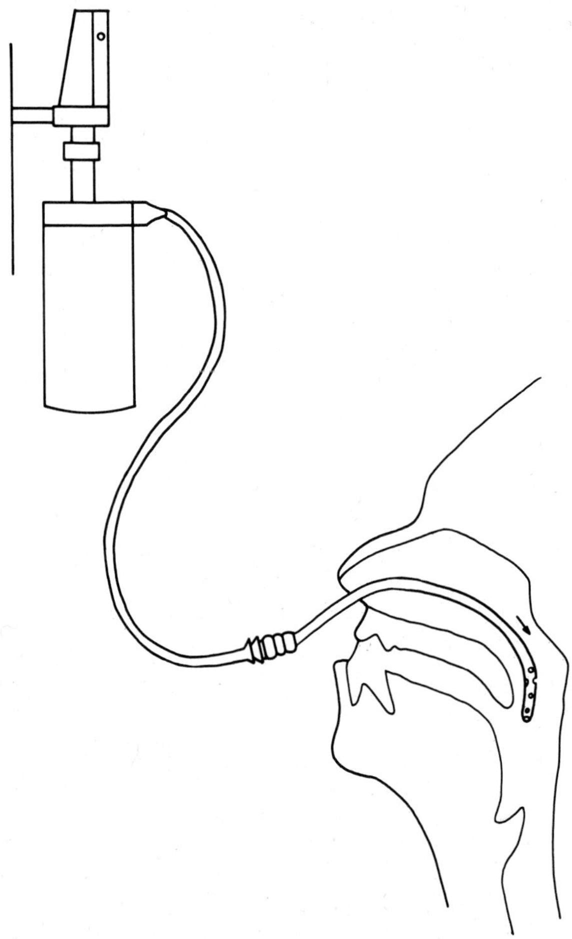

Fig. 7-4. Assembled nasal catheter.

Exercise C: Identification and Assembly of a Simple Mask

1. Select a simple mask. Examine the primary components of a simple mask using the following diagram (Fig. 7-5).
2. Identify the following components:
   A. Gas inlet
   B. Exhalation ports
   C. Malleable metal nose piece
   D. Air dilution inlet (if applicable)
   E. Transparent plastic mask
3. Connect a flowmeter to a wall outlet, or connect a regulator to a gas cylinder.
4. Wash your hands.
5. Connect the humidifier to the flowmeter.
6. Connect small-bore oxygen tubing to the humidifier outlet.
7. Attach the mask to the oxygen tubing.
8. Adjust the flowrate to a minimum of 6 liters/minute.
9. Check the system for proper function.
10. Apply the mask to a simulated patient. Ensure that the mask is fitted snugly against the face (Fig. 7-6).
11. Verify that a no-smoking sign is posted.
12. Dissassemble all equipment.

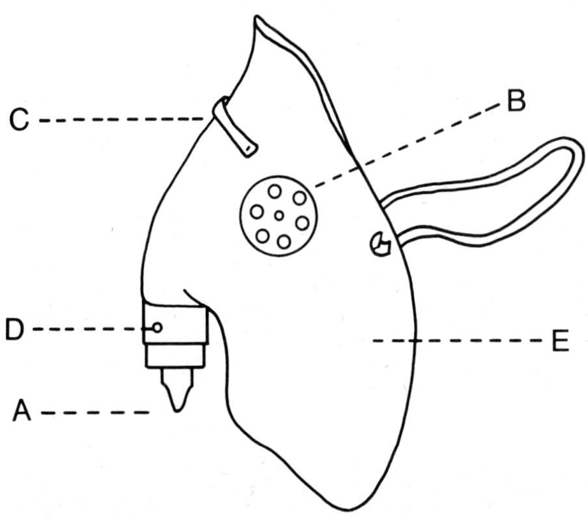

Fig. 7-5. Simple oxygen mask components.

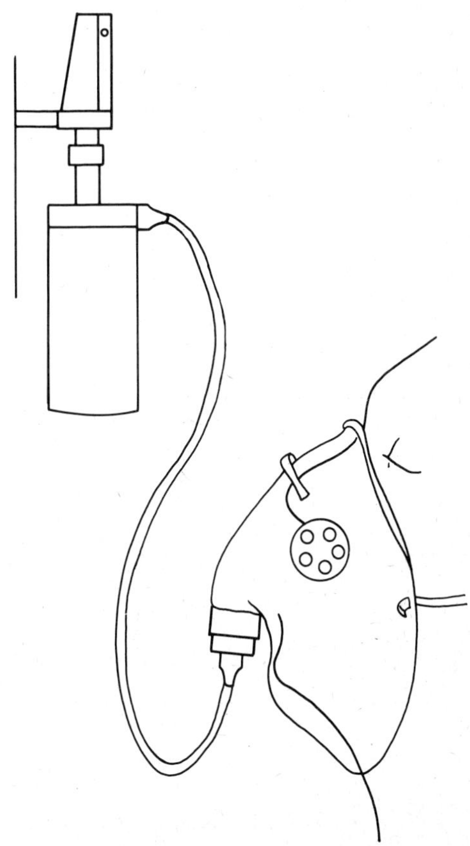

Fig. 7-6. Assembled simple oxygen mask.

Exercise D: Identification and Assembly of a Partial Rebreathing Mask

1. Select a partial rebreathing mask. Examine the primary components of a partial rebreathing mask using the following diagram (Fig. 7-7).
2. Identify the following components:
   A. Gas inlet
   B. Exhalation ports
   C. Reservoir bag
   D. Malleable metal nose piece
3. Connect a flowmeter to a wall outlet, or connect a regulator to a gas cylinder.
4. Wash your hands.
5. Connect the humidifier to the flowmeter.
6. Connect the small-bore oxygen tubing to the humidifier outlet.
7. Attach the mask to the humidifier with the tubing connected to a humidifier.
8. Adjust the flowrate to a minimum of 6 liters/minute.
9. Check the system for proper function.
10. Apply the mask to a laboratory partner (Fig. 7-8).
11. Adjust the flowrate so that the bag remains at least one-third full when your laboratory partner inhales. Note this flowrate on the laboratory report.
12. Disassemble all equipment.
    Note: In clinical use, the partial rebreathing mask is intended to give high oxygen concentrations. Therefore, the oxygen flowrate should be adequate to prevent complete collapse of the reservoir bag during inspiration.

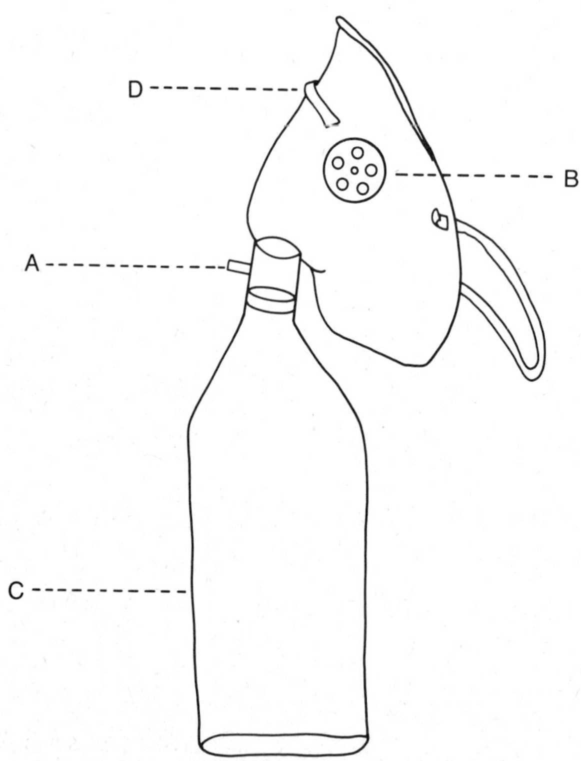

Fig. 7-7. Partial rebreathing mask components.

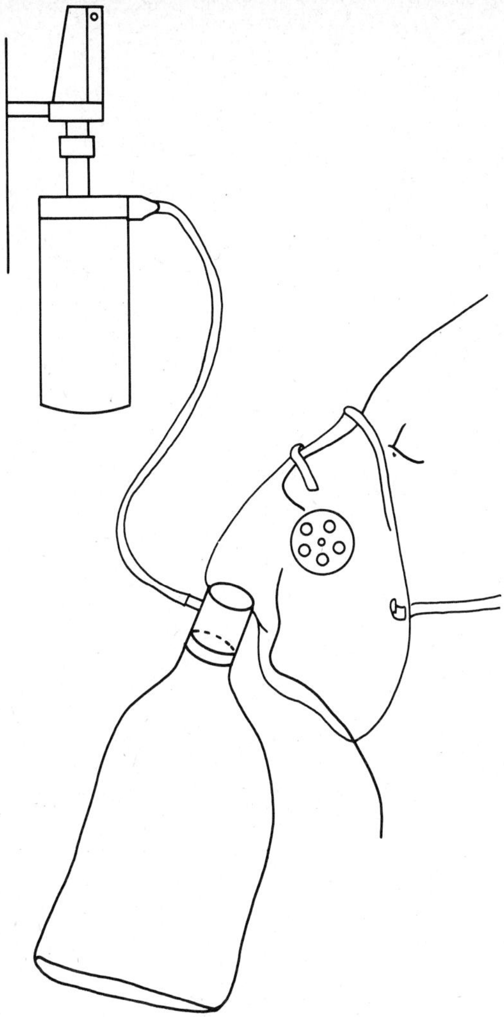

Fig. 7-8. Assembled partial rebreathing mask.

Exercise E: Identification and Assembly of a Nonrebreathing Mask

1. Select a nonrebreathing mask. Examine the components of a nonrebreathing mask using the following diagram (Fig. 7-9).
2. Identify the following components:
   - **A.** Gas inlet
   - **B.** Inspiratory one-way valve
   - **C.** One-way exhalation valves
   - **D.** Reservoir bag
   - **E.** Emergency air intake valve (if applicable)
3. Connect a flow meter to a wall outlet, or connect a regulator to a gas cylinder.
4. Wash your hands.
5. Connect the humidifier to the flowmeter.
6. Connect small-bore oxygen tubing to the humidifier outlet.
7. Attach the mask to the humidifier with the tubing.

8. Adjust the flowrate to a minimum of 6 liters/minute.
9. Check the system for proper function.
10. Apply the mask to a laboratory partner (Fig. 7-10).
11. Adjust the flowrate so that the bag remains at least one-third full when your laboratory partner inhales. Note this flowrate on the laboratory report.
12. Dissassemble all equipment.
13. Review the usual operating flowrate and range of oxygen concentrations delivered during a normal resting ventilatory pattern by the nasal cannula, nasal catheter, simple mask, partial rebreathing mask, and nonrebreathing mask in Table 7-1.

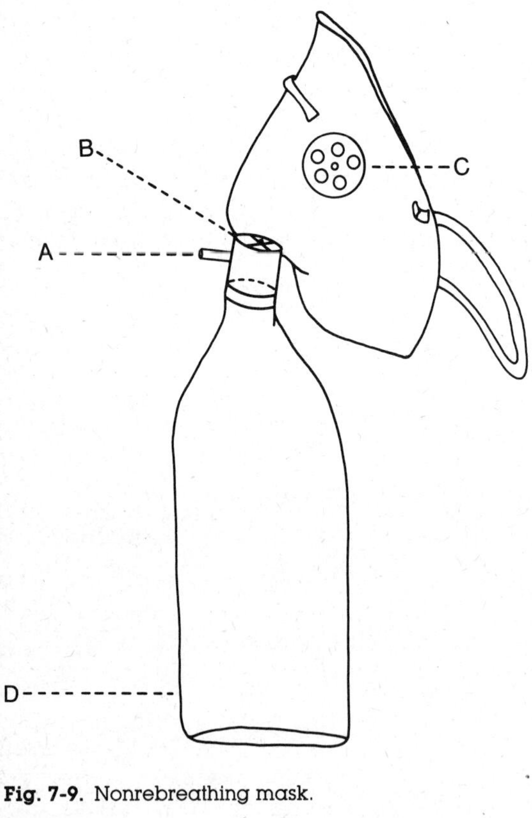

Fig. 7-9. Nonrebreathing mask.

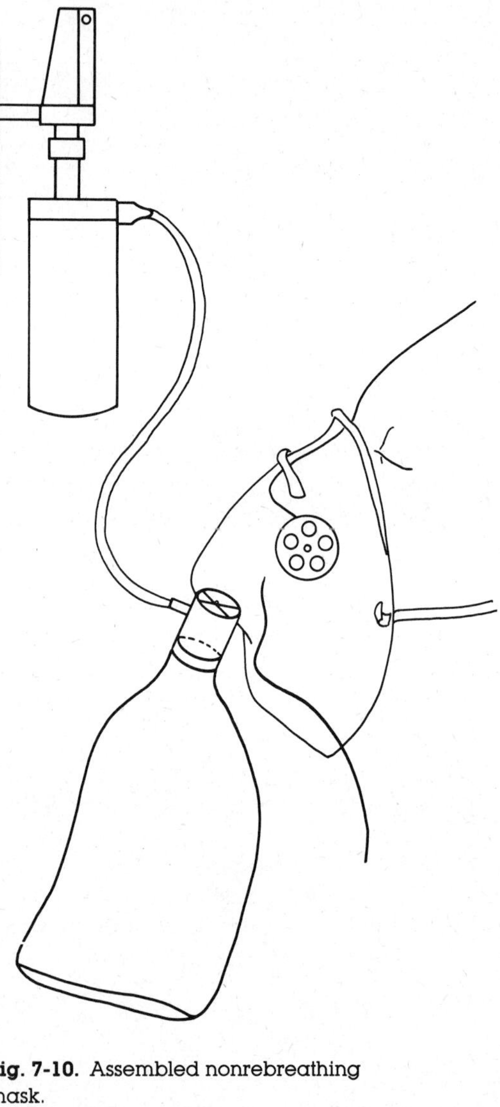

Fig. 7-10. Assembled nonrebreathing mask.

Table 7-1. Oxygen Flowrates and Range of Delivered F_{IO_2} from Oxygen Delivery Devices

Device	Oxygen Source Liters/Minute	Range of F_{IO_2}*
Nasal Cannula and nasal catheter	1	0.24
	2	0.28
	3	0.32
	4	0.36
	5	0.40
	6	0.44
	>6	>0.44
Simple mask	5–6	0.40
	6–7	0.50
	7–8	0.60
Partial rebreathing mask	6	0.60
	7	0.70
	8	0.80
	9	>0.80
Nonrebreathing mask	6–10	>0.90

(Reproduced with permission from Shapiro BA et al: Clinical Application of Respiratory Care, 3rd ed. Copyright © 1985 by Year Book Medical Publishers, Inc., Chicago)
* All ranges of F_{IO_2} are approximate. The delivered F_{IO_2} applies to the situation in which a normal, resting ventilatory pattern is assumed. With abnormal ventilatory patterns, which frequently accompany cardiopulmonary disease, the F_{IO_2} may differ significantly from those stated in Table 7-1. With masks, the delivered F_{IO_2} is dependent upon the tightness of the fit of the mask with the face.

Exercise F: Identification and Assembly of an Air Entrainment (Venturi) Mask

1. Select an air entrainment mask. Using the following diagram, examine the primary components (Fig. 7-11).

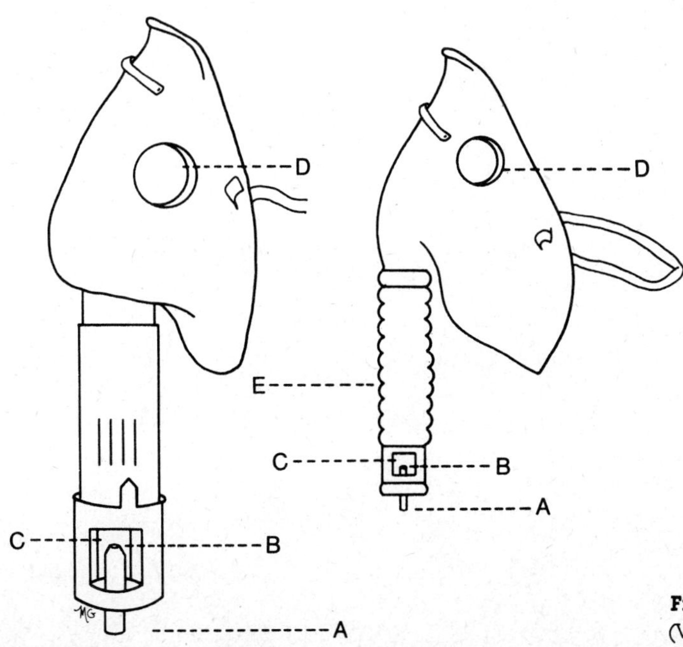

Fig. 7-11. Air-entrainment (Venturi) mask components.

2. Identify the following components:
   A. Gas inlet connection
   B. Jet
   C. Entrainment ports
   D. Mask exhalation ports
   E. Large-bore aerosol tubing adapter (if applicable)
3. Connect a flowmeter to a wall outlet, or connect a regulator to a gas cylinder.
4. Wash your hands.
5. Connect the humidifier to the flowmeter.
6. Connect small-bore oxygen tubing to the humidifier outlet.
7. Attach the mask to the tubing.
8. Adjust the flowrate according to the delivered oxygen concentration.
   Note: $F_{I_{O_2}} < 30\%$, use flow of 3 liters/minute, or as stated on adapter.
   $F_{I_{O_2}} \geq 30\%$, use flow of 6 liters/minute, or as stated on adapter.
9. Check the system for proper function.
10. Apply the mask to your laboratory partner (Fig. 7-12).

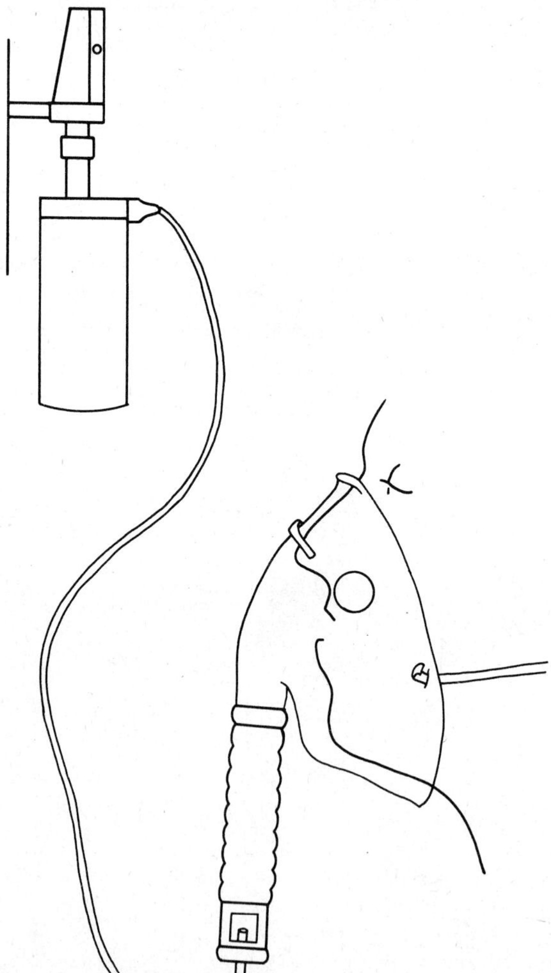

Fig. 7-12. Assembled Venturi mask.

Table 7-2. Entrainment Ratios and Total Gas Flowrates of the Venturi System

FI_{O_2}	Oxygen Flowrate	Entrainment Ratio	Total Gas Flowrate
0.24	3	25/1	78
0.28	3	10/1	33
0.31	3	7/1	24
0.35	6	5/1	36
0.40	6	3/1	24
0.60	10	1/1	20
0.70	10	0.6/1	16

(Reproduced with permission from Kacmarek RM et al: Essentials of Respiratory Therapy, 2nd ed. Copyright © 1985 by Year Book Medical Publishers, Inc., Chicago)
Note: To prevent inadvertent dilution of the desired oxygen concentration, the total flowrate should exceed the subject's peak inspiratory flowrate. The peak inspiratory flowrate of a healthy resting adult is about 15 to 30 liters/minute. Patients with cardiopulmonary disease may have higher peak inspiratory flowrates and require total gas flowrates in excess of 40 liters/minute.

11. Adjust either the jet or entrainment ports to administer an FI_{O_2} of
    A. 0.24
    B. 0.28
    C. 0.40
    D. 0.50
12. Verify the presense of no-smoking signs.
13. Disassemble all equipment.
14. Review the entrainment ratio and total gas flowrate delivered at various oxygen concentrations using a Venturi mask in Table 7-2.

Exercise G: Administration of Oxygen Therapy to a Simulated Patient

After completing the previous exercises, practice administering oxygen administration to a simulated patient. Either a mannequin or a laboratory partner may be the simulated patient.

1. Review the order. Verify the appropriateness of therapy.
2. Obtain the appropriate equipment.
3. Introduce yourself to the "patient."
4. Identify the patient by wrist band.
5. Simply and clearly explain the therapy to the patient. Confirm patient understanding.
6. Wash your hands.
7. Properly assemble the equipment.
8. Correctly adjust the oxygen flowrate or concentration.
9. Pretest the equipment function before patient application.
10. Apply the device to the patient.
11. Evaluate the patient's response to therapy.
12. Inform the patient of the fire hazard of oxygen.
13. Assemble a no-smoking sign.
14. Document the procedure, including the date, time, device, flowrate or FI_{O_2}, and patient response.

RECOMMENDED READING

Burgess WR, Chernick V: Respiratory Therapy in Newborn Infants and Children. New York, Thieme–Stratton, 1982

Burton GG, Hodgkin JE: Respiratory Care. A guide to Clinical Practice, 2nd ed. Philadelphia, JB Lippincott, 1984

Kacmarek RM, Dimas S, Mack C: Essentials of Respiratory Therapy, 2nd ed. Chicago, Year Book Medical Publishers, 1985

McPherson SP, Spearman CB: Respiratory Therapy Equipment, 3rd ed. St Louis, CV Mosby, 1985

Rarey KP, Youtsey JW: Respiratory Patient Care. Englewood Cliffs, Prentice-Hall, 1981

Rau J, Rau M: Fundamental Respiratory Therapy Equipment: Principles of Use and Operation. Sarasota, Glenn Educational Medical Services, 1977

Shapiro BA, Harrison RA, Kacmarek RM, Cane RD: Clinical Application of Respiratory Care, 3rd ed. Chicago, Year Book Medical Publishers, 1985

Spearman CB, Sheldon RL: Egan's Fundamentals of Respiratory Therapy, 4th ed. St. Louis, CV Mosby, 1982

Laboratory Performance Evaluation (#7)

Topic: Oxygen Therapy Delivery Devices

Student ______________________ Course ______________________

Date ______________________ Section ______________________

Performance Elements	Acceptable	Unacceptable	Not Applicable	Comments
1. Reviews the order				
2. Obtains the appropriate equipment				
3. Introduces self to simulated patient				
4. Identifies the "patient"				
5. Explains procedure to simulated patient				
6. Washes hands				
7. Assembles equipment properly				
8. Adjusts device to prescribed flowrate or concentration				
9. Pretests equipment function before patient application				
10. Applies device to patient				
11. Evaluates patient response.				
12. Instructs patient in oxygen fire hazards				
13. Posts a no-smoking sign				
14. Documents procedure				

Knowledge of Procedure

- ☐ Good; student is knowledgeable about rationale and theory related to procedure
- ☐ Fair; student has adequate understanding of rationale and theory related to procedure
- ☐ Poor; student has inadequate understanding of rationale and theory related to procedure

Performance Deficiencies (check those that apply)

- ☐ Excessive time needed to complete procedure
- ☐ Broke aseptic or sterile technique
- ☐ Gross inaccuracy noted
- ☐ Technique may be harmful to patient
- ☐ Incorrect dosage or gas concentration
- ☐ Incorrect equipment assembly/use
- ☐ Unable to answer questions correctly about rationale and/or theory related to procedure
- ☐ Other ______________________________

Evaluation Summary

- ☐ Satisfactory performance
- ☐ Unsatisfactory performance

Recommendations of Evaluator

- ☐ Skills may be applied/observed in clinical setting
- ☐ Specific evaluation deficiencies require correction
- ☐ Complete re-evaluation required
- ☐ Additional laboratory practice required

Signatures:

Evaluator ______________________ Date ______________________

Student ______________________ Date ______________________

Laboratory Report

Student ______________________ Acceptable ______________________

Date ______________________ Unacceptable ______________________

Course ______________________

Topic: Oxygen Therapy Delivery Devices

Experimental Data

Exercise C = __________ liters/minute

Exercise D = __________ liters/minute

Scenario: The patient, a young female, arrives in the emergency room via the local rescue squad. Enroute, she has received 2 liters/minute of oxygen by means of a nasal cannula. Because of her clinical appearance, it is decided that until blood gas results are available, she will probably benefit from a partial rebreathing mask set up at 8 liters/minute of oxygen.

You became involved in this fascinating case when the pulmonary physician, as part of his consultation, asks you the following questions about oxygen therapy and delivery devices:

1. Why are oxygen administrative devices transparent?

2. Why is the minimum flowrate administered with an oxygen mask greater than 6 liters/minute?

3. What is the purpose of
   A. a reservoir bag on a partial rebreathing mask?

B. inspiratory and expiratory valves on a nonrebreathing mask?

4. Identify three potential hazards of oxygen administration by mask, and give a method for avoiding these hazards.

5. Define the following terms:

A. Fractional inspired oxygen concentration

B. High-flow system

C. Low-flow system

chapter 8

Environmental and gas mixing systems

INTRODUCTION

The respiratory care of patients may require environmental control of the atmosphere. Environmental variables that may be controlled in the inspired atmosphere include gas temperature, relative humidity, and respired gas concentrations. Gas temperature may be either heated or cooled and measured with a thermometer. The relative humidity of inspired gas may be increased by using either a humidifier or a nebulizer. Inspired oxygen concentration may be controlled by using a Venturi jet, gas blender, or air and oxygen mixing system. Carbon dioxide concentrations may be minimized by providing adequate gas flowrates to flush out gas reservoirs. The purpose of this chapter is to introduce you to gas blenders, mixing systems, oxygen hoods, and tent systems.

OBJECTIVES

After completing this chapter, you should be able to do the following:

1. *Identify the environmental variables controlled by an oxygen tent and oxygen hood.*
2. *State the minimum total gas flowrate administered to an oxygen tent or hood.*
3. *Classify an oxygen tent, hood, and mixing system as a high- or low-flow system.*
4. *State the oxygen concentration provided by oxygen hoods, tents, and mixing systems.*
5. *Completely assemble an oxygen hood, tent, or gas mixing system.*
6. *Trace the flow of gas through the system.*
7. *Manipulate the oxygen concentration delivered by a hood, tent, or mixing system.*

EQUIPMENT NEEDED

- ☐ Oxygen Hood
  - Oxyhood
  - Aerosol tubing
  - Flowmeters (air and oxygen)
  - Nebulizer or humidifier
  - Heating probe
  - Thermometer
  - Sterile H_2O
  - Oxygen analyzer
- ☐ Tent
  - Frame
  - Tent
  - Nebulizer jar
  - Oxygen analyzer
  - Thermometer
- ☐ Mixing Systems
  - Jet nebulizer
  - Flowmeters (air and oxygen)
  - Aerosol tubing
  - Aerosol delivery device
  - T-tube
  - Endotracheal tube adapter
  - Oxygen analyzer
  - Venturi
- ☐ Gas Blender
  - Air high-pressure hose
  - Oxygen high-pressure hose
  - Flowmeter

ACTIVITIES

Exercise A: Identification and Assembly of a Gas Mixing System

1. Using the following diagram, examine the primary components of a gas mixing system (Fig. 8-1).
2. Identify the following components of a gas mixing system:
   - **A.** Air flowmeter
   - **B.** Oxygen flowmeter
   - **C.** T-tube
   - **D.** 15 mm adapter
   - **E.** Small-bore tubing
   - **F.** Oxygen analyzer
   - **G.** Nebulizer or humidifier

Assembly of a Gas Mixing System

1. Plug flowmeters (air and O_2) into wall and attach a nebulizer.
2. Fill the nebulizer with sterile H_2O.
3. Close the entrainment ports on the nebulizer.
4. Attach a T-tube to the nebulizer.
5. Plug an endotracheal tube (3.5 mm) adapter into the T-tube.
6. Attach aerosol tubing to the T-tube.

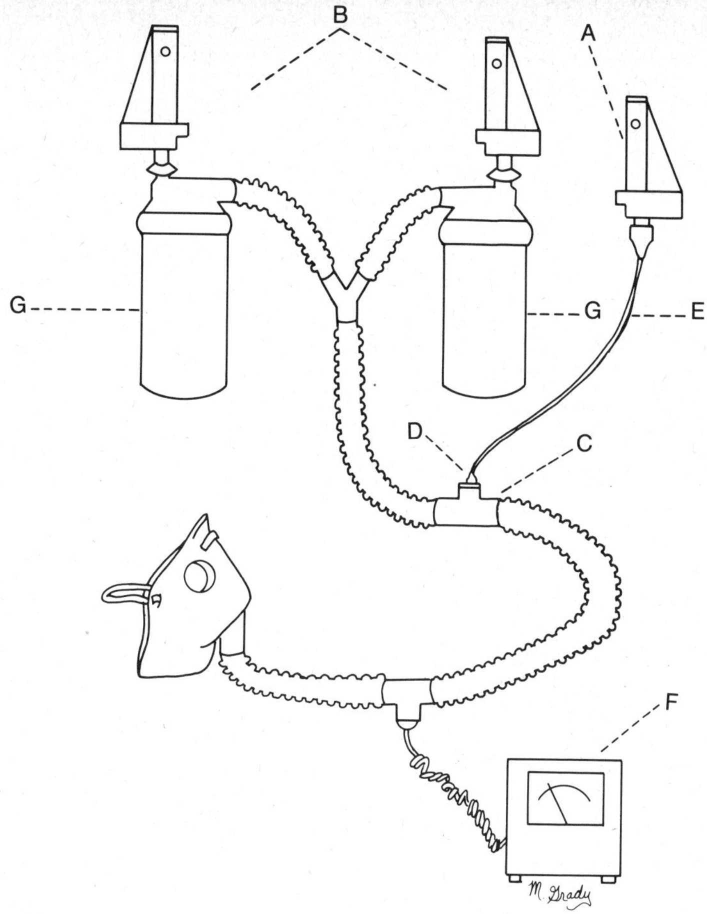

Fig. 8-1. Components and assembly of a gas mixing system.

7. Connect an aerosol delivery device to the aerosol tubing.
8. Adjust the oxygen concentration by adjusting the air or oxygen flowmeter. *Note:* When attempting to deliver oxygen concentrations in excess of 0.60, drive the nebulizer with flow from the oxygen flowmeter, and titrate or mix in the necessary flow of air. In a gas mixing system, a consistent oxygen concentration may be delivered only when the total gas flow exceeds the patient's peak inspiratory flowrate.
9. Analyze the oxygen concentration delivered by inserting the analyzer probe proximal to the aerosol delivery device.
10. Obtain the following oxygen concentrations:
    - **A.** 30%
    - **B.** 35%
    - **C.** 40%
    - **D.** 60%
    - **E.** 80%
11. Determine the total gas flowrate delivered by the addition of the flowrates set on the air and oxygen flowmeters.
12. Document on the laboratory report the flowrates of air and oxygen required to deliver the specified oxygen concentrations. Be sure to determine the total gas flowrate.

Exercise B: Identification and Assembly of a Gas Blender

1. Using the diagram provided, examine the primary components of a gas blender (Fig. 8-2).
2. Identify the following components:
   A. 50 psi air inlet
   B. 50 psi oxygen inlet
   C. Oxygen concentration selector
   D. Flowmeter
   E. 50 psi air and oxygen lines

Assembly of a Gas Blender

1. Attach one end of a high-pressure air hose to the air inlet on the blender. Connect the other end of the hose to a 50 psi air source (wall outlet).
2. Attach one end of a high-pressure oxygen hose to the oxygen inlet on the blender. Connect the other end of the hose to a 50 psi oxygen source (wall outlet).
3. Adjust the flowmeter to a sample flowrate of 10 liters/minute.
4. Attach small-bore oxygen tubing to the flowmeter.
5. Adjust the oxygen concentration selector to obtain the following concentrations:
   A. 21%
   B. 30%
   C. 45%
   D. 65%
   E. 100%
6. Verify the selected oxygen concentrations by analysis. See your laboratory instructor for assistance in oxygen analysis.

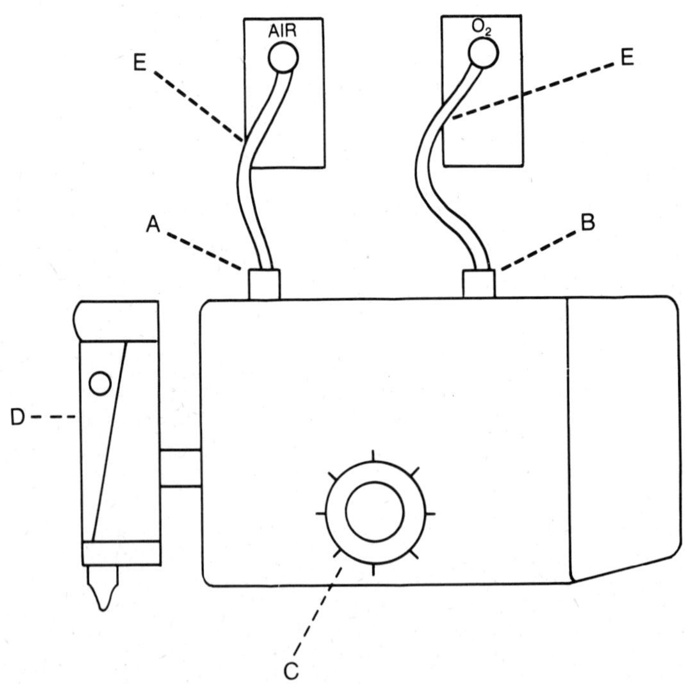

Fig. 8-2. Components and assembly of a gas blender.

7. Compare the set oxygen concentration on the selector with the analyzed concentration. Assuming analytical accuracy, does the gas blender provide precise (within ± 2%) oxygen concentrations? Record your observations on the laboratory report.

Exercise C: Identification and Assembly of an Oxygen Tent

1. Obtain the equipment necessary to assemble an oxygen tent. Examine the primary components of an oxygen tent (Fig. 8-3).
2. Identify the following components of an oxygen tent.
   - A. Ice chamber or refrigeration unit
   - B. Nebulizer (not shown)
   - C. Gas inlet connection
   - D. Plastic tent
   - E. Frame
   - F. No-smoking signs
   - G. Filter

Assembly of an Oxygen Tent

1. Obtain the tent, frame, and air or oxygen flowmeter.
2. Attach the frame to the bed.
3. Attach the tent to the frame.
4. Connect the portholes in the tent to the frame.

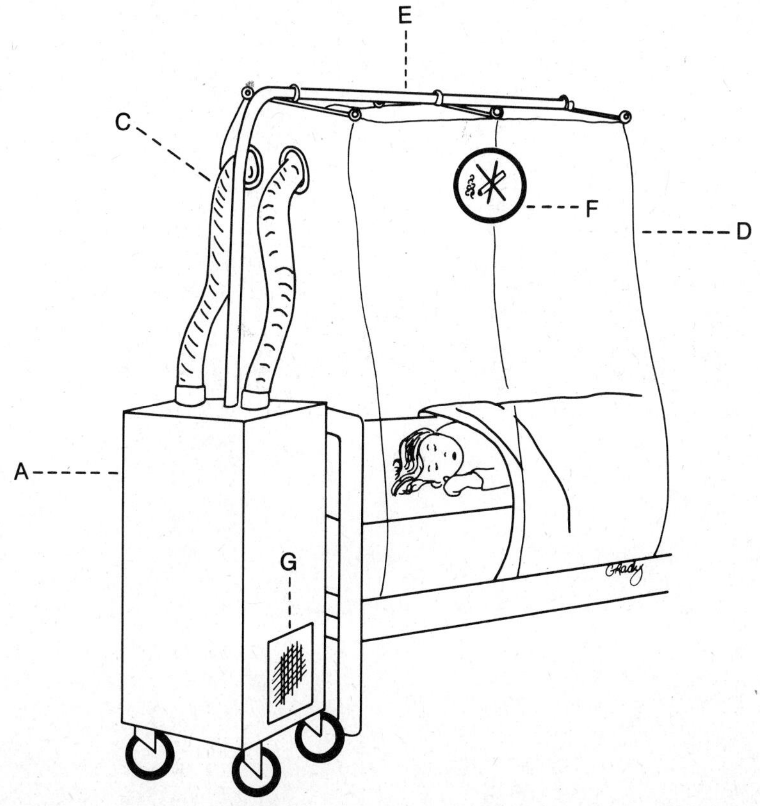

Fig. 8-3. Oxygen tent system.

5. Attach drain hose to the base of the ice chamber, and be certain that it is closed or clamped.
6. Fill the nebulizer with sterile H_2O.
7. Fill the chamber with ice if needed, or activate the refrigeration unit.
8. Connect the oxygen tubing to the nebulizer jar.
9. Turn on the gas flowmeter. Use a flow of at least 10 liters/minute.
10. Monitor the oxygen concentration. If the desired oxygen concentration cannot be obtained, secure possible leaks in the system.
11. Place a thermometer inside the tent.
12. After the tent has been in operation for 15 to 20 minutes, analyze the oxygen concentration.
13. If you are using oxygen as the gas source, record the highest possible delivered oxygen concentration. Record your results on the laboratory report, including the measured temperature within the tent.

Exercise D: Identification and Assembly of an Oxygen Hood

1. Obtain the equipment necessary to assemble an oxygen hood.
   Note: A humidifier may replace a nebulizer, and a gas blender may be used to mix gases.
2. Examine the components of an oxygen hood system (Fig. 8-4).

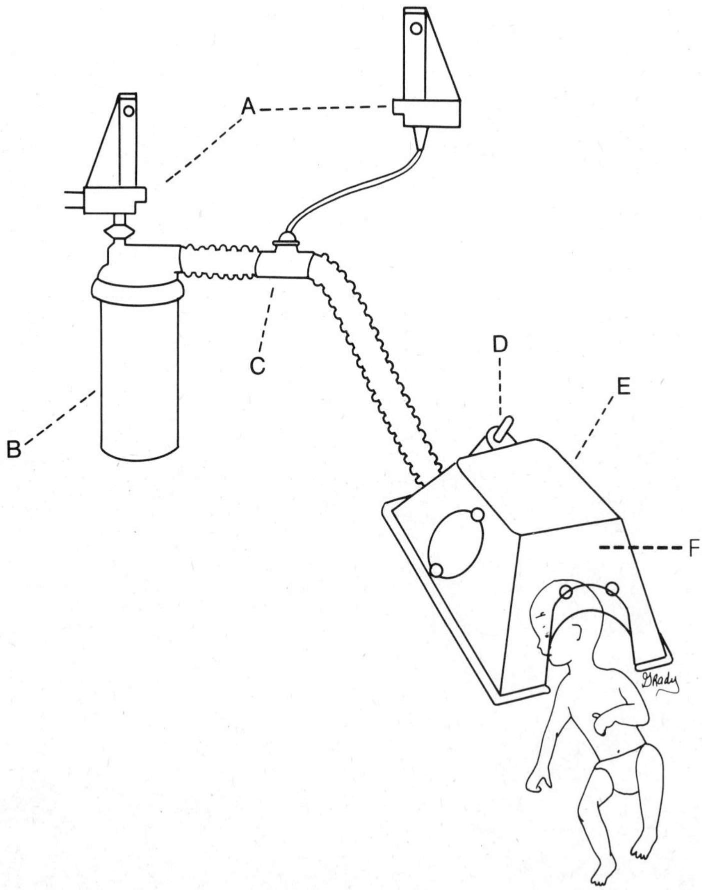

Fig. 8-4. Components of an oxygen hood system.

3. Identify the following components of an oxygen hood system:
   A. Air and oxygen flowmeters or gas blender
   B. Heated humidifier or nebulizer
   C. T-Tube
   D. Thermometer
   E. Baffle (not shown)
   F. Oxyhood

Assembly of an Oxygen Hood

1. Plug flowmeters (air and O_2) into the wall and attach a nebulizer or humidifier.
2. Place heating probe in nebulizer or humidifier. Plug into wall outlet.
3. Fill nebulizer with sterile H_2O.
4. Adjust oxygen concentration by closing the entrainment ports on the nebulizer and adjusting the flowmeters, or adjust the oxygen blender.
5. Attach the aerosol tubing to the nebulizer and to the hood.
6. Place a thermometer in the oxygen hood.
7. Check for adequate aerosol output or humidity and gas flow. A minimum flow of 7 liters/minute is needed.
8. Calibrate the oxygen analyzer and analyze the oxygen concentration.
9. Monitor the temperature in the hood. Adjust the temperature to 36.5°C or a neutral thermal temperature for a simulated neonatal patient.
10. Place the infant in the hood. Obtain the following oxygen concentrations:
    A. 30% D. 25%
    B. 45% E. 100%
    C. 60%

    Note: In clinical practice, the oxygen concentration is analyzed proximal to an infant's airway because neonates are obligate nasal breathers and because of the layering effect of gaseous oxygen within a hood. In other words, oxygen is more dense than air and may layer out in a hood, causing wide variance in the concentration measured at different locations within the hood.

Exercise E: Assembly of an Air Injector (Venturi) for Use with Aerosol Generating System

1. A variety of specific oxygen concentrations may be administered during aerosol therapy by the incorporation of either a gas mixing system or a Venturi jet into the system.
2. Examine the components of an aerosol generating system in which a Venturi jet is utilized to provide a specific oxygen concentration using the following diagram (Fig. 8-5).
3. Identify the following components:
   A. Air injector
   B. Ultrasonic nebulizer
   C. Water trap
   D. Aerosol tubing
4. If a Venturi is used to deliver specific oxygen concentrations with an ultrasonic nebulizer, a water trap will help prevent inadvertent fluctuations (increases) in the oxygen concentration owing to condensate collecting in the aerosol tubing.
5. Assemble an aerosol generating system incorporating a Venturi. Obtain the following oxygen concentrations:
   A. 0.24
   B. 0.28
   C. 0.40

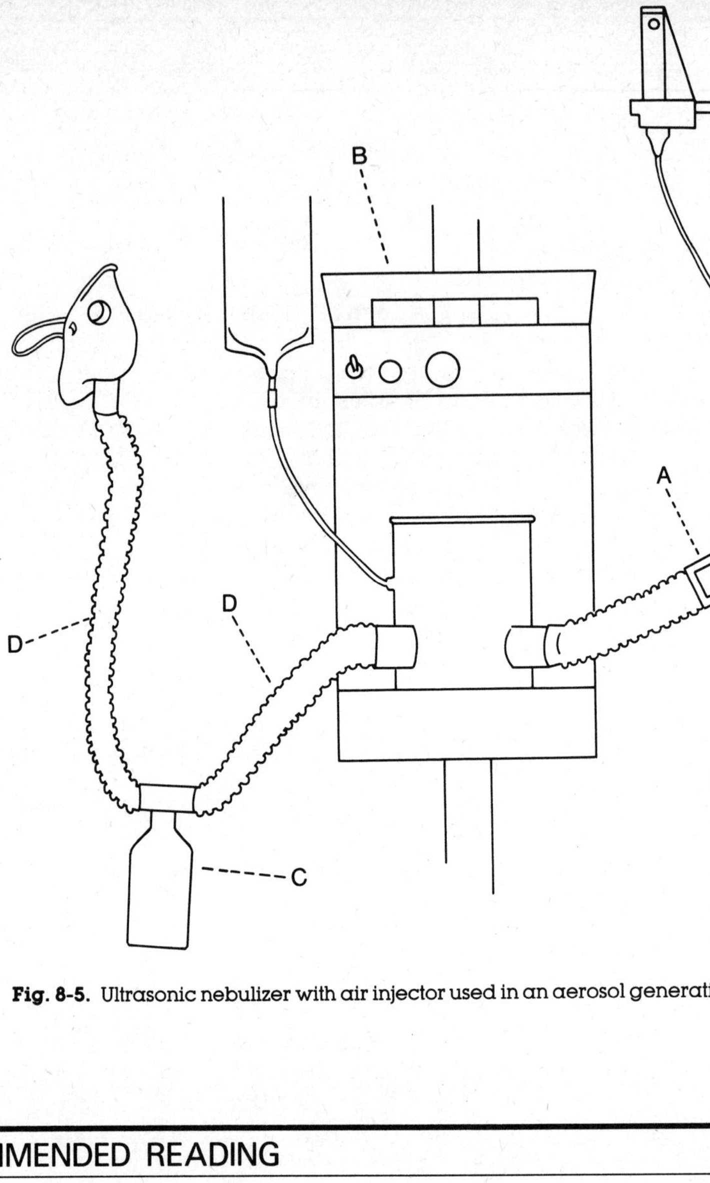

Fig. 8-5. Ultrasonic nebulizer with air injector used in an aerosol generating system.

RECOMMENDED READING

Burgess WR, Chernick V: Respiratory Therapy in Newborn Infants and Children. New York, Thieme-Stratton, 1982

Burton GG, Hodgkin JE: Respiratory Care. A Guide to Clinical Practice, 2nd ed. Philadelphia, JB Lippincott, 1984

Kacmarek RM, Dimas S, Mack C: Essentials of Respiratory Therapy, 2nd ed. Chicago, Year Book Medical Publishers, 1985

McPherson SP, Spearman CB: Respiratory Therapy Equipment, 3rd ed. St Louis, CV Mosby, 1985

Rarey KP, Youtsey JW: Respiratory Patient Care. Englewood Cliffs, Prentice-Hall, 1981

Rau J, Rau M: Fundamental Respiratory Equipment: Principles of Use and Operation. Sarasota, Glenn Educational Medical Services, 1977

Shapiro BA, Harrison RA, Kacmarek RM, Cane RD: Clinical Application of Respiratory Care, 3rd ed. Chicago, Year Book Medical Publishers, 1985

Spearman CB, Sheldon RL: Egan's Fundamentals of Respiratory Therapy, 4th ed. St Louis, CV Mosby, 1982

Laboratory Performance Evaluation (#8a)

Topic: Environmental and Gas Mixing Systems

Student ______________________ Course ______________________

Date ______________________ Section ______________________

Performance Elements	Acceptable	Unacceptable	Not Applicable	Comments
1. Reviews the order				
2. Obtains proper equipment				
3. Washes hands				
4. Assembles equipment correctly				
5. Administers adequate total gas flowrate				
6. Administers prescribed FI_{O_2}				
7. Analyzes FI_{O_2}				
8. Provides adequate humidification or nebulization				
9. Assures appropriate gas temperature				
10. Checks equipment function				
11. Applies system to simulated patient				
12. Documents procedure				

Knowledge of Procedure

- ☐ Good; student is knowledgeable about rationale and theory related to procedure
- ☐ Fair; student has adequate understanding of rationale and theory related to procedure
- ☐ Poor; student has inadequate understanding of rationale and theory related to procedure

Performance Deficiencies (check those that apply)

- ☐ Excessive time needed to complete procedure
- ☐ Broke aseptic or sterile technique
- ☐ Gross inaccuracy noted
- ☐ Technique may be harmful to patient
- ☐ Incorrect dosage or gas concentration
- ☐ Incorrect equipment assembly/use
- ☐ Unable to answer questions correctly about rationale and/or theory related to procedure
- ☐ Other ____________________

Evaluation Summary

- ☐ Satisfactory performance
- ☐ Unsatisfactory performance

Recommendations of Evaluator

- ☐ Skills may be applied/observed in clinical setting
- ☐ Specific evaluation deficiencies require correction
- ☐ Complete re-evaluation required
- ☐ Additional laboratory practice required

Signatures:

Evaluator ____________________ Date ____________________

Student ____________________ Date ____________________

Laboratory Performance Evaluation (#8b)

Topic: Oxygen Hood

Student ______________________ Course ______________________

Date ______________________ Section ______________________

Performance Elements	Acceptable	Unacceptable	Not Applicable	Comments
1. Reviews the order				
2. Obtains proper equipment				
3. Washes hands				
4. Assembles equipment correctly				
5. Administers adequate total gas flowrate				
6. Administers prescribed FI_{O_2}				
7. Analyzes FI_{O_2}				
8. Provides adequate humidification or nebulization				
9. Assures appropriate gas temperature				
10. Monitors temperature				
11. Checks equipment function				
12. Applies system to simulated patient				
13. Documents procedure				

Knowledge of Procedure

- ☐ Good; student is knowledgeable about rationale and theory related to procedure
- ☐ Fair; student has adequate understanding of rationale and theory related to procedure
- ☐ Poor; student has inadequate understanding of rationale and theory related to procedure

Performance Deficiencies (check those that apply)

- ☐ Excessive time needed to complete procedure
- ☐ Broke aseptic or sterile technique
- ☐ Gross inaccuracy noted
- ☐ Technique may be harmful to patient
- ☐ Incorrect dosage or gas concentration
- ☐ Incorrect equipment assembly/use
- ☐ Unable to answer questions correctly about rationale and/or theory related to procedure
- ☐ Other ______________________________

Evaluation Summary

- ☐ Satisfactory performance
- ☐ Unsatisfactory performance

Recommendations of Evaluator

- ☐ Skills may be applied/observed in clinical setting
- ☐ Specific evaluation deficiencies require correction
- ☐ Complete re-evaluation required
- ☐ Additional laboratory practice required

Signatures:

Evaluator ______________________ Date ______________________

Student ______________________ Date ______________________

Laboratory Performance Evaluation (#8c)

Topic: Oxygen Tent

Student ______________________ Course ______________________

Date ______________________ Section ______________________

Performance Elements	Acceptable	Unacceptable	Not Applicable	Comments
1. Reviews the order				
2. Obtains proper equipment				
3. Washes hands				
4. Assembles equipment correctly				
5. Administers adequate total gas flow				
6. Administers prescribed FI_{O_2}				
7. Analyzes FI_{O_2}				
8. Provides adequate nebulization				
9. Assures appropriate gas temperature				
10. Checks equipment function				
11. Applies system to simulated patient				
12. States fire hazards of oxygen				
13. Posts no-smoking signs				
14. Documents procedure				

Knowledge of Procedure

- ☐ Good; student is knowledgeable about rationale and theory related to procedure
- ☐ Fair; student has adequate understanding of rationale and theory related to procedure
- ☐ Poor; student has inadequate understanding of rationale and theory related to procedure

Performance Deficiencies (check those that apply)

- ☐ Excessive time needed to complete procedure
- ☐ Broke aseptic or sterile technique
- ☐ Gross inaccuracy noted
- ☐ Technique may be harmful to patient
- ☐ Incorrect dosage or gas concentration
- ☐ Incorrect equipment assembly/use
- ☐ Unable to answer questions correctly about rationale and/or theory related to procedure
- ☐ Other ______________________________

Evaluation Summary

- ☐ Satisfactory performance
- ☐ Unsatisfactory performance

Recommendations of Evaluator

- ☐ Skills may be applied/observed in clinical setting
- ☐ Specific evaluation deficiencies require correction
- ☐ Complete re-evaluation required
- ☐ Additional laboratory practice required

Signatures:

Evaluator ____________________ Date ____________________

Student ____________________ Date ____________________

Laboratory Report

Student ______________________ Acceptable ______________________

Date ______________________ Unacceptable ______________________

Course ______________________

Topic: Oxygen Hoods, Tents, and Mixing Systems

Data and Measurements

Gas Mixing System

FI_{O_2}	Air Flowrate	Oxygen Flowrate	Total Delivered Flowrate
0.30			
0.35			
0.40			
0.60			
0.80			

Gas Blender

Set FI_{O_2}	Analyzed FI_{O_2}	Observations
21%		
30%		
45%		
65%		
100%		

Oxygen Tent

Maximum FI_{O_2} obtained ______________________

Flowrate ______________________

Temperature ______________________

Scenario: Today you have been assigned to the pediatrics unit. Your specific area of responsibility includes the following patient modalities: one oxyhood, two T-tube patients, one oxygen tent, and a tracheostomy collar. Gas mixing for the oxyhood has been achieved by using an oxygen blender. The fraction of inspired oxygen being delivered to the T-tube and to tracheostomy patients is controlled by an air and oxygen mixture (*i.e.*, an air flowmeter and oxygen flowmeter, the lines of which merge in a reservoir).

Please answer the following questions:

1. What is the minimally acceptable total gas flowrate for an

   A. oxygen hood? ______________________

   B. oxygen tent? ______________________

   C. oxygen mixing system? ______________________

2. How may the delivered FI_{O_2} be affected by an inadequate total gas flowrate?

3. Classify as a high- or low-flow system:

A. Oxygen hood ______________________________

B. Oxygen tent ______________________________

C. Mixing system ______________________________

4. An oxygen tent controls what environmental factors?

5. What is the highest $F_{I_{O_2}}$ an oxygen tent system can deliver?

6. The physician has ordered that the $F_{I_{O_2}}$ of the T-tube patient be decreased from 0.40 to 0.35.

What ratio of air to oxygen in liters per minute will be needed to accomplish this? Air __________

Oxygen __________

7. The tracheostomy patient is receiving 4 liters/minute of oxygen and 12 liters/minute of air. What is his $F_{I_{O_2}}$?

8. What variables, other than $F_{I_{O_2}}$, are controllable when using an oxyhood?

chapter 9

Atmospheric oxygen analysis

INTRODUCTION

Under most clinical conditions, oxygen is a colorless, odorless, tasteless, and transparent gas. The concentration of oxygen in the atmosphere or gas mixture inhaled by a patient is impossible to detect without the use of special apparatus. An oxygen analyzer is one type of apparatus that measures the percentage or partial pressure of oxygen in a gaseous mixture. The purpose of this chapter is to introduce you to the analysis of gaseous oxygen.

OBJECTIVES

After completing this chapter, you should be able to do the following:

1. *Identify four types of oxygen analyzers.*
2. *Classify a given oxygen analyzer according to the principle of operation.*
3. *Explain the purpose of oxygen analysis.*
4. *Verify the delivered oxygen concentration provided by any oxygen/aerosol device.*
5. *Identify the primary components of an oxygen analyzer.*
6. *Properly calibrate the oxygen analyzer.*
7. *Demonstrate the correct operation of an oxygen analyzer.*
8. *Measure the oxygen concentration of an "unknown" gas mixture within an accuracy range of ± 2%.*

EQUIPMENT NEEDED

- ☐ Oxygen hood system
- ☐ Oxygen tent system
- ☐ Gas mixing system
- ☐ Jet nebulizer and aerosol tubing
- ☐ Paramagnetic (Beckman D-2) analyzer

☐ Thermal conductivity (MIRA) analyzer
☐ Galvanic (Hudson) analyzer
☐ Polarographic analyzer

ACTIVITIES

Exercise A: Identification and Operation of a Paramagnetic Analyzer

1. Examine the components of a paramagnetic analyzer (Beckman D-2) using the following diagram (Fig. 9-1).
2. Identify the following components:
   A. Read-out scale
   B. Aspiration bulb
   C. Sampling inlet tip
   D. Power switch
   E. Silica gel crystal desiccant (not shown)
3. Prepare the analyzer for use. Check the battery function by depressing the power switch and observing the light beam on the read-out scale.
4. Check the color of the silica gel crystals. The crystals should have a blue appearance in order to act as a desiccant by removing water vapor from the gas sample.
5. Place the analyzer on a flat, level surface before use. Ideally, the read-out scale should be located at eye level.

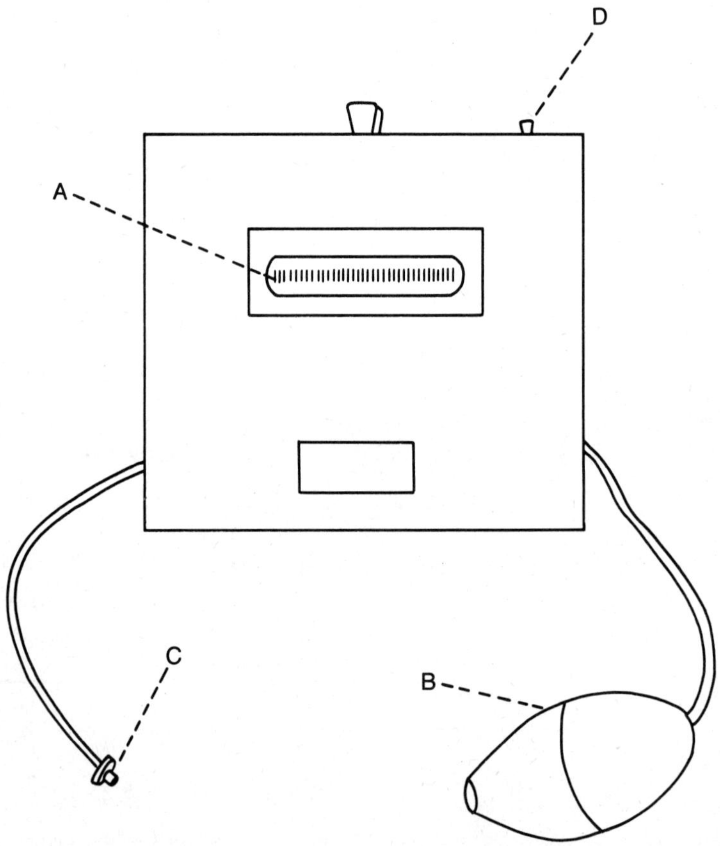

Fig. 9-1. Physical analyzer (paramagnetic) components.

6. To sample an atmosphere, place the sampling inlet in the gas. Aspirate the sample by squeezing the bulb 10 to 12 times. Depress the power switch.
7. Read the oxygen percentage and partial pressure on the readout scale.
8. After taking a reading, aspirate air ($FI_{O_2} = 21\%$) into the sample chamber.

Exercise B: Identification and Operation of a Thermal Conductivity Analyzer

1. Examine the components of a thermal conductivity analyzer using the following diagram (Fig.9-2).
2. Identify the following components:
   A. Read-out scale
   B. Sample inlet
   C. Power switch
   D. Aspiration bulb
   E. Calibration screw
3. Prepare the analyzer for use by doing the following:
   A. Calibrate the analyzer.
   B. Check color of silica gel crystals (pink).
   C. Check battery function by lifting the power switch and observing the meter needle.
   D. Place the analyzer on a flat surface for use.
4. To sample gas, place the sampling inlet in the gas. Aspirate the contents by squeezing the bulb 8 to 10 times. Lift the power switch.
5. Read the oxygen percentage on the read-out scale.
6. After sampling a gas mixture, aspirate air ($FI_{O_2} = 21\%$) into the sample chamber.

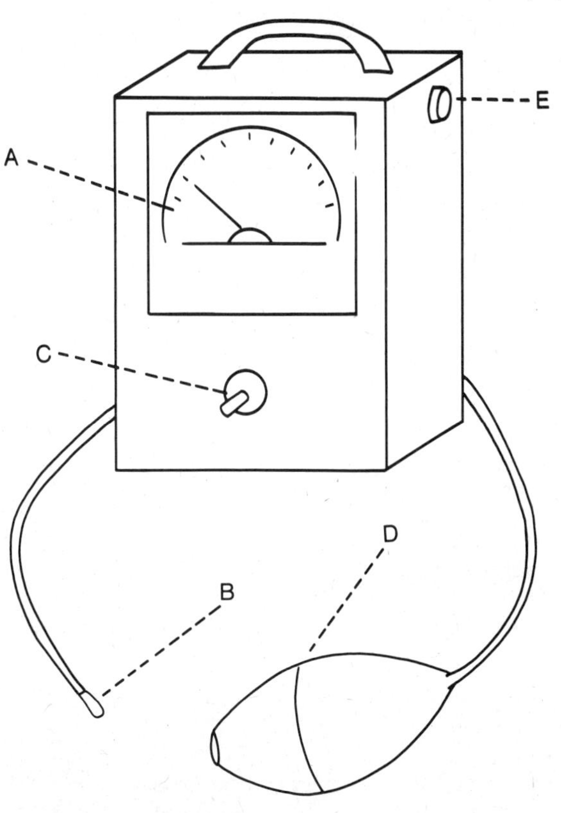

Fig. 9-2. Thermal conductivity analyzer components.

Exercise C: Identification and Operation of a Galvanic Analyzer

1. Obtain a galvanic analyzer. Using the following diagram, examine the components (Fig. 9-3).
2. Identify the following components:
   A. Oxygen sensor
   B. Read-out scale
   C. Sensor plug (if applicable)
   D. Calibration dial
   E. Wide-bore aerosol tubing adapter
3. Prepare the analyzer for use by doing the following:
   A. Calibrate the analyzer (see Exercise E).
   B. Place analyzer on a flat surface.
   C. Plug in the sensor (if applicable).
4. To sample gas, attach the wide-bore aerosol tubing adapter to the sensor, and connect the sensor to the aerosol tubing.
5. Observe the oxygen percentage on the read-out scale. *Note:* The analyzer provides a continuous reading of $F_{I_{O_2}}$ while the sensor is plugged into the rear of the unit.
6. Please disconnect the sensor plug when not in use.

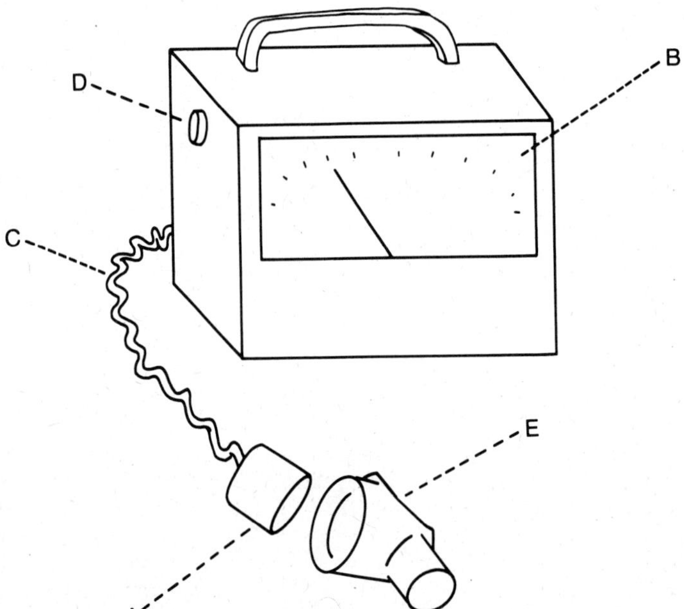

Fig. 9-3. Galvanic analyzer components.

Exercise D: Identification and Operation of a Polarographic Analyzer

1. Obtain a polarographic analyzer. Using the following diagram (Fig. 9-4), examine the primary components.
2. Identify the following components:
   A. Read-out scale
   B. Calibration knob
   C. Sensor or electrode

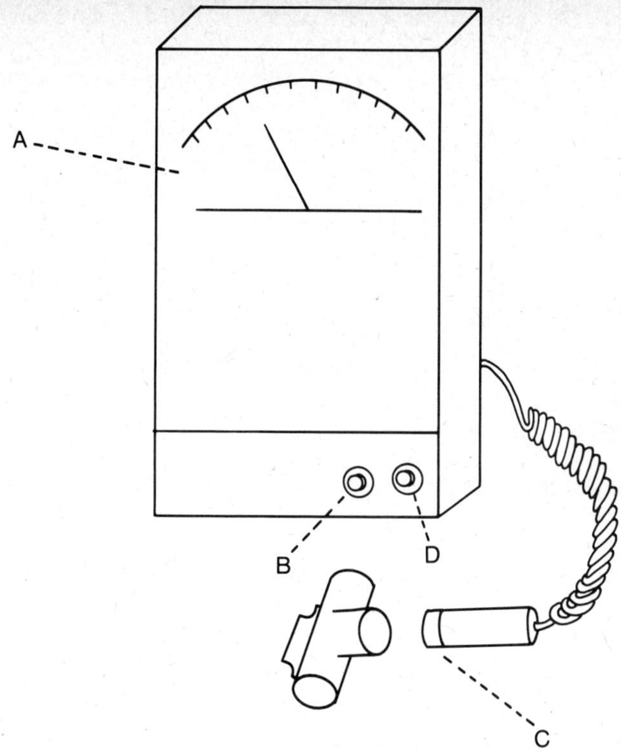

Fig. 9-4. Polarographic analyzer components.

D. On/off switch
E. Batteries (not shown)
F. Alarms (if applicable)

3. Prepare the analyzer for use by doing the following:
   A. Calibrate the analyzer (see Exercise E).
   B. Place the analyzer on a flat surface.
   C. Test the battery function by activating the battery check switch.
   D. Test the alarms (if applicable) by turning the analyzer on and setting the alarm limits outside the indicated oxygen concentration.
4. To sample gas, expose the sensor to the gaseous mixture. *Note:* An adapter may be necessary for use in a mechanical ventilator circuit.
5. Observe the oxygen percentage on the read-out scale after turning the analyzer power switch on.
6. Turn the power switch off after a measurement has been made and recorded.

Exercise E: Calibration of an Oxygen Analyzer

1. To ensure accuracy, calibration of some oxygen analyzers is recommended before measuring the oxygen concentration of a gas mixture. Calibration refers to exposing the analyzer sensor to a predetermined, known oxygen concentration and adjusting the analyzer reading accordingly. A two-point calibration refers to the exposure of the analyzer to two different known values of oxygen with subsequent adjustment of the reading to each value.
2. Some analyzers have been factory calibrated and usually require no further adjustment before analysis (unless the analyzer is used at high altitudes). The para-

magnetic analyzer is one type that usually does not routinely require calibration before use.

3. Other analyzers, such as some polarographic types, may require a periodic check of the zero reading when the analyzer is in operation. To check the zero reading, expose the analyzer sensor to 100% nitrogen and adjust accordingly to zero percent oxygen.
4. For many electrochemical analyzers, accuracy of the measurement may be improved if the analyzer is calibrated according to the concentration of oxygen measured.

Low Oxygen Concentration Calibration

1. For delivered gas concentrations ≤ 50%, calibrate the analyzer to an FI_{O_2} of 21%.
2. Depending on the type of analyzer, either expose the sensor to room air or aspirate air into the measuring chamber.
3. Using the calibration dial, adjust the meter needle to read precisely 21%.

High Oxygen Concentration Calibration For gas concentration > 50%, calibrate the analyzer to 100% oxygen.

1. Depending on the type of analyzer, either aspirate pure oxygen into the sample chamber or place both the sensor and small-bore oxygen tubing into a plastic bag.
2. Provide a gas flow of 5 liters/minute of dry 100% oxygen into the bag, and "flush" the air out of the bag by squeezing it several times.
3. Allow the bag to refill with pure oxygen so that the analyzer sensor is exposed to 100% oxygen. Allow about 20 to 30 seconds for stabilization to occur.
4. While the analyzer sensor is exposed to 100% oxygen, adjust the read-out needle to read precisely 100% (Fig. 9-5).
5. After the calibration to 100% oxygen, the analyzer may be read slightly higher than 21% (± 2–5%) when the sensor is re-exposed to air.
6. The analyzer is ready for the analysis of oxygen concentrations in excess of 50%.

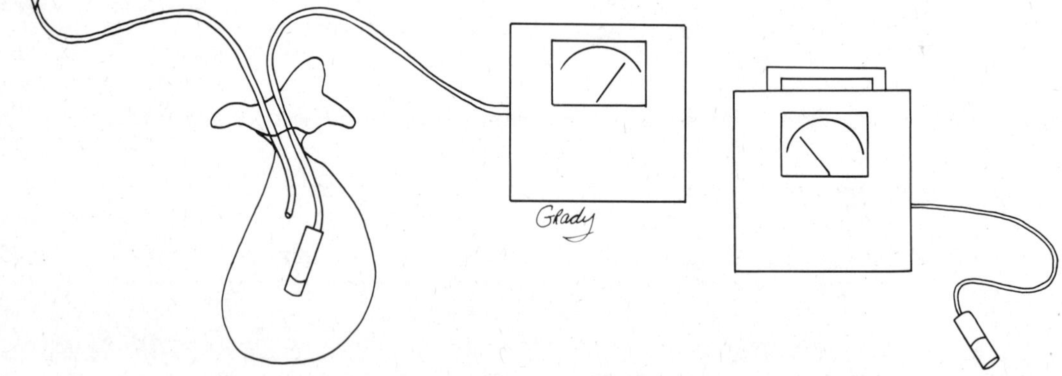

Fig. 9-5. Two-point calibration of an oxygen analyzer to room air (FI_{O_2} = 0.21) and pure oxygen (FI_{O_2} = 1.0).

7. Practice the calibration of an oxygen analyzer according to the manufacturer's recommendations. See your laboratory instructor for assistance regarding the calibration of specific brands of analyzers.
8. Review the information on the principles of operation, calibration procedure, and factors affecting the measurement of oxygen in Tables 9-1 and 9-2.

Table 9-1. List of Analyzer Principles and Their Respective Calibration Procedure

Principle of Operation	Calibration
Paramagnetic	Does not require calibration (are factory calibrated). Should be checked for accuracy with known O_2 concentration. Return to factory if recalibration is necessary.
Thermal conductivity	These units require a two-point calibration (21% and 100%).
Galvanic fuel cell	Normally requires only a single-point calibration (21%); however, if desired, a two-point calibration (21% and 100%) can be used.
Polarographic (Clark electrode)	Normally requires only a single-point calibration (21%); however, if desired, can use a two-point calibration (21% and 100%)

(Rarey, Youtsey: Respiratory Patient Care. Englewood Cliffs, Prentice-Hall, 1981. Used with permission)

Table 9-2. List of Various Factors on Operation of Oxygen Analyzers

Principle of Operation	Factors: Pressure	Factors: Humidity	Factors: Temperature
Paramagnetic (Beckman D2)	Accuracy affected by ambient pressure	Read dry gases	Not affected by ambient temperature
Thermal conductivity	Generally unaffected by ambient pressure ranges	Can read wet or dry gases depending on the unit	Compensated through the calibration process
Polarographic	Will read higher % under increasing pressure	Unaffected by humidity unless condensate forms on electrodes	Electrically compensated
Galvanic fuel cell	Will read higher % under increasing pressure	Unaffected by humidity unless condensate forms on electrodes	Electrically compensated

(Rarey Youtsey: Respiratory Patient Care. Englewood Cliffs, Prentice-Hall, 1981. Used with permission)

Exercise F: Determination of "Unknown"

1. Your instructor will assemble an oxygen, aerosol, or gas mixing system(s) with a known analyzed oxygen concentration. You will be informed if the oxygen concentration of the system exceeds 50% oxygen so that proper calibration of the analyzer may be performed.

2. Analyze the "unknown" gas mixture(s) provided by your instructor. Record your results on the laboratory report. Acceptable results must be within ± 2% of the oxygen concentration measured by your instructor.
3. For analysis of the oxygen concentration delivered to an oxygen hood, obtain the sample proximal to a simulated infant's airway. For analysis of the oxygen concentration in an aerosol or gas mixing system, be sure to locate the analyzed sensor or sampling tip downstream from the point of gas mixing (Fig. 9-6).
   Note: Some analyzer sensors should not be positioned so that condensate will collect on the sensor in an aerosol system.

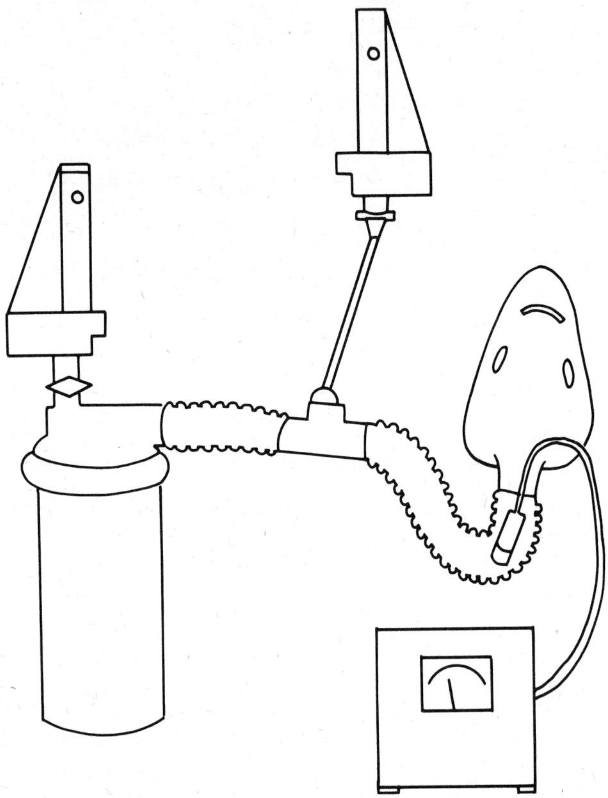

Fig. 9-6. Location of analyzer sensor in a gas mixing system.

RECOMMENDED READING

Burgess WR, Chernick V: Respiratory Therapy in Newborn Infants and Children. New York, Thieme-Stratton, 1982

Kacmarek RM, Dimas S, Mack C: Essentials of Respiratory Therapy, 2nd ed. Chicago, Year Book Medical Publishers, 1985

McPherson SP, Spearman CB: Respiratory Therapy Equipment, 3rd ed. St Louis, CV Mosby, 1985

Rarey KP, Youtsey JW: Respiratory Patient Care. Englewood Cliffs, Prentice-Hall, 1981

Spearman CB, Sheldon RL: Egan's Fundamentals of Respiratory Therapy, 4th ed. St Louis, CV Mosby, 1982

Laboratory Performance Evaluation (#9)

Topic: Atmospheric Oxygen Analysis

Student ______________________ Course ______________________

Date ______________________ Section ______________________

Performance Elements	Acceptable	Unacceptable	Not Applicable	Comments
1. Identifies the following types of oxygen analyzers: A. Physical B. Electrical C. Electrochemical D. Polarographic				
2. States operative principle of each type of analyzer				
3. Checks battery function				
4. Calibrates the analyzer properly				
5. Places analyzer on a flat surface				
6. Demonstrates proper procedure for analyzing a gas sample				
7. Verifies delivered oxygen concentration				
8. Documents obtained results				

Knowledge of Procedure

- ☐ Good; student is knowledgeable about rationale and theory related to procedure
- ☐ Fair; student has adequate understanding of rationale and theory related to procedure
- ☐ Poor; student has inadequate understanding of rationale and theory related to procedure

Performance Deficiencies (check those that apply)

- ☐ Excessive time needed to complete procedure
- ☐ Broke aseptic or sterile technique
- ☐ Gross inaccuracy noted
- ☐ Technique may be harmful to patient
- ☐ Incorrect dosage or gas concentration
- ☐ Incorrect equipment assembly/use
- ☐ Unable to answer questions correctly about rationale and/or theory related to procedure
- ☐ Other ______________________________

Evaluation Summary

- ☐ Satisfactory performance
- ☐ Unsatisfactory performance

Recommendations of Evaluator

- ☐ Skills may be applied/observed in clinical setting
- ☐ Specific evaluation deficiencies require correction
- ☐ Complete re-evaluation required
- ☐ Additional laboratory practice required

Signatures:

Evaluator ______________________ Date ______________________

Student ______________________ Date ______________________

Laboratory Report

Student ______________________ Acceptable ______________________

Date ______________________ Unacceptable ______________________

Course ______________________

Topic: Atmospheric Oxygen Analysis

Data and Measurements

Results of analysis of "unknown" gas mixtures

A = __________ %

B = __________ %

C = __________ %

Scenario: Today you have been assigned to the intensive care nursery. All except one of the patients are receiving oxygen by means of one delivery system or another: nasal CPAP, oxyhood, infant ventilator, and Isolettes.

The following types of analyzers are available: one paramagnetic, one thermal conductivity, three galvanic fuel cell, and two polarographic. Please answer the following questions:

1. Which analyzers need to be recalibrated when analysis of an oxygen concentration greater than 0.60 is required?

2. Which analyzer(s) provide a continuous measurement of FI_{O_2}

3. Which analyzers must not be used with flammable anesthetics, and why?

4. Which analyzer(s) measure the partial pressure of oxygen?

5. Which analyzer(s) measure the percentage of oxygen in the atmosphere?

6. Why does the Beckman D-2 analyzer contain blue silica gel?

7. Which type of oxygen analyzer gives a "true" oxygen percentage?

chapter 10

Humidity therapy devices

INTRODUCTION

Humidity may be defined as evaporated liquid water or as water vapor present in gas. In respiratory care, increased humidity or water vapor is added to inspired gas that may be dry or that may bypass the upper airway. Devices that add water vapor to inspired gas are called humidifiers. The purpose of this chapter is to introduce you to humidity therapy devices.

OBJECTIVES

After completing this chapter, you should be able to do the following:

1. *Describe the purpose of a humidifier.*
2. *Identify the primary components of a humidifier.*
3. *Discuss the mechanisms by which humidifier components increase evaporation.*
4. *Identify five types of humidifiers.*
5. *Explain how humidification may be increased or decreased with a humidifier.*

EQUIPMENT NEEDED

- ☐ Pass-over humidifier (blow-by)
- ☐ Bubble humidifier
- ☐ Jet humidifier
- ☐ Underwater jet humidifier
- ☐ Cascade humidifier
- ☐ Oxygen tubing
- ☐ Aerosol tubing

ACTIVITIES

Exercise A: Identification and Assembly of a Pass-over Humidifier

1. Select a pass-over humidifier. Examine the components of a pass-over humidifier using the following diagram (Fig. 10-1).
2. Identify the following components:
   - A. Gas inlet
   - B. Gas outlet
   - C. Heating mechanism
   - D. Pressure relief valve
3. Fill with sterile distilled water.
4. Connect the appropriate size tubing to the flowmeter and gas inlet and outlet.
5. Adjust the gas flow to 10 liters/minute.
6. Trace gas flow through the device.
7. On the laboratory report, discuss the mechanism(s) by which water vapor is added to gas.

Exercise B: Identification and Assembly of Bubble Humidifier

1. Select a bubble humidifier. Examine the components of a bubble humidifier (Fig.10-2).
2. Identify the following parts:
   - A. Gas inlet
   - B. Gas outlet
   - C. Pressure relief valve
   - D. Porous stone filter or diffuser head
   - E. Capillary tube
3. Fill with sterile water (if applicable).

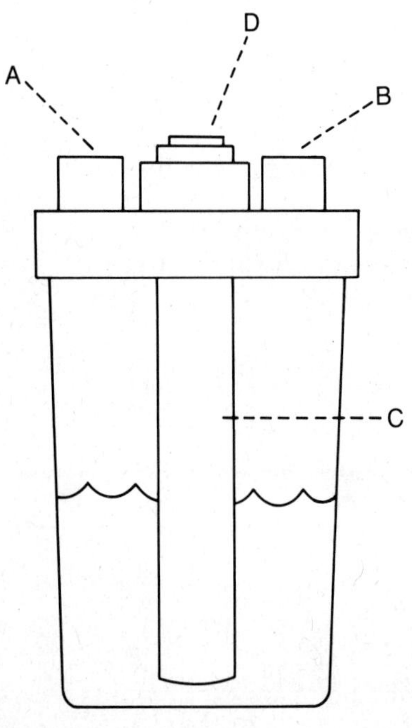

Fig. 10-1. Pass-over humidifier.

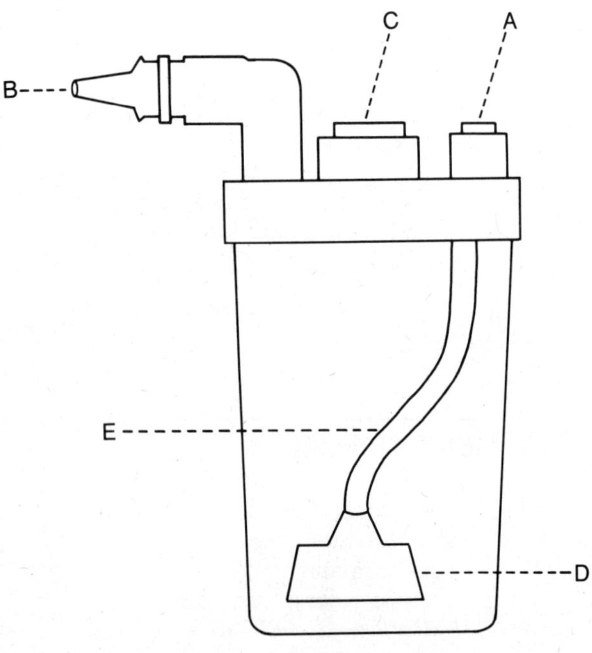

Fig. 10-2. Bubble diffusion humidifier.

4. Attach the humidifier to a flowmeter. *Caution:* Be certain that the humidifier is properly connected to the flowmeter. Improperly connected humidifiers may cause large gas leaks and inadequate gas flow to a patient. Connect small-bore oxygen tubing to the humidifier outlet.
5. Adjust the gas flowmeter to 5 liters/minute.
6. Check the pressure relief valve function by occluding or kinking the oxygen tubing. The pressure valve should be activated.
7. Trace gas flow through the device.
8. On the laboratory report, discuss the mechanism(s) by which water vapor is added to gas.

Exercise C: Identification and Assembly of a Jet and Underwater Jet Humidifier

1. Select either a jet or an underwater jet humidifier. Examine the primary components of a jet or an underwater jet humidifier using the following diagram (Fig. 10-3).
2. Identify the following components:
   A. Gas inlet
   B. Gas outlet
   C. Capillary tube
   D. Baffle
   E. Pressure relief valve
3. Fill the unit with sterile water (if applicable).
4. Attach the humidifier to an oxygen flowmeter.
5. Adjust the flow to 6 liters/minute.
6. Verify the proper function of the pressure relief valve (if present) by occluding the gas outlet.
7. Trace the gas flow through the device.

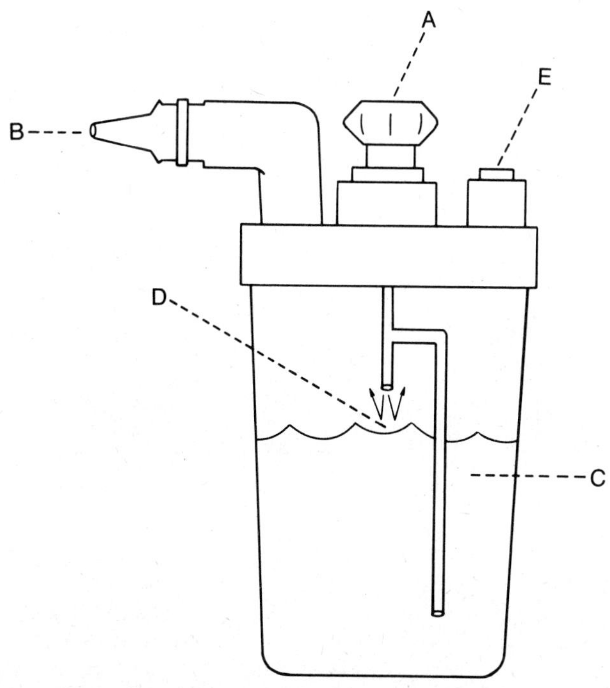

Fig. 10-3. Jet and underwater jet humidifiers.

8. On the laboratory report, discuss the mechanism(s) by which water vapor is added to gas.

Exercise D: Identification and Assembly of a Cascade Humidifier

1. Select a heated cascade humidifier. Using the following diagram, examine the components of a cascade humidifier (Fig. 10-4).
2. Identify the following components:
   A. Gas inlet
   B. Gas outlet
   C. Bubble grid
   D. Tower
   E. One-way valve
   F. Heater
   G. Temperature control
   H. Sensing porthole
3. Fill with sterile distilled water.
4. Assemble the cascade.
5. Replace the top of the cascade.
6. Attach gas tubing to inlet. Turn on the gas flow to 10 liters/minute.
7. Trace gas flow through the device.
8. Adjust the heating probe control. Monitor the temperature. Adjust the heater control to provide a temperature of 37°C.
9. On the laboratory report, discuss the mechanism(s) by which water vapor is added to gas.

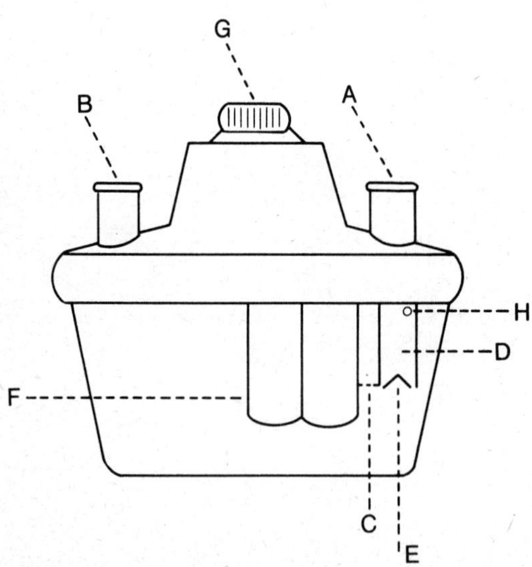

Fig. 10-4. Cascade humidifier.

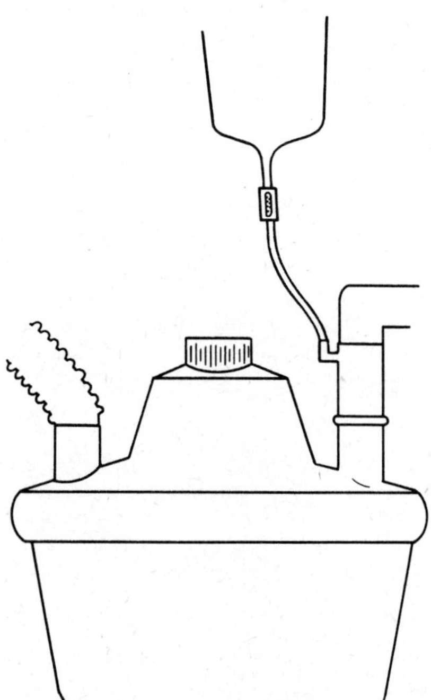

Fig. 10-5. Sterile feed system for use with a cascade humidifier with a mechanical ventilator.

10. Many adult mechanical ventilators use a heated cascade humidifier to provide approximately 100% relative humidity to inspired gas. Because interruptions in continuous mechanical ventilation may be deleterious to patients, a sterile feed type of system may be used to allow the inevitable refilling of the humidifier with sterile water without causing an interruption in ventilation.
11. Examine a sterile feed system for a cascade humidifier (Fig. 10-5).
12. Practice refilling the cascade humidifier during continuous ventilation without causing interruptions in ventilation (do not allow more than three breaths to be missed). Your instructor will provide you with an operatonal mechanical ventilator.
13. A heated cascade humidifier may also be used to provide heated humidified gas to a neonate when used with an oxygen hood (Fig. 10-6).
14. Practice the assembly of an oxygen hood system using a heated cascade humidifier.

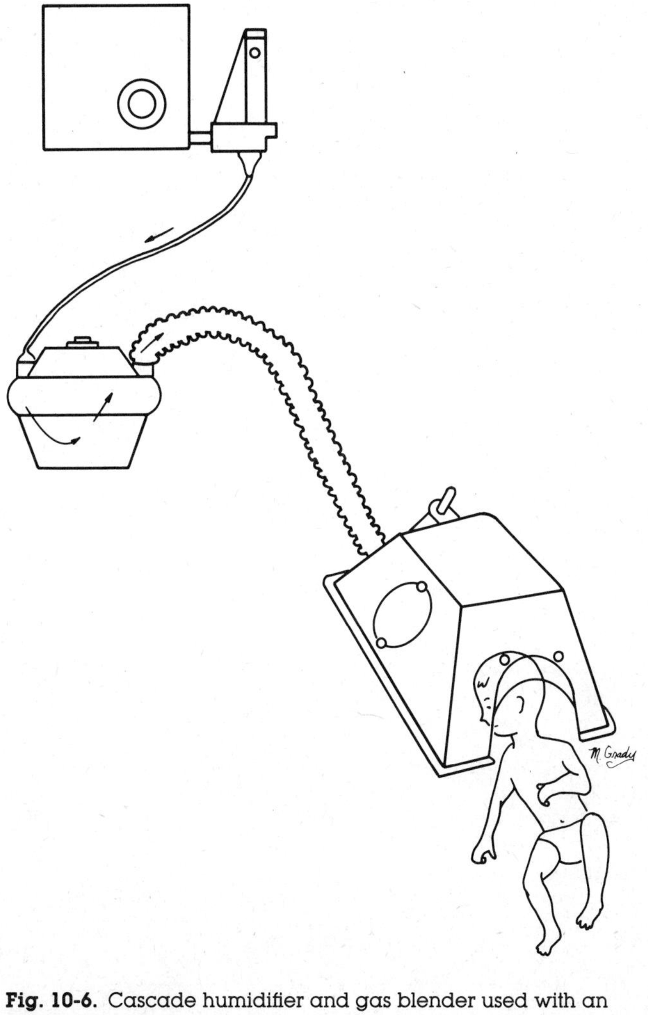

Fig. 10-6. Cascade humidifier and gas blender used with an oxygen hood system.

Exercise E: Identification and Assembly of a Wick Humidifier

1. Obtain a wick humidifier. Examine the primary components (Fig. 10-7).
2. Identify the following parts of a wick humidifier:
   A. Gas inlet
   B. Gas outlet
   C. Heater
   D. Wick
3. Assemble the wick humidifier.
4. If used with a mechanical ventilator, connect the appropriate tubes to the gas inlet and outlet.
5. Fill the wick with sterile water.
6. Adjust the heater to provide a temperature of 37°C.

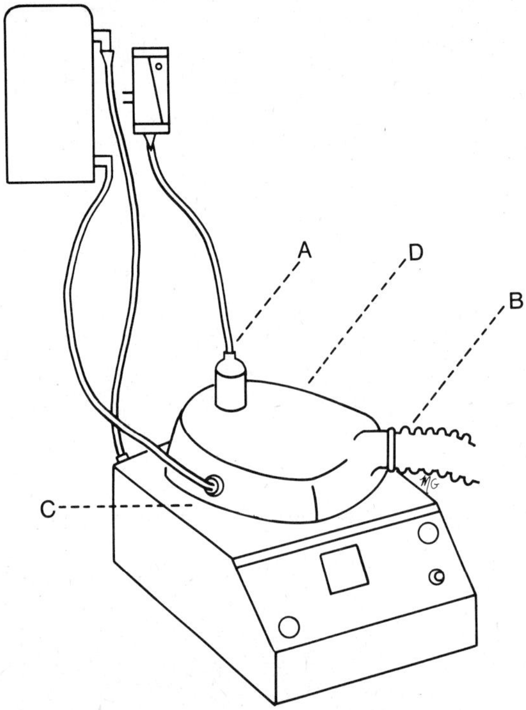

Fig. 10-7. Wick humidifier components.

RECOMMENDED READING

Burton GG, Hodgkin JE: Respiratory Care. A Guide to Clinical Practice, 2nd ed. Philadelphia, JB Lippincott, 1984

Kacmarek RM, Dimas S, Mack C: Essentials of Respiratory Therapy, 2nd ed. Chicago, Year Book Medical Publishers, 1985

McPherson SP, Spearman CB: Respiratory Therapy Equipment, 3rd ed. St Louis, CV Mosby, 1985

Spearman B, Sheldon RL: Egan's Fundamentals of Respiratory Therapy, 4th ed. St Louis, CV Mosby, 1982

Laboratory Performance Evaluation (#10)

Topic: Humidity Therapy Devices

Student ____________________ Course ____________________

Date ____________________ ____ Section ____________________

Performance Elements	Acceptable	Unacceptable	Not Applicable	Comments
1. Identifies the following types of humidifiers: Pass-over Bubble Jet Underwater jet Cascade				
2. Washes hands				
3. Fills humidifier with sterile H_2O				
4. Attaches flowmeter to gas outlet				
5. Attaches humidification device to flowmeter				
6. Attaches O_2 connecting tubing and O_2 administration device to humidifier				
7. Turns gas source on				
8. Checks pressure relief valve				
9. Verifies proper function of device				
10. Replaces water in cascade humidifier during continous operation of mechanical ventilator				
11. Accomplishes step 10 in less than three ventilator cycles				

Knowledge of Procedure

- ☐ Good; student is knowledgeable about rationale and theory related to procedure
- ☐ Fair; student has adequate understanding of rationale and theory related to procedure
- ☐ Poor; student has inadequate understanding of rationale and theory related to procedure

Performance Deficiencies (check those that apply)

- ☐ Excessive time needed to complete procedure
- ☐ Broke aseptic or sterile technique
- ☐ Gross inaccuracy noted
- ☐ Technique may be harmful to patient
- ☐ Incorrect dosage or gas concentration
- ☐ Incorrect equipment assembly/use
- ☐ Unable to answer questions correctly about rationale and/or theory related to procedure
- ☐ Other ______

Evaluation Summary

- ☐ Satisfactory performance
- ☐ Unsatisfactory performance

Recommendations of Evaluator

- ☐ Skills may be applied/observed in clinical setting
- ☐ Specific evaluation deficiencies require correction
- ☐ Complete re-evaluation required
- ☐ Additional laboratory practice required

Signatures:

Evaluator ______ Date ______

Student ______ Date ______

Laboratory Report

Student ____________________ Acceptable ____________________

Date ____________________ Unacceptable ____________________

Course ____________________

Topic: Humidity Therapy Devices

Scenario: Today, you are assigned to an adult critical care unit. Several patients are receiving continuous mechanical ventilation. Two patients have recently been weaned from ventilators and are receiving oxygen by means of a tracheostomy mask and T-tube, respectively. Another patient, who is being transferred to a step-down unit, is receiving low-flow oxygen by means of a nasal cannula. Please answer the following questions:

1. What types of humidification devices would be best suited for the patient being transferred to the step-down unit?

2. What type of humidifier would you recommend for the patient with a tracheostomy?

3. What types of humidification devices are suitable for those patients receiving continuous mechanical ventilation?

4. Describe the function of a wick humidifier.

5. Briefly describe the purposes of a humidifier.

6. What is the most efficient type of humidifier, and why?

7. Define humidity.

chapter 11

Aerosol generators

INTRODUCTION

In respiratory care, one of the most commonly used therapeutic techniques is aerosol therapy. An aerosol is a visible suspension of particles in a gas stream. For therapeutic use, the particles usually consist of sterile water, saline, or drug solutions. The gas stream that transports therapeutic particles usually consists of air or oxygen mixtures. A device that can generate an aerosol is called a nebulizer.

Five types of nebulizers can be used for producing aerosols, including the large-reservoir (jet), Babbington, ultrasonic, centrifugal, and various small-reservoir nebulizers. Small-reservoir nebulizers are frequently used on an intermittent basis, whereas other nebulizers may be operated continuously. The purpose of this chapter is to introduce you to aerosol generators or nebulizers.

OBJECTIVES

After completing this chapter, you should be able to do the following:

1. *Describe the purpose of a nebulizer.*
2. *Identify the primary components of a nebulizer.*
3. *Cite five types of nebulizers.*
4. *Completely assemble and operate a nebulizer.*
5. *Trace the flow of gas through a nebulizer.*

EQUIPMENT NEEDED

- ☐ Gas source
- ☐ Flowmeter
- ☐ Wide-bore aerosol tubing
- ☐ Small-bore tubing

☐ Nebulizers

Jet
Ultrasonic
Centrifugal
Babbington
Medication

ACTIVITIES

Exercise A: Identification and Assembly of a Large-Reservoir Nebulizer

1. Examine the primary components of a jet nebulizer (Fig. 11-1).
2. Identify the following components:
   - A. Gas inlet
   - B. Jet
   - C. Entrainment ports
   - D. Capillary tube
   - E. Pressure relief valve
   - F. Gas outlet
   - G. Heating probe (if applicable)
3. Fill the reservoir with sterile water.
4. Assemble the nebulizer by connecting the gas inlet to a flowmeter.
5. Attach wide-bore aerosol tubing to the gas outlet. Attach an aerosol delivery device to the wide-bore tubing.
6. Turn the flowmeter to a minimum flow of 10 liters/minute. (The flowmeter is usually set at 10 to 15 liters/minute or more, depending on the total gas flowrate required.)
7. Trace the flow of gas and water particles through the device (Fig. 11-2).
8. Adjust the entrainment port to deliver an FI_{O_2} of 0.40. Observe the aerosol density produced. Increase the FI_{O_2} to 1.0 by adjusting the entrainment ports. Again, observe the aerosol density. Record your observation on the laboratory report.
9. Note the FI_{O_2} range that the nebulizer can deliver. Select an oxygen concentration, and analyze the delivered concentration. Is the oxygen concentration setting accurate? Record your observation on the laboratory report.

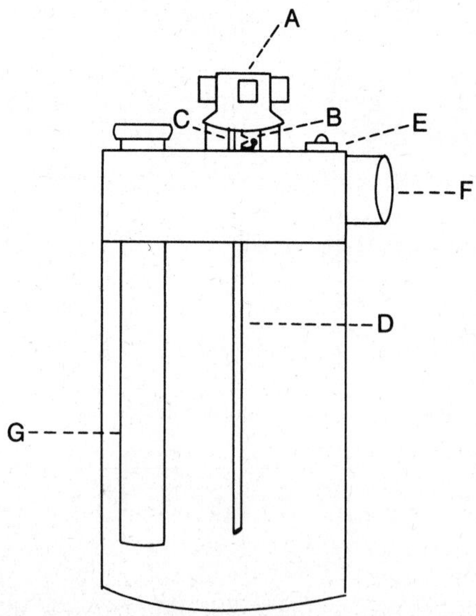

Fig. 11-1. Components of a large-reservoir (jet) nebulizer.

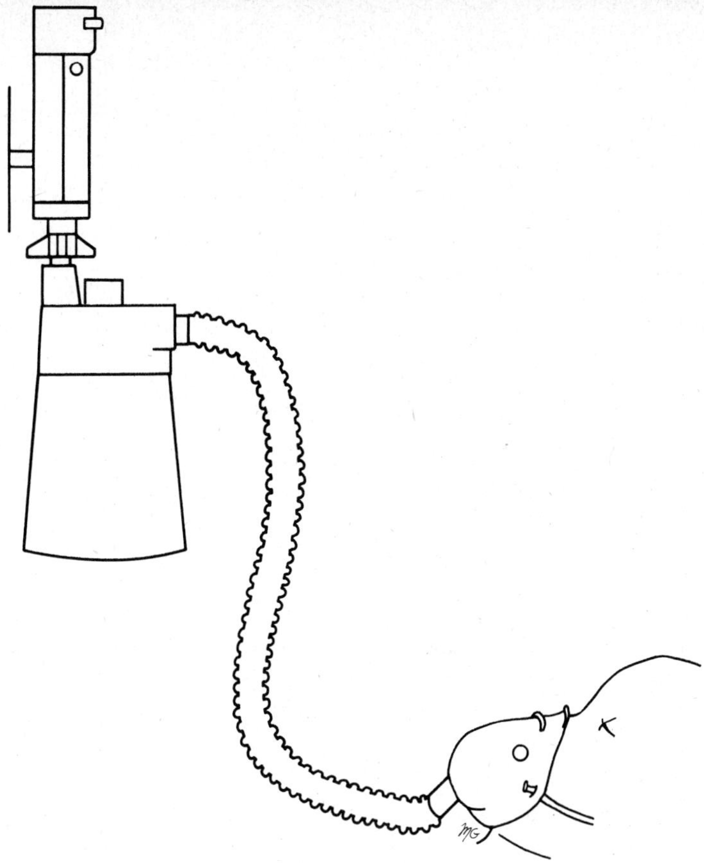

Fig. 11-2. Assembly of a jet nebulizer.

Exercise B: Identification and Assembly of a Babbington Nebulizer

1. Select a Babbington nebulizer for use with an oxygen tent or used as a large reservoir and driven by a flowmeter. Examine the primary components of a Babbington nebulizer (Fig. 11-3).
2. Identify the following components:
   A. Gas outlet
   B. Water reservoir
   C. Hollow sphere
   D. Baffle
   E. Entrainment ports
   F. Flowmeter or high-pressure (50 psi) gas hose connection
3. Connect the nebulizer to a flowmeter, or, if using the nebulizer component to an oxygen tent, attach a high-pressure gas hose to the DISS wall outlet.
4. Trace the flow of gas and water particles through the device.
5. If using a flowmeter, adjust the oxygen flowrate to a minimum of 10 liters/ minute.
6. Manipulate the delivered FI_{O_2} by adjusting the entrainment ports.
7. Determine the effect of changing the oxygen concentration from 0.40 to 1.0 on the aerosol density. Record your observations on the laboratory report.
8. Note the oxygen concentrations available with the Babbington nebulizer.

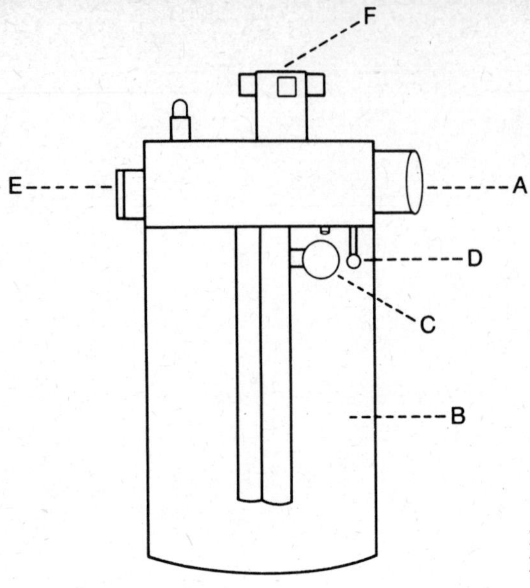

Fig. 11-3. Components of a Babbington hydrosphere nebulizer.

9. Select an oxygen concentration, and analyze the delivered concentration. Is the delivered oxygen concentration accurate? Record your results on the laboratory report.

Exercise C: Identification and Assembly of Medication Nebulizers

1. Your instructor will provide you with several types of medication nebulizers.
2. Identify the gas inlet, gas outlet, jet, baffle, and medication reservoir.
3. Place 1 to 4 ml of sterile water in the nebulizer.
4. Attach small-bore oxygen tubing to the gas inlet. Apply an aerosol mask to nebulizer outlet.
5. Turn on gas flow (minimum flow of 6–8 liters/minute). Refer to the following illustration for the assembly of a medication nebulizer (Fig. 11-4).
6. Check the nebulizer for adequte function.
7. Trace the gas flow through the device.
8. Attach small-bore gas tubing to the gas inlet of a medication nebulizer used with an intermittent positive pressure breathing or mechanical ventilator circuit. Observe the nebulizer for aerosol production.
9. Disassemble the equipment.

Exercise D: Identification and Assembly of an Ultrasonic Nebulizer

1. Select an ultrasonic nebulizer for either intermittent or continuous aerosol therapy. Examine the components of the ultrasonic nebulizer (Fig. 11-5).
2. Identify the following components:
   - **A.** Medication chamber
   - **B.** Couplant
   - **C.** Piezoelectric disk
   - **D.** Diaphragm
   - **E.** Gas inlet
   - **F.** Gas outlet
3. Other important components of an ultrasonic nebulizer not shown include a gas source or fan, air filter, on/off switch, and amplitude adjustment.

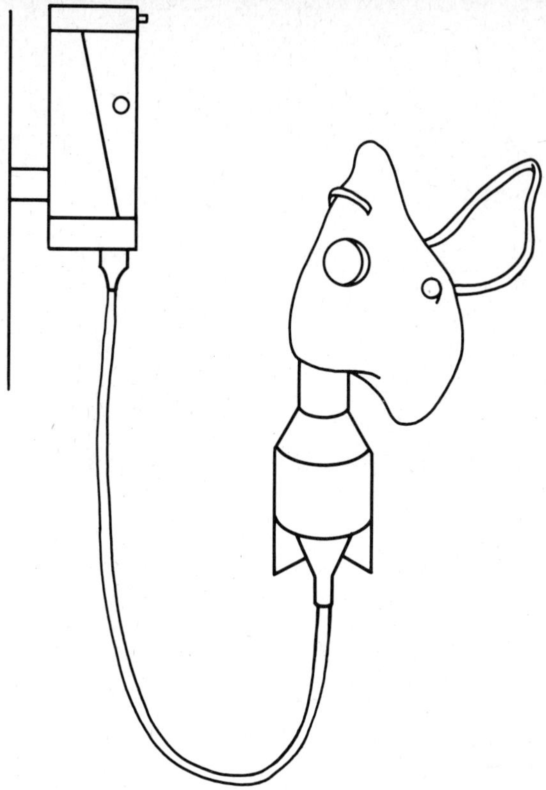

Fig. 11-4. Assembly of an intermittent medication nebulizer.

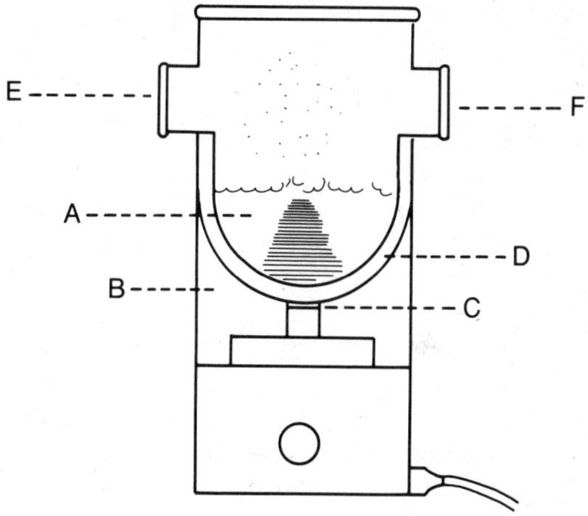

Fig. 11-5. Components of an ultrasonic nebulizer.

4. Check the couplant for adequate water levels.
5. Fill the medication chamber with sterile water or saline.
6. Assemble the nebulizer for use by attaching a gas hose from the fan to the inlet.
7. Attach large-bore aerosol tubing to the chamber outlet.
8. Turn on the nebulizer.
9. Adjust the amplitude to regulate the aerosol density.
10. Trace the flow of gas and water particles through the device (Fig. 11-6).
11. Turn the amplitude control to the minimum setting and then to the maximum setting. How is aerosol density affected? Record your observations on the laboratory report.

Exercise E: Identification and Assembly of a Centrifugal Nebulizer

1. Select a centrifugal nebulizer.
2. Identify and label the gas outlet, baffle, spinning disk, and water reservoir.
3. Fill the reservoir with water.
4. Plug the power cord into an electrical outlet.
5. Trace the flow of gas and water particles through the device (Fig. 11-7).
   Note: Although the centrifugal (impeller) nebulizer can generate an aerosol, the primary purpose of the device is to allow evaporation of the aerosolized particles and to act as a humidifier.
6. Disassemble the electrical cord.

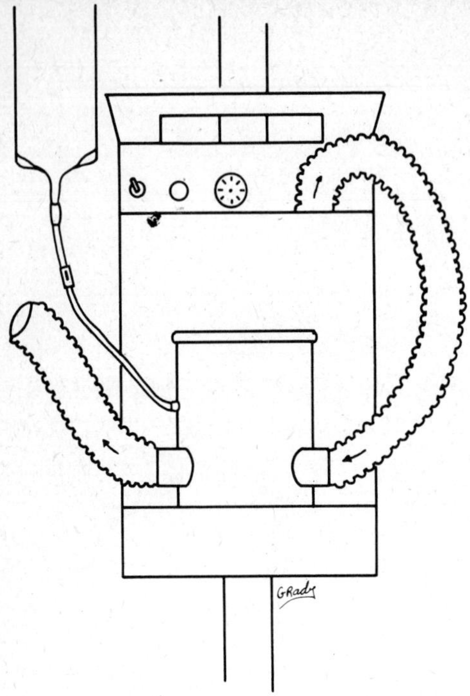

Fig. 11-6. Assembled ultrasonic nebulizer.

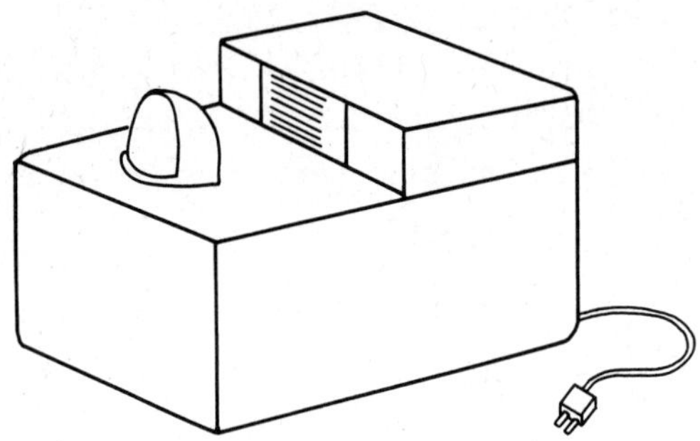

Fig. 11-7. Assembled centrifugal nebulizer.

RECOMMENDED READING

Burton GG, Hodgkin JE: Respiratory Care. A Guide to Clinical Practice, 2nd ed. Philadelphia, JB Lippincott, 1984

Kacmarek RM, Dimas S, Mack C: Essentials of Respiratory Therapy, 2nd ed. Chicago, Year Book Medical Publishers, 1985

McPherson SP, Spearman CB: Respiratory Therapy Equipment, 3rd ed. St Louis, CV Mosby, 1985

Spearman CB, Sheldon RL: Egan's Fundamentals of Respiratory Therapy, 4th ed. St Louis, CV Mosby, 1982

Laboratory Performance Evaluation (#11)

Topic: Aerosol Generators

Student ______________________ Course ______________________

Date ______________________ Section ______________________

Performance Elements	Acceptable	Unacceptable	Not Applicable	Comments
1. Reviews order				
2. Obtains proper equipment				
3. Washes hands				
4. Fills nebulizers with sterile H_2O or medication				
5. Assembles equipment properly				
6. Attaches appropriate aerosol delivery device				
7. Adjusts source gas to appropriate flowrate				
8. Checks aerosol device for appropriate function				
9. Applies aerosol generating system to simulated patient				
10. Adjusts aerosol to prescribed FI_{O_2}				
11. Analyzes oxygen concentration				
12. Documents procedure and results				

Knowledge of Procedure

- ☐ Good; student is knowledgeable about rationale and theory related to procedure
- ☐ Fair; student has adequate understanding of rationale and theory related to procedure
- ☐ Poor; student has inadequate understanding of rationale and theory related to procedure

Performance Deficiencies (check those that apply)

- ☐ Excessive time needed to complete procedure
- ☐ Broke aseptic or sterile technique
- ☐ Gross inaccuracy noted
- ☐ Technique may be harmful to patient
- ☐ Incorrect dosage or gas concentration
- ☐ Incorrect equipment assembly/use
- ☐ Unable to answer questions correctly about rationale and/or theory related to procedure
- ☐ Other ______________________________

Evaluation Summary

- ☐ Satisfactory performance
- ☐ Unsatisfactory performance

Recommendations of Evaluator

- ☐ Skills may be applied/observed in clinical setting
- ☐ Specific evaluation deficiencies require correction
- ☐ Complete re-evaluation required
- ☐ Additional laboratory practice required

Signatures:

Evaluator ______________________ Date ______________________

Student ______________________ Date ______________________

Laboratory Report

Student ______________________ Acceptable ______________________

Date ______________________ Unacceptable ______________________

Course ______________________

Topic: Aerosol Generators

Data and Measurements

	Available Ranges of FI_{O_2}	Set FI_{O_2}	Analyzed FI_{O_2}
Jet Nebulizer	________	________	________
Babbington Nebulizer	________	________	________

Scenario: An elderly COPD patient who is routinely seen in the outpatient clinic has arrived for his scheduled appointment. While waiting to be seen, he begins experiencing some mild bronchospasm. You have been asked to treat the patient with a nebulized solution of Bronkosol and saline. Please respond to the following questions:

1. Assuming the outpatient clinic has piped-in air and oxygen, what equipment and supplies will be needed to administer the medication.

2. Specifically, what type of aerosol device would you use?

Later that same day, the patient is admitted to Ward 8A, at which time his physician has decided that he would benefit from a heated aerosol and 0.30 oxygen. You have been asked to provide the patient with the aforementioned. Please answer the following questions:

3. What specific nebulizer would you use?

4. How is the nebulizer you have chosen classified?

5. What hazards, if any, are associated with the system you have chosen?

6. Please describe the method you would use to deliver an FI_{O_2} of 0.30.

7. How does a nebulizer differ from a humidifier?

8. How may aerosol density be increased with a jet nebulizer?

9. How may aerosol output be increased with a
   A. jet nebulizer?

   B. ultrasonic nebulizer?

chapter 12

Aerosol delivery systems

INTRODUCTION

Aerosol delivery devices are designed to interface aerosol generating equipment with a patient's airway. Four aerosol delivery devices are commonly used in the clinical setting: the face tent, aerosol mask, Briggs adapter (T-tube), and tracheostomy mask. The face tent and aerosol mask are used to deliver aerosols (and oxygen mixtures) to the face. The face tent may be used in cases of severe facial trauma, burns, or after cranial surgery. The face tent may also allow rapid access to the airway in unconscious patients who need aerosol therapy. The aerosol mask may be used for the routine delivery of intermittent or continuous aerosols.

The Brigg's adapter and tracheostomy mask are used to deliver aerosol (and oxygen) therapy to patients with an artificial airway. The Brigg's adapter primarily is used to deliver aerosols to an endotracheal tube, and the tracheostomy mask allows aerosol delivery to a tracheostomy tube. The purpose of this chapter is to introduce you to aerosol delivery devices. Before attempting completion of these exercises, you should perform the previous exercises on aerosol generators.

OBJECTIVES

After completing this chapter, you should be able to do the following:

1. *Identify and assemble an aerosol mask, face tent, Brigg's adapter, and tracheostomy mask.*
2. *Understand the purpose of aerosol delivery devices.*
3. *Describe the advantages and disadvantages of aerosol delivery devices.*
4. *Identify methods of adding an aerosol or oxygen reservoir to a Brigg's adapter or aerosol mask.*
5. *Assemble nebulizers in tandem to increase the total gas flowrate.*

EQUIPMENT NEEDED

- ☐ Gas source
- ☐ Flowmeters (air and oxygen)
- ☐ Jet nebulizer
- ☐ Aerosol delivery devices
  - Aerosol mask
  - Face tent
  - Brigg's adapter
  - Tracheostomy mask
- ☐ Mannequin
- ☐ Oxygen analyzer
- ☐ Endotracheal and tracheostomy tube

ACTIVITIES

Exercise A: Identification and Assembly of a Face Tent

1. Obtain a face tent.
2. Identify the gas inlet, aerosol tubing connector, and elastic strap.
3. Attach a large-reservoir jet nebulizer to an oxygen-flowmeter.
4. Fill the nebulizer with sterile water (tap water may be used when working with a mannequin).
5. Connect large-bore aerosol tubing to the nebulizer outlet.

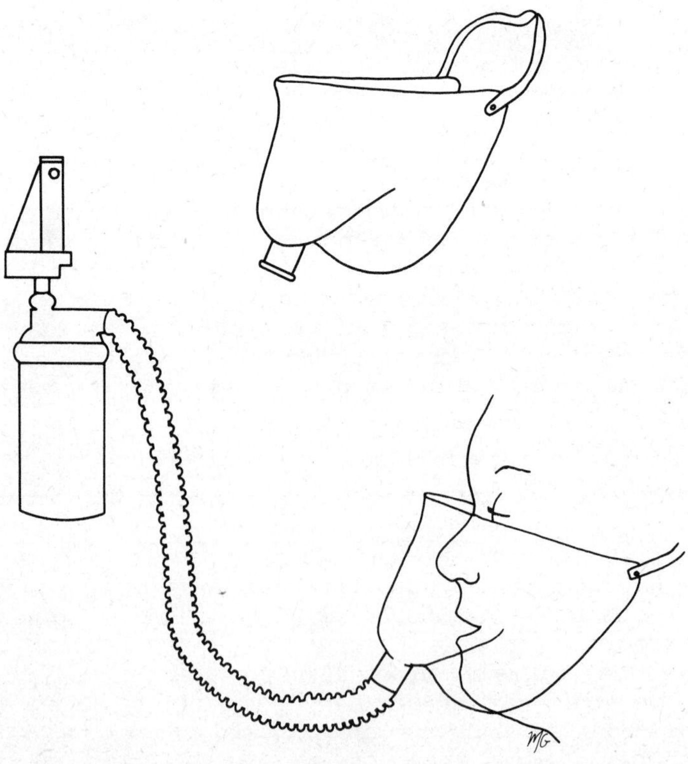

Fig. 12-1. Face tent and assembled face tent.

6. Attach the face tent to the large-bore tubing. Verify that a tight fit exists between the face tent tubing connector and the aerosol tubing.
7. Adjust the gas flowrate to a minimum of 10 liters/minute. Set the oxygen concentration at 0.40 or at an FI_{O_2} designated by your laboratory instructor. *Note:* In clinical use, the gas flowrate and FI_{O_2} must meet or exceed the peak inspiratory flowrate of the patient. To determine the total gas flowrate delivered at a given oxygen concentration, review Chapter 7: Oxygen Delivery Devices.
8. Before applying the face tent, check the system for adequate aerosol output and gas flow. Analyze the oxygen concentration.
9. Using a mannequin, connect the assembled face tent to the mannequin by adjusting the elastic strap (Fig. 12-1).
10. Post a no-smoking sign.
11. Disassemble the equipment.

Exercise B: Identification and Assembly of an Aerosol Mask

1. Obtain an aerosol mask.
2. Identify the gas inlet, aerosol tubing connector, exhalation ports, and elastic strap.
3. Attach a large-reservoir jet nebulizer to an oxygen flowmeter.
4. Fill the nebulizer with sterile water.
5. Connect large-bore aerosol tubing to the nebulizer outlet.
6. Attach the aerosol mask to the large-bore tubing. Verify that a tight fit exists between the aerosol tubing and the tubing connector.
7. Adjust the flowmeter to provide an adequate total gas flowrate. Set the FI_{O_2} at 0.40 or at the concentration designated by your laboratory instructor.
8. Before applying the aerosol mask, check the system for adequate aerosol output and gas flow. Verify the delivered oxygen concentration by analysis.
9. Using a mannequin, connect the assembled aerosol mask to the face by adjusting both the elastic strap and the malleable metal nosepiece (Fig. 12-2).

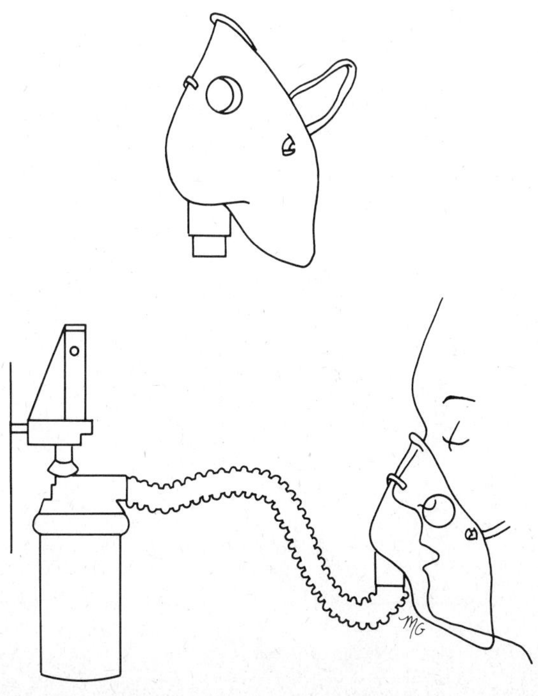

Fig. 12-2. Aerosol mask and assembled aerosol mask.

10. Ensure that the mask fits snugly to the face.
11. Post a no-smoking sign.
12. Disassemble the equipment.

Exercise C: Identification and Assembly of a Tracheostomy Collar

Your instructor will provide you with a mannequin having a tracheostomy tube in place. When properly positioned and with the cuff inflated, you may assume that breathing occurs through the tracheostomy tube.

1. Obtain a tracheostomy collar.
2. Identify the aerosol tubing connector, exhalation port, and elastic strap.
3. Attach a large-reservoir jet nebulizer to an oxygen flowmeter.
4. Fill the nebulizer reservoir with sterile water.
5. Connect large-bore aerosol tubing to the nebulizer outlet.
6. Attach the tracheostomy collar to the large-bore tubing. Verify that a tight connection exists between the tracheostomy mask tubing connector and the aerosol tubing.
7. Adjust the flowmeter to provide an adequate total gas flowrate. Set the FI_{O_2} at 0.50 or at the concentration designated by your laboratory instructor.
8. Before applying the tracheostomy mask, check the system for adequate aerosol output and gas flow. Verify the delivered oxygen concentration by analysis.
9. Using the mannequin provided by your instructor, place the tracheostomy mask over the tracheostomy tube. While stabilizing the mask, adjust the elastic strap around the neck to provide an adequate fit (Fig. 12-3).
10. Ensure that the tracheostomy mask is adequately stabilized.
11. Post a no-smoking sign.
12. Disassemble the equipment.

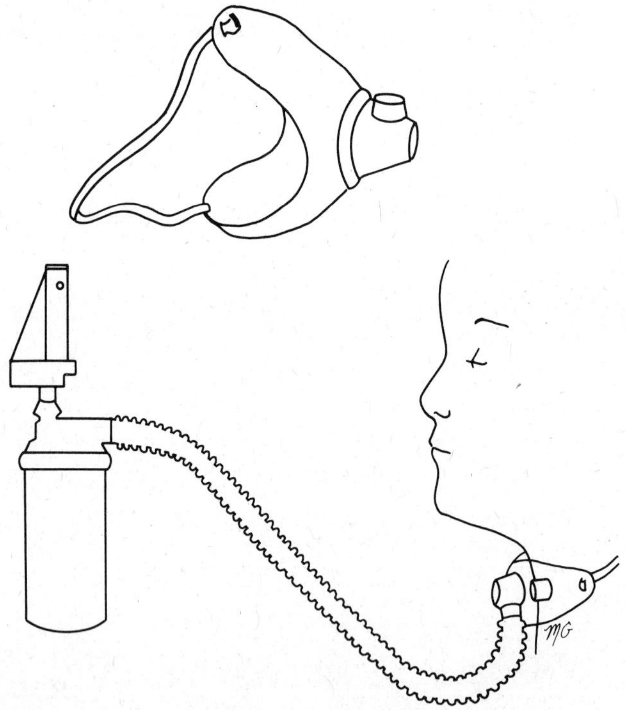

Fig. 12-3. Tracheostomy mask and assembled tracheostomy mask.

Exercise D: Identification and Assembly of a T-tube (Brigg's Adapter)

Your instructor will provide you with an intubated mannequin having either an oral or a nasal endotracheal tube in place. When properly positioned and with the tube cuff inflated, you may assume that breathing occurs only through the endotracheal tube.

1. Obtain a T-tube.
2. Identify the aerosol tubing connectors and 15 mm inner diameter endotracheal tube adapter.
3. Assemble a large-reservoir jet nebulizer by connecting the nebulizer to an oxygen flowmeter.
4. Fill the nebulizer with sterile water.
5. Connect large-bore aerosol tubing to the nebulizer outlet.
6. Attach the T-tube to the large-bore tubing. The aerosol tubing is *not* connected to the 15 mm adapter.
7. Attach a small (6 – 8 inch) piece of aerosol tubing to the other side of the T-tube. The small piece of aerosol tubing acts as an oxygen reservoir to prevent inadvertent air dilution and should maintain a consistent oxygen concentration.
8. Adjust the flowmeter to provide an adequate total gas flowrate. Set the FI_{O_2} at 0.45 or at the concentration designated by your laboratory instructor.
9. Before connecting the T-tube to the endotracheal tube, check the system for adequate aerosol output and gas flowrate. Verify the delivered oxygen concentration by analysis.
10. Using the intubated mannequin provided by your instructor, connect the T-tube system to the endotracheal tube. The 15 mm endotracheal tube adapter should tightly fit the 15 mm adapter on the T-tube (Fig. 12-4).
11. *Note:* In clinical use, an adequate total gas flowrate through the T-tube and reservoir may be estimated by osberving the aerosol mist during spontaneous

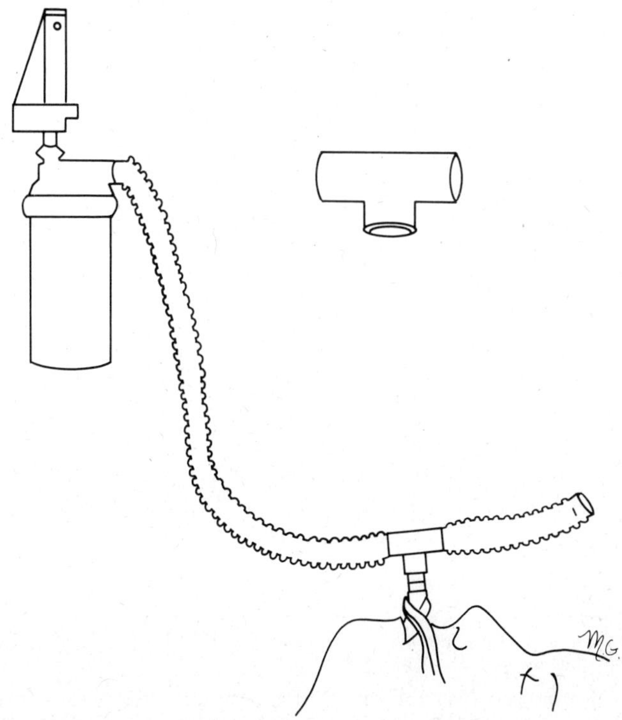

Fig. 12-4. T-tube (Brigg's adapter) and assembled T-tube.

ventilation. If the aerosol is not visible during inhalation, the total flowrate through the system may be inadequate. In other words, the flow of aerosol mist should be continuous.

12. Practice the assembly of an aerosol mask, face tent, tracheostomy mask, and T-tube using an ultrasonic or Babbington nebulizer.
13. Disassemble and organize the equipment.

Exercise E: Assembly of Combined Nebulizers for Increased Flow

1. When the total flowrate provided from a single nebulizer is inadequate (especially with high oxygen concentrations), the gas flowrate may be increased by incorporating a second flowmeter and nebulizer into the system (Fig. 12-5).
2. Obtain the increased flowrate from two nebulizers by connecting the aerosol tubing from the nebulizers with a "wye" connector. *Note:* If a T-tube is used to connect the tubing, be certain that opposing flow does not occur. Air may be mixed into the system to obtain specific oxygen concentrations. Be certain to analyze the oxygen concentration downstream from the point of gas mixing.
3. Using the aerosol delivery devices described on a mannequin, practice the assembly of combined nebulizers to obtain the following oxygen concentrations:
   A. 40% oxygen by face tent
   B. 55% oxygen by aerosol mask
   C. 68% oxygen by tracheostomy mask
   D. 75% oxygen by T-tube
4. Analyze the FI_{O_2} before application to the mannequin.

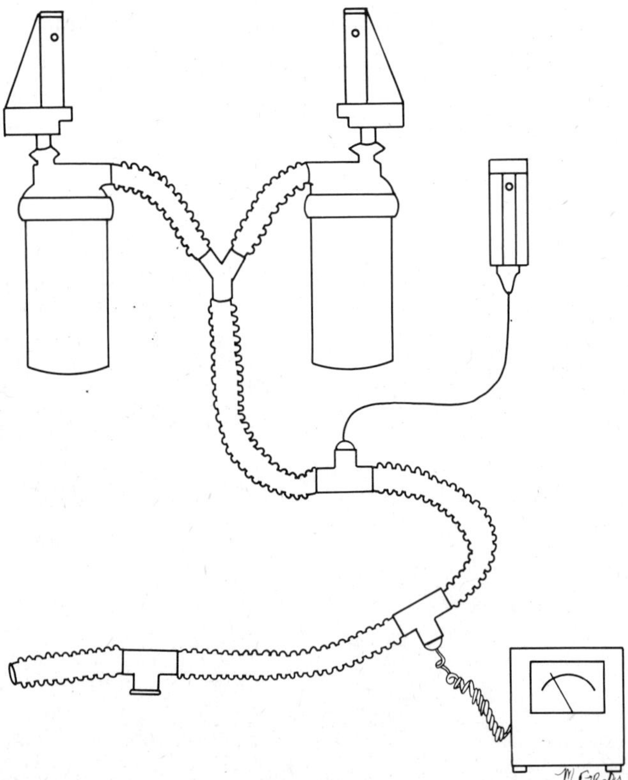

Fig. 12-5. Nebulizers in tandem for augmenting total gas flow.

5. An additional technique may be used to add a reservoir of aerosol tubing or "tusks" to the exhalation ports on the aerosol mask (Fig. 12-6).
6. If reservoirs are added to an aerosol mask, it is imperative that an adequate total gas flowrate be used to prevent rebreathing of carbon dioxide.
7. Practice the assembly of reservoirs added to an aerosol mask. Disassemble and properly store all equipment.

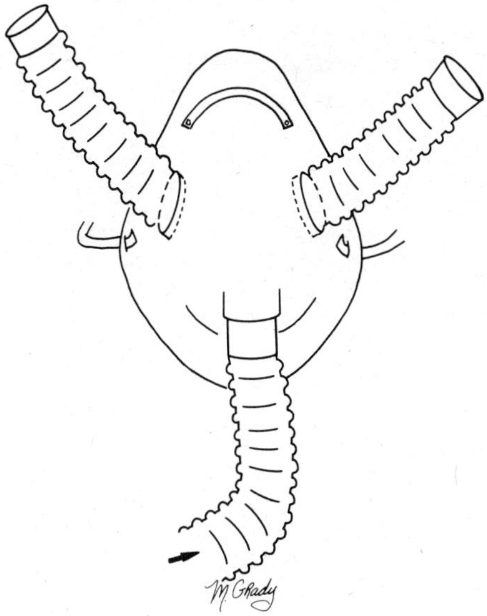

Fig. 12-6. Oxygen reservoir or "tusks" added to aerosol mask.

RECOMMENDED READING

Blodgett D: Manual of Pediatric Respiratory Care Procedures. Philadelphia, JB Lippincott, 1982

Burton GG, Hodgkin JE: Respiratory Care. A Guide to Clinical Practice, 2nd ed. Philadelphia, JB Lippincott, 1984

Rarey KP, Youtsey JW: Respiratory Patient Care. Englewood Cliffs, Prentice-Hall, 1981

Spearman CB, Sheldon RL: Egan's Fundamentals of Respiratory Therapy, 4th ed. St Louis, CV Mosby, 1982

Laboratory Performance Evaluation (#12)

Topic: Aerosol Delivery Systems

Student ______________________ Course ______________________

Date ______________________ Section ______________________

Performance Elements	Acceptable	Unacceptable	Not Applicable	Comments
1. Confirms order				
2. Obtains appropriate equipment				
3. Washes hands				
4. Assembles equipment properly				
5. Confirms proper equipment function				
6. Assures adequate total gas flow				
7. Adjusts oxygen concentration to prescribed FI_{O_2}				
8. Analyzes oxygen concentration				
9. Applies functioning system to simulated patient				
10. Evaluates system				
11. Documents procedure				

Knowledge of Procedure

- ☐ Good; student is knowledgeable about rationale and theory related to procedure
- ☐ Fair; student has adequate understanding of rationale and theory related to procedure
- ☐ Poor; student has inadequate understanding of rationale and theory related to procedure

Performance Deficiencies (check those that apply)

- ☐ Excessive time needed to complete procedure
- ☐ Broke aseptic or sterile technique
- ☐ Gross inaccuracy noted
- ☐ Technique may be harmful to patient
- ☐ Incorrect dosage or gas concentration
- ☐ Incorrect equipment assembly/use
- ☐ Unable to answer questions correctly about rationale and/or theory related to procedure
- ☐ Other ______________________________

Evaluation Summary

- ☐ Satisfactory performance
- ☐ Unsatisfactory performance

Recommendations of Evaluator

- ☐ Skills may be applied/observed in clinical setting
- ☐ Specific evaluation deficiencies require correction
- ☐ Complete re-evaluation required
- ☐ Additional laboratory practice required

Signatures:

Evaluator ______________________ Date ______________________

Student ______________________ Date ______________________

Laboratory Report

Student ______________________ Acceptable ______________________

Date ______________________ Unacceptable ______________________

Course ______________________

Topic: Aerosol Delivery Systems

Scenario: You have been assigned to the neurosurgical unit. The following aerosol delivery systems are in use: three tracheostomy masks, four T-tubes, and two face tents. Two of the tracheostomy patients are being weaned from their tracheostomy tubes and are allowed to breathe through their upper airway. Please answer the following questions:

1. When in the weaning process, would you provide the patients with a device other than the tracheostomy mask for effective aerosol delivery?

2. What aerosol delivery system would you use?

3. In what way(s) can you determine the adequacy of the total flow of an aerosol delivery system?

4. When using an aerosol delivery system in conjunction with oxygen therapy, how do you determine the delivered FI_{O_2}?

5. Compare and contrast an aerosol mask with a simple oxygen mask.

6. When used for a spontaneously breathing patient, how may an adequate total gas flowrate through a T-tube be estimated?

7. Which aerosol delivery device is most appropriate for the patient with

   A. facial burns?

   B. nasal endotracheal tube?

   C. a tracheostomy tube?

   D. recent neurosurgery?

chapter 13

Chest physiotherapy

INTRODUCTION

Chest physiotherapy consists of therapeutic techniques that are used to maintain tracheobronchial hygiene, such as postural drainage, percussion, and vibration. Postural drainage is the positioning of the body to facilitate the drainage of mucus by using the force of gravity. In postural drainage, the lobar or segmental bronchus is geometrically positioned so that secretions will flow down into a larger airway for removal. Chest percussion and vibration are mechanical means of mucokinesis in which force is applied to the chest wall for the purpose of loosening mucus within the airways.

Postural drainage, percussion, and vibration have been compared by Frownfelter to the techniques used to remove ketchup from a bottle. Ketchup, like mucus, may be thick, tenacious, and viscous. To remove the ketchup, the bottle is inverted (postural drainage), struck with the hand (percussion), and shaken (vibration). In this chapter, you will become familiar with chest physiotherapy.

OBJECTIVES

After completing this chapter, you should be able to do the following:

1. *Cite the lobes and segments of the lungs.*
2. *Identify the position used to drain a specific lung segment.*
3. *Perform the techniques of postural drainage, chest percussion, and vibration.*

EQUIPMENT NEEDED

☐ Hospital bed or postural drainage table

ACTIVITIES

Exercise A: Identification of Lung Lobes and Segments

1. Using the following diagram, identify the lung lobes (Fig. 13-1).
2. Label the lung lobes with the corresponding number from the following list:

Right Lung	Left Lung
1. Upper Lobe	4. Upper Lobe
2. Middle Lobe	5. Lower Lobe
3. Lower Lobe	

3. Using the following diagram, identify the pulmonary segments (Fig. 13-2).
4. Label the pulmonary segments with the corresponding number from the following list:

Lung	Lobe	Segment
Right	Upper	1. Apical
		2. Anterior
		3. Posterior
	Middle	4. Medial
		5. Lateral
Right	Lower	6. Superior
		7. Medial basal (not shown)
		8. Anterior basal
		9. Lateral basal
		10. Posterior basal (not shown)

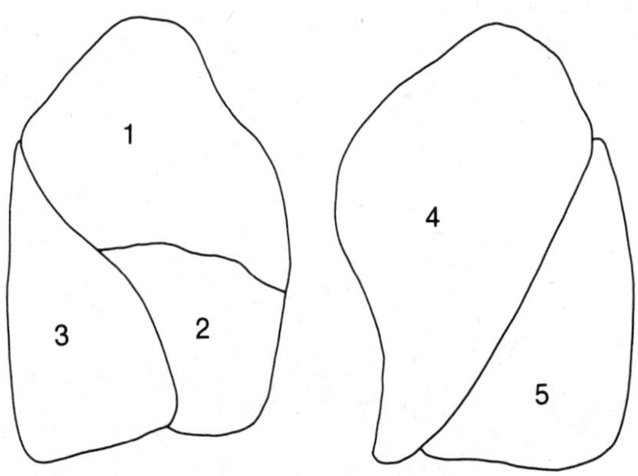

Fig. 13-1. Lung lobes.

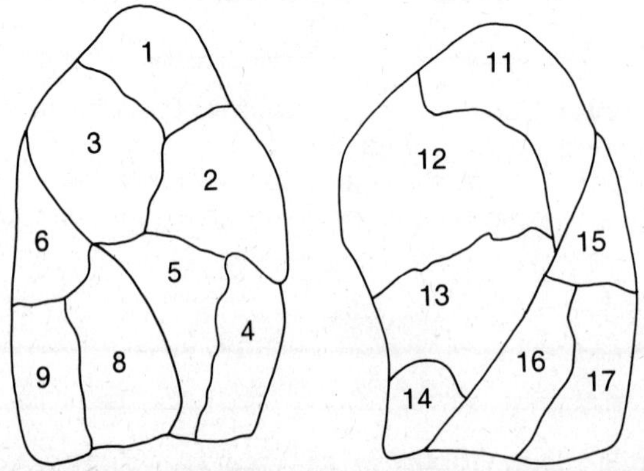

Fig. 13-2. Pulmonary segments.

Lung	Lobe	Segment
Left lung	Upper	11. Apical posterior
		12. Anterior
	Lingula	13. Superior
		14. Inferior
		15. Superior
		16. Anterior–medial basal
		17. Lateral basal
		18. Posterior basal (not shown)

Exercise B: Administration of Postural Drainage

1. Have a laboratory partner act as a simulated patient.
2. In the clinical setting, as with nearly all respiratory care procedures, the patient's chart is thoroughly reviewed for verification of orders for therapy, history and physical results, working diagnosis, diagnostic test results, chest radiograph interpretation, segments recommended for drainage, medications, and precautions prior to administering therapy.
3. Identify the patient and introduce yourself.
4. Explain the procedure to the patient and confirm patient understanding.
5. Position the patient by placing the desired lung segment to be drained in the uppermost position relative to the other lung segments.
6. Place a laboratory partner in the appropriate drainage position for each lung segment. *Note:* For middle lobes, elevate the feet 14 inches or 15°. For lower lobes, elevate the feet 18 inches or 30°. The exception to these generalizations is the position used to drain the superior segments of the lower lobes. To drain the superior segments of the lower lobes, place the patient prone with the bed flat.
7. Perform postural drainage for all the lung segments on a laboratory partner using the following diagrams (Figs. 13-3 through 13-14).

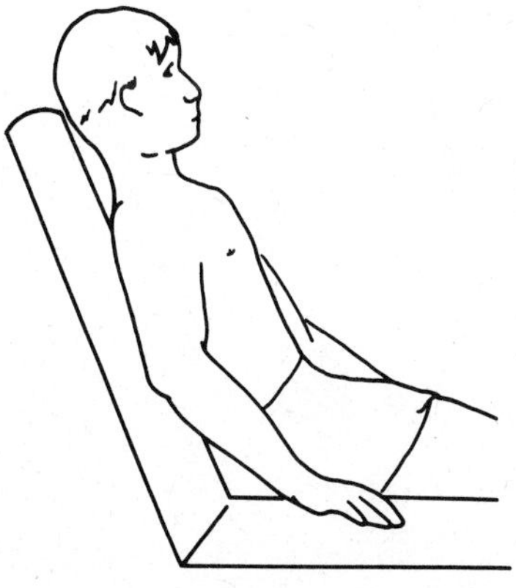

Fig. 13-3. Drainage of upper lobes, apical segments.

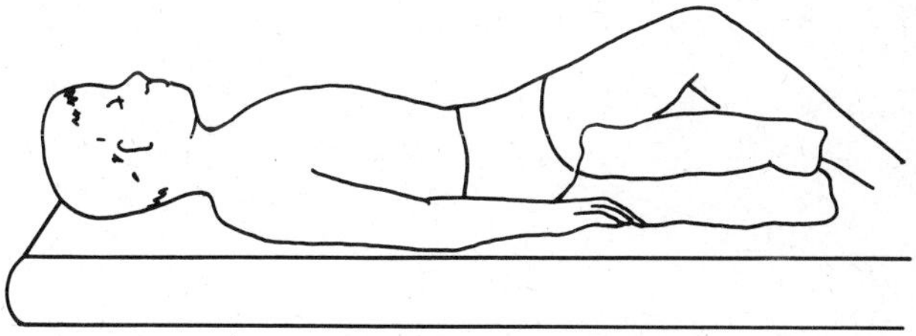

Fig. 13-4. Drainage of upper lobes, anterior segments.

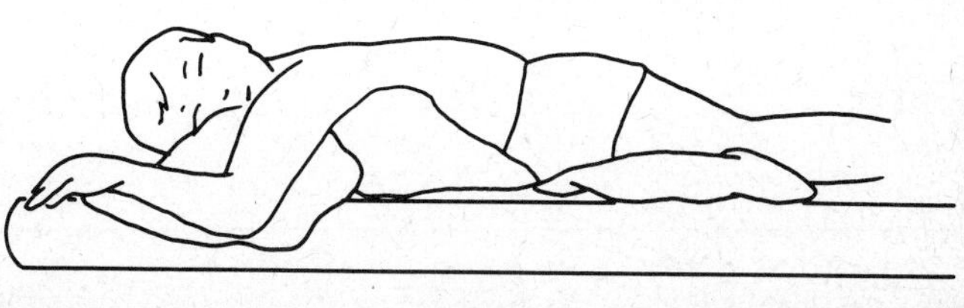

Fig. 13-5. Drainage of right upper lobe, posterior segment.

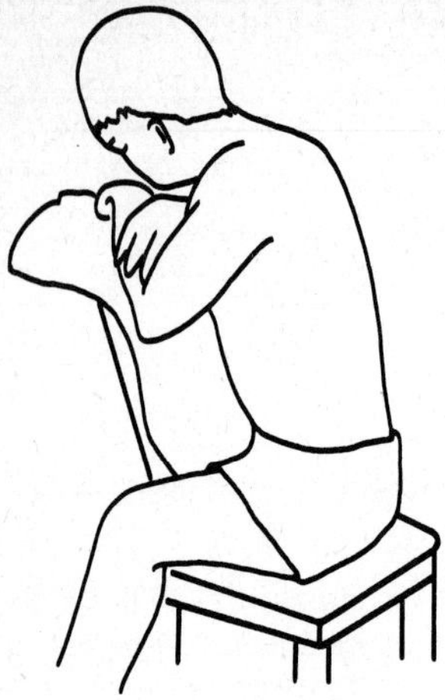

Fig. 13-6. Drainage of left upper lobe, posterior segment.

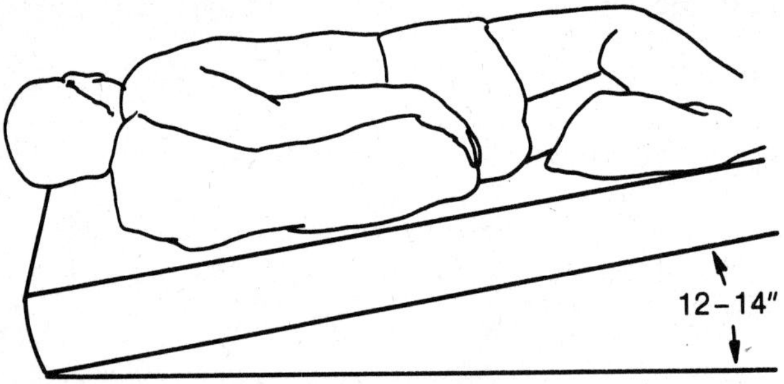

Fig. 13-7. Drainage of right middle lobe.

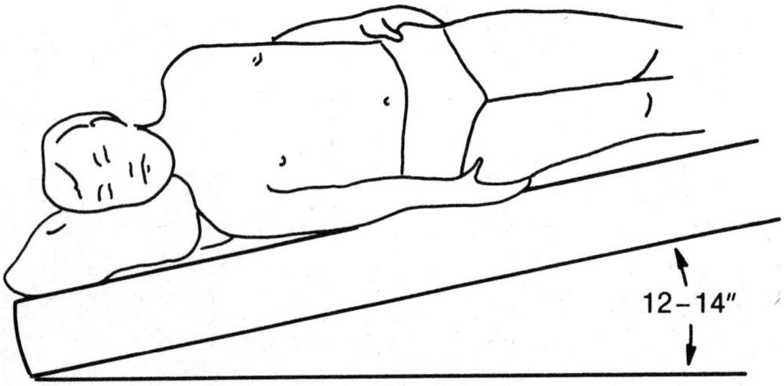

Fig. 13-8. Drainage of lingula.

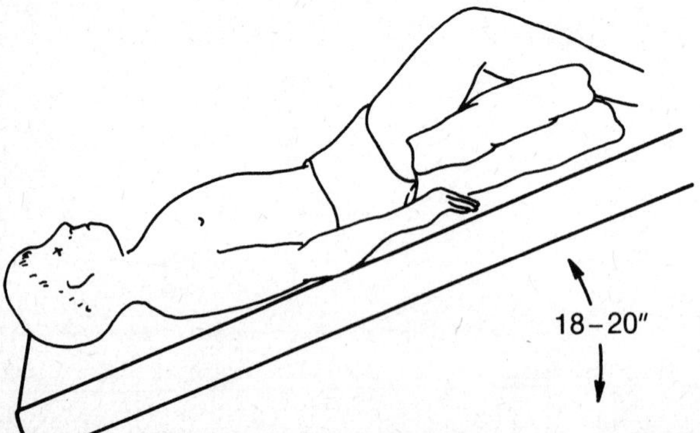

Fig. 13-9. Drainage of both lower lobes, anterior segments.

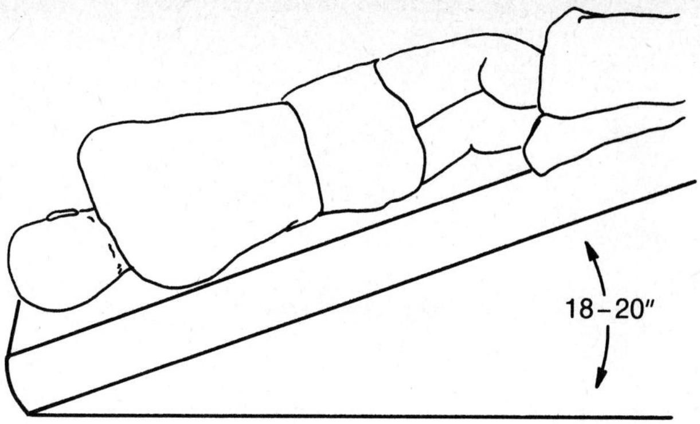

Fig. 13-10. Drainage of right lower lobe, medial and lateral segment.

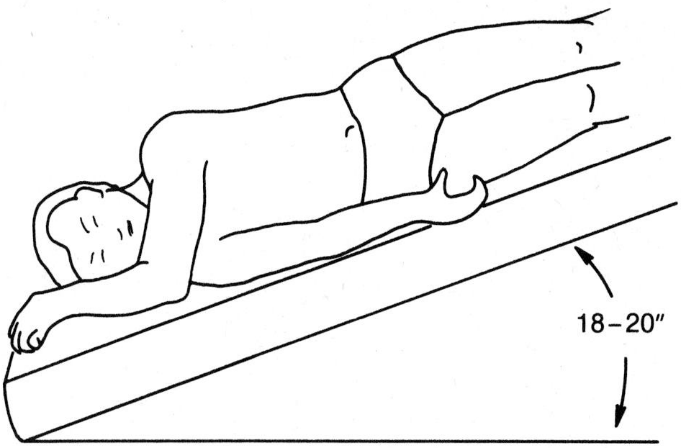

Fig. 13-11. Drainage of left lower lobe, lateral segment.

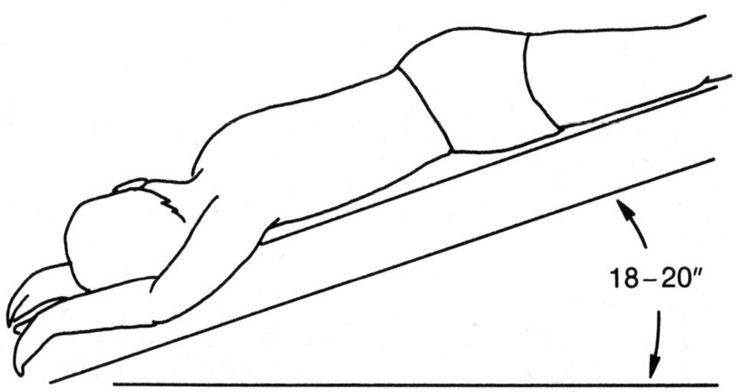

Fig. 13-12. Drainage of lower lobes, posterior segment.

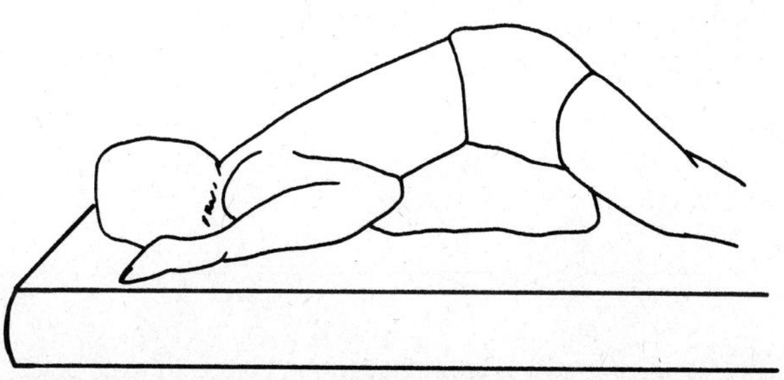

Fig. 13-13. Drainage of both lower lobes, superior segments.

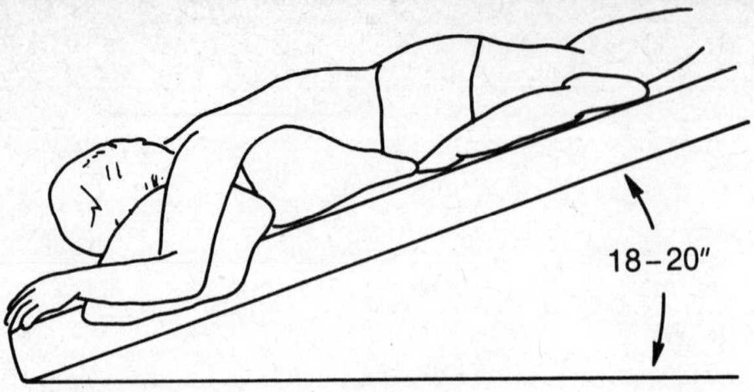

Fig. 13-14. Drainage of left lower lobe, posterior segments.

Exercise C: Administration of Chest Percussion

1. Position a laboratory partner for postural drainage.
2. Percuss the chest wall by cupping the hands, and make a "popping" noise as the cupped hand strikes the chest wall (Fig. 13-15).
3. Avoid percussion over the sternum, spine, scapula, kidney area, abdomen, and female breasts.
4. Perform percussion during both inspiration and expiration on all lung segments of a laboratory partner.

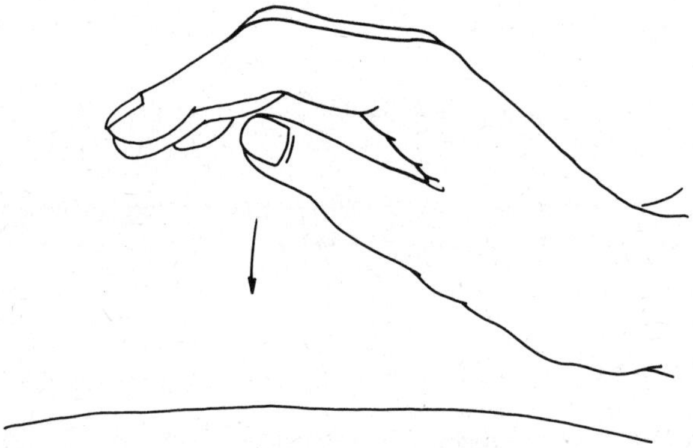

Fig. 13-15. Cupping of hand for chest percussion.

Exercise D: Administration of Chest Vibration

1. Position a laboratory partner for postural drainage.
2. Perform percussion on each lung segment for about 5 minutes.
3. After performing chest percussion, place the hand flat against the chest wall.
4. During exhalation, strong, rapid, repetitive isometric contractions of the shoulder and forearm cause vibrations on the chest wall (Fig. 13-16).
5. Following the sequence of postural drainage, percussion, and vibration, request a deep breath and a cough.

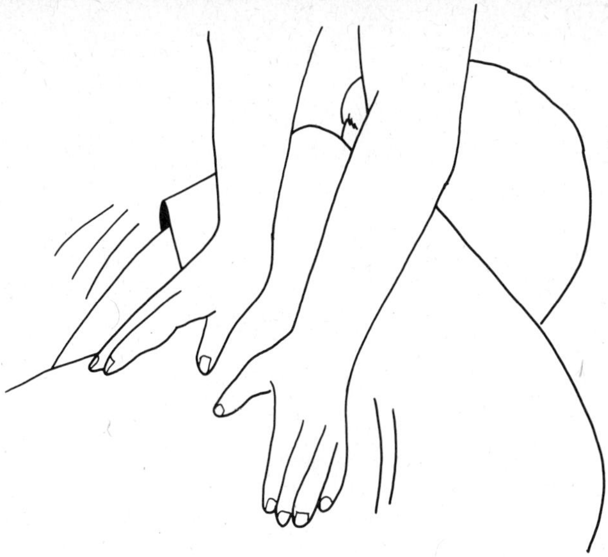

Fig. 13-16. Vibration of chest during exhalation.

Exercise E: Determination of "Unknown"

1. Your instructor will provide you with a mannequin or model placed in a special position(s) for postural drainage. Identify the segment(s) drained by each position.

RECOMMENDED READING

Burton GG, Hodgkin JE: Respiratory Care. A Guide to Clinical Practice, 2nd ed. Philadelphia, JB Lippincott, 1984

Frownfelter D: Chest Physical Therapy and Pulmonary Rehabilitation: An Interdisciplinary Approach. Chicago, Year Book Medical Publishers, 1978

Gaskell DV, Webber BA: The Brompton Hospital Guide to Chest Physiotherapy, 4th ed. St Louis, Blackwell Scientific, 1980

Kacmarek RM, Dimas S, Mack C: Essentials of Respiratory Therapy, 2nd ed. Chicago, Year Book Medical Publishers, 1985

Laboratory Performance Evaluation (#13)

Topic: Chest Physiotherapy

Student ______________________ Course ______________________

Date ______________________ Section ______________________

Performance Elements	Acceptable	Unacceptable	Not Applicable	Comments
1. Identifies simulated patient				
2. Introduces self to simulated patient				
3. Explains procedure to patient				
4. Confirms patient understanding of procedure				
5. Washes hands				
6. Positions patient for prescribed segmental drainage				
7. Applies appropriate chest wall percussion				
8. Applies appropriate chest wall vibration				
9. Monitors patient status throughout procedures				
10. Modifies therapy, if necessary				
11. Encourages simulated patient to breathe deeply and cough				
12. Documents procedure				

Knowledge of Procedure

☐ Good; student is knowledgeable about rationale and theory related to procedure

☐ Fair; student has adequate understanding of rationale and theory related to procedure

☐ Poor; student has inadequate understanding of rationale and theory related to procedure

Performance Deficiencies (check those that apply)

☐ Excessive time needed to complete procedure

☐ Broke aseptic or sterile technique

☐ Gross inaccuracy noted

☐ Technique may be harmful to patient

☐ Incorrect dosage or gas concentration

☐ Incorrect equipment assembly/use

☐ Unable to answer questions correctly about rationale and/or theory related to procedure

☐ Other ____________________

Evaluation Summary

☐ Satisfactory performance

☐ Unsatisfactory performance

Recommendations of Evaluator

☐ Skills may be applied/observed in clinical setting

☐ Specific evaluation deficiencies require correction

☐ Complete re-evaluation required

☐ Additional laboratory practice required

Signatures:

Evaluator ____________________ Date ____________________

Student ____________________ Date ____________________

Laboratory Report

Student ______________________ Acceptable ______________________

Date ______________________ Unacceptable ______________________

Course ______________________

Topic: Chest Physiotherapy

Data and Measurements

	Area of Postural Drainage		
Unknown	Lung	Lobe	Segment
Position 1	________	________	________
Position 2	________	________	________
Position 3	________	________	________
Position 4	________	________	________
Position 5	________	________	________

Scenario: Mr. Watson, an 85-year-old who, 72 hours ago, underwent a right-sided total hip replacement, has been placed on chest physiotherapy for treatment of bilateral lower lobe pneumonia. Please answer the following questions:

1. Which segments would you percuss in this situation?

2. How would you position him for effective drainage?

3. Would you modify your approach (positioning and so forth) if he complained of pain on his right side? Yes ________ No ________

4. If yes, specifically what modifications would you enact?

5. Name two other therapeutic modalities that complement chest physiotherapy.

6. List four hazards associated with chest physiotherapy.

7. What are the goals of chest physical therapy?

8. What anatomical areas are avoided during chest percussion?

9. Vibration is performed during which phase of the ventilatory cycle?

chapter 14

Incentive spirometry and breathing exercises

INTRODUCTION

In respiratory care, a variety of techniques may be used to encourage deep breathing, maintain bronchial hygiene, or improve respiratory muscular efficiency. Incentive spirometry is a technique used to encourage deep breathing in order to optimize lung inflation. An incentive spirometer is a device that may be used to provide a "reward" for inhaling a specified flow or volume of air. Respiratory muscle training and breathing exercises are intended to increase respiratory muscular strength in order to improve the ventilatory pattern. Splinting of the chest and controlled coughing are used to maintain bronchial hygiene. In this chapter, you are introduced to incentive spirometry and breathing exercises.

OBJECTIVES

After completing this chapter, you should be able to do the following:

1. *Identify an inspiratory volume that may act as a goal during incentive spirometry.*
2. *Demonstrate diaphragmatic, lateral costal, segmental, pursed-lip, and movement-coordinated breathing exercises.*
3. *Demonstrate chest splinting and controlled coughing.*

EQUIPMENT NEEDED

- ☐ Incentive spirometers
- ☐ Mouthpieces
- ☐ Fixed orifice muscle training device

ACTIVITIES

Exercise A: Administration of Incentive Spirometry

1. Obtain an incentive spirometer.
2. Locate and identify the volume or flow increments. Adjust the volume scale or goal as needed. *Note:* For an adult, a minimum goal of three times the tidal volume or 1500 ml is recommended.
3. Using a laboratory partner as a simulated patient, explain the purpose of incentive spirometry.
4. Position the patient in a sitting or upright position.
5. Instruct the simulated patient to exhale normally and inhale maximally through the mouthpiece (Fig. 14-1). A goal may be set that is slightly higher than the maximal inspired volume.
6. Instruct the simulated patient to perform a breath-hold following the maximal inhalation. Ideally, the breath-hold is performed for 3 to 10 seconds.
7. Monitor the frequency of maximal inhalations. To prevent inadvertent hyperventilation, limit the number of maximal inspiratory attempts to a few each minute.
8. Increase the goal by volume increments as needed.

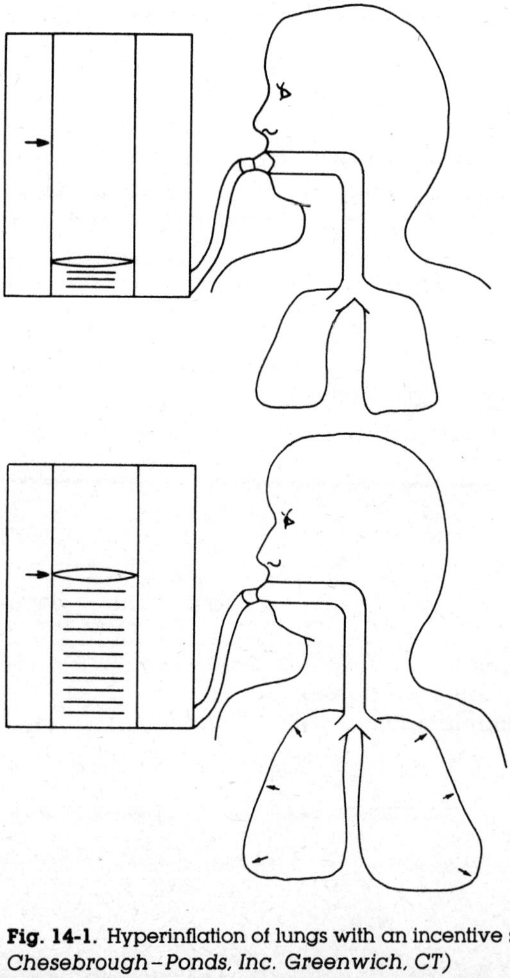

Fig. 14-1. Hyperinflation of lungs with an incentive spirometer. *(Modified from Chesebrough–Ponds, Inc. Greenwich, CT)*

9. Inform the patient of the treatment frequency. Incentive spirometry is recommended at least once during each waking hour.
10. Monitor the patient's progress and provide encouragement as needed.
11. Document the results of the procedure. Be sure to include the following:
    Date and time
    Patient position
    Volume or flow goal
    Number of times goal was reached
    Number of attempts
    Frequency of treatment
    Patient effort

Exercise B: Respiratory Muscle Training

1. Obtain a respiratory muscle training device. Identify the fixed orifice diameter settings, one-way valves, and mouthpiece (Fig. 14-2).
2. Practice inhaling through the largest diameter setting. Perform several inhalations.
3. Practice inhaling through the smallest diameter setting. Perform several inhalations.
4. *Note:* For optimal results, the device should be used for several weeks beginning with the largest diameter and progressing gradually to the smallest diameter setting. As with any type of training, scheduled practice sessions and consistency yield the most productive results.
5. Disassemble the device.

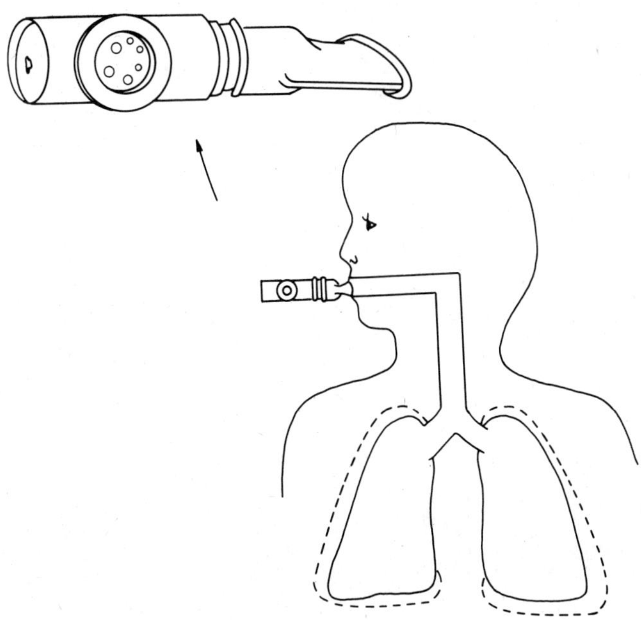

Fig. 14-2. Respiratory muscle exerciser. *(Modified from Healthscan Inc, Upper Montclair, NJ)*

Exercise C: Diaphragmatic and Pursed-Lip Breathing Exercises

1. Demonstrate diaphragmatic breathing by placing a hand in the epigastric triangle immediately below the xiphoid process. Assume the supine Trendelenburg

(feet-up) position. By inhaling through the nose or "sniffing" slowly, the hand is lifted gently from the epigastrium (Fig. 14-3).

2. Arching of the back and abdominal protrusion may mimic diaphragmatic breathing and must be avoided. The lower lateral rib cage should also expand with proper diaphragmatic breathing. Practice diaphragmatic breathing in supine, sitting, standing, and walking positions.
3. Measurement of Diaphragmatic Muscular Strength
   A. Obtain the following weights:
      2 lb
      5 lb
      10 lb
   B. Assume the supine Trendelenburg position.
   C. Place a 2 lb weight in the epigastrium.
   D. Attempt to displace the weight maximally by sniffing slowly.
   E. Document the total weight displaced in the Laboratory Report. *Note:* A "functional" diaphragmatic breather may displace a 10 lb. weight.
4. Demonstrate pursed-lip breathing to a laboratory partner by inhaling and slowly exhaling through pursed lips in a relaxed, prolonged manner.

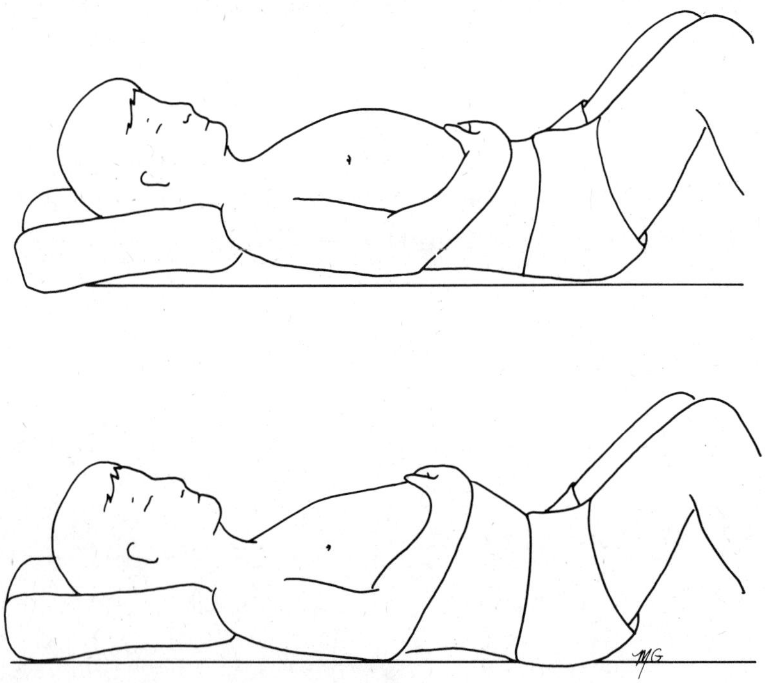

Fig. 14-3. Diaphragmatic breathing.

Exercise D: Lateral Costal Breathing Exercises

1. Demonstrate lateral costal breathing by placing the hands at the base of the rib cage near the midaxillary line (Fig. 14-4).
2. Request a slow, deep inspiration. Apply a slight pressure to the rib cage at the beginning of inspiration to stimulate expansion of the lower rib cage and lung bases.

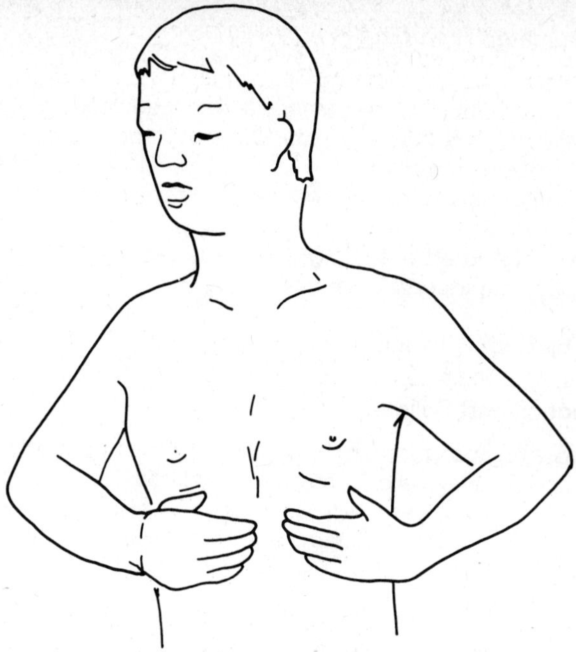

Fig. 14-4. Lateral costal breathing.

Exercise E: Segmental Breathing Exercises

1. After surgery, expansion of the chest may be needed proximal to an incision.
2. Demonstrate segmental breathing by placing a hand over the chest wall where expansion of a selected lung segment is desired. Inhale, and concentrate on expanding the chest where the hand is located (Fig. 14-5).

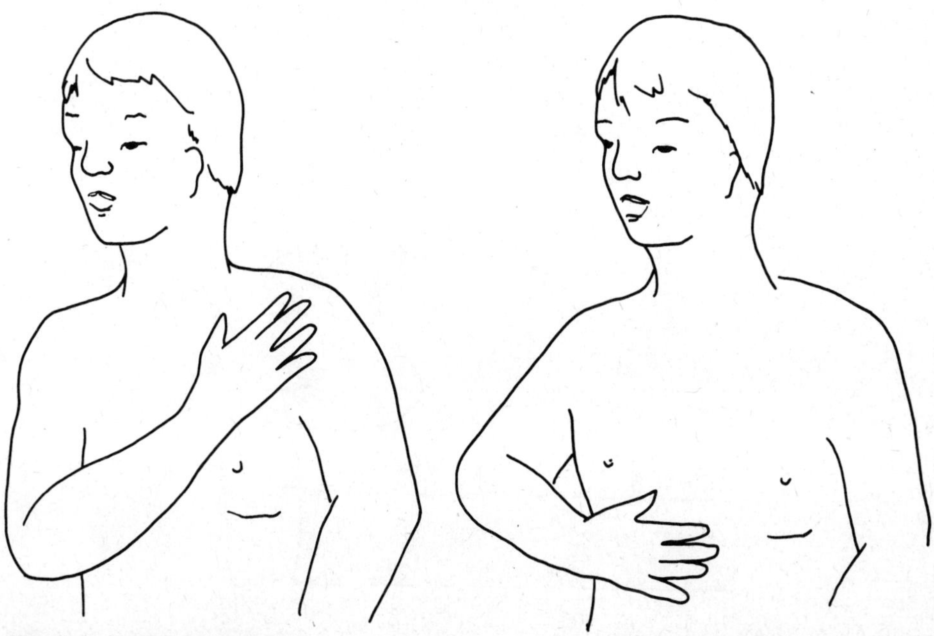

Fig. 14-5. Segmental breathing

Exercise F: Movement Coordinated Breathing Exercises

1. Demonstrate movement-coordinated breathing by exhaling during any activity that causes increased proximity between the knees and chest or activity that causes abdominal muscular contraction. Inhalation should accompany forward flexion of the arms or abduction above the head. Breath-holding while bending over is to be avoided by inhaling before bending and exhaling slowly during a bend.
2. Practice movement-coordinated breathing during the following activities:
   - A. Reaching for an object placed above your head
   - B. Sit-ups
   - C. Picking up an object from the floor

Exercise G: Coughing Instruction and Splinting

1. After surgery, a cough may produce extreme pain at the site of the incision. "Splinting" of a surgical incision may be accomplished by tightly gripping a pillow or towel and applying adequate pressure to an incision (Fig. 14-6).
2. Practice splinting the chest for incisions made in the following locations:
   - A. Medial sternotomy
   - B. Upper epigastric incision
   - C. Lower abdominal incision
3. Demonstrate proper coughing by inhaling deeply, momentarily holding the breath, and explosively coughing in a controlled manner. If a cough is nonproductive and mucus is present in the airways, relax and take a series of deep breaths before the next controlled cough. For postoperative patients, positioning should

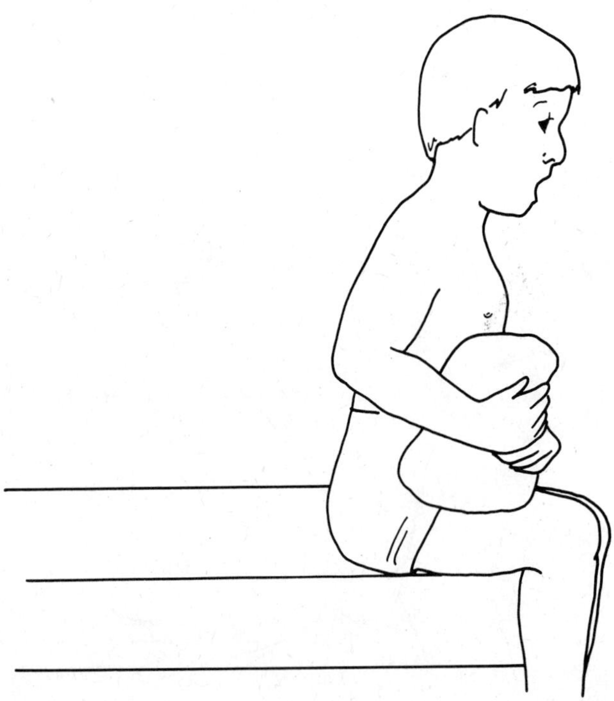

Fig. 14-6. Postoperative splinting of an incision.

minimize traction on the incision site. The hands may be placed on either side of an incision to produce pressure and "splinting" during coughing.

Note: In clinical practice, patients with chronic airway obstruction and air trapping should cough from the midinspiratory position rather than a maximum inspiratory position. The cough should be expelled in short controlled bursts rather than in a single, explosive blast.

RECOMMENDED READING

Burton GG, Hodgkin JE: Respiratory Care. A Guide to Clinical Practice, 2nd ed. Philadelphia, JB Lippincott, 1984

Kacmarek RM, Dimas S, Mack C: Essentials of Respiratory Therapy, 2nd ed. Chicago, Year Book Medical Publishers, 1985

Shapiro BA, Harrison RA, Kacmarek RM, Cane RD: Clinical Application of Respiratory Care, 3rd ed. Chicago, Year Book Medical Publishers, 1985

Spearman CB, Sheldon RL: Egan's Fundamentals of Respiratory Therapy, 4th ed. St Louis, CV Mosby, 1982

Laboratory Performance Evaluation (#14)

Topic: Incentive Spirometry/Breathing Exercises

Student ______________________ Course ______________________

Date ______________________ Section ______________________

Performance Elements	Acceptable	Unacceptable	Not Applicable	Comments
1. Confirms order				
2. Obtains any necessary equipment				
3. Validates patient's identification				
4. Introduces self to simulated patient				
5. Washes hands				
6. Assembles equipment				
7. Confirms patient's understanding of the procedure				
8. Positions simulated patient properly				
9. Instructs simulated patient to inspire deeply through mouthpiece				
10. Instructs patient in breath hold at peak inspiration when signaled				
11. Evaluates simulated patient's progress				
12. Assesses effectiveness of therapy				
13. Documents procedure				

Knowledge of Procedure

- ☐ Good; student is knowledgeable about rationale and theory related to procedure
- ☐ Fair; student has adequate understanding of rationale and theory related to procedure
- ☐ Poor; student has inadequate understanding of rationale and theory related to procedure

Performance Deficiencies (check those that apply)

- ☐ Excessive time needed to complete procedure
- ☐ Broke aseptic or sterile technique
- ☐ Gross inaccuracy noted
- ☐ Technique may be harmful to patient
- ☐ Incorrect dosage or gas concentration
- ☐ Incorrect equipment assembly/use
- ☐ Unable to answer questions correctly about rationale and/or theory related to procedure
- ☐ Other ____________________

Evaluation Summary

- ☐ Satisfactory performance
- ☐ Unsatisfactory performance

Recommendations of Evaluator

- ☐ Skills may be applied/observed in clinical setting
- ☐ Specific evaluation deficiencies require correction
- ☐ Complete re-evaluation required
- ☐ Additional laboratory practice required

Signatures:

Evaluator ____________________ Date ____________________

Student ____________________ Date ____________________

Laboratory Report

Student ______________________ Acceptable ______________________

Date ______________________ Unacceptable ______________________

Course ______________________

Topic: Incentive Spirometry and Breathing Exercises

Scenario: Mr. Eliot suffers from, among other ailments, asthmatic bronchitis. His acute episode has passed, and he has derived so much benefit from aerosol therapy, incentive spirometry, and other bronchial hygiene modalities that he is only a few hours away from being discharged to home. Before he leaves, however, you have been asked to stop by and teach him some breathing exercises. Please answer the following questions:

1. In order to teach Mr. Eliot diaphragmatic breathing, he needs to know how to locate his diaphragm. How can you accomplish this?

2. What benefit can be gained from pursed-lip breathing?

3. Why is movement-coordinated breathing advantageous?

4. How would you describe to Mr. Eliot "proper coughing technique"?

5. Assume Mr. Eliot has been diligently performing his breathing exercises for the past few months. Is there a method for determining whether he has increased the efficiency of his diaphragm?

6. What is the purpose of incentive spirometry?

7. What is an incentive spirometer, and how does it work?

8. What type of patient may benefit from incentive spirometry?

9. How can the effectiveness of the therapy be determined?

chapter 15

Intermittent positive pressure breathing

INTRODUCTION

Many techniques may be used to promote lung hyperinflation. In addition to using voluntary deep breathing and incentive spirometry, lung inflation may be optimized using a mechanical ventilator. With current mechanical ventilators, lung inflation occurs when positive pressure is applied to the airway and a pressure gradient is created between the mouth and alveoli. Treatments of short duration (10–30 minutes) incorporating positive pressure to achieve lung inflation are referred to as intermittent positive pressure breathing (IPPB).

In clinical practice, IPPB is frequently used as one of several methods for delivering medication. Because simpler, less complicated, and less expensive methods of medication administration are available, however, the primary purpose of IPPB is to deliver a larger tidal volume of gas than can be generated spontaneously. In this chapter, you are introduced to intermittent positive pressure breathing.

OBJECTIVES

After completing this chapter, you should be able to do the following:

1. *Assemble and operate a mechanical ventilator for IPPB therapy.*
2. *Understand the primary IPPB ventilator controls.*
3. *Understand the cycling mechanism (inspiration to expiration) for an IPPB ventilator.*
4. *Administer an IPPB treatment to a simulated patient.*
5. *Measure the exhaled tidal volume during IPPB.*

EQUIPMENT NEEDED

- ☐ IPPB ventilator (Bird Mark 7, Bennett AP-5, or Bennett PR-2)
- ☐ IPPB circuit (disposable or nondisposable)
- ☐ Single-dose sterile water medication

☐ Spirometer
☐ Stethoscope
☐ Mouthpiece or mask
☐ 50 psi gas source

ACTIVITIES

Exercise A: Identification of Ventilator Components

1. Your instructor will provide you with a ventilator that will be used to administer IPPB. You should become familiar with the operator's manual for the ventilator before performing these exercises.
2. Examine a Bird Mark 7 ventilator (Fig. 15-1).
   Identify and label the following controls on the Bird ventilator:
   A. Flowrate control
   B. Pressure limit
   C. Air mix plunger
   D. Inspiratory effort control (sensitivity)
   E. Expiratory timer
   F. Manometer
   G. Gas inlet
   H. Large-bore mainstream tubing connection
   I. Small-bore nebulizer and exhalation valve tubing connection
   J. Ambient pressure chamber
   K. Positive pressure chamber
   L. Center body (not shown)
      Magnets and clutch plates
      Brass filter
      Automatic or hand cycling control
3. Examine a Bennett PR-2 ventilator (Fig. 15-2).
   Identify and label the following controls on the Bennett PR-2 ventilator:
   A. Pressure limit
   B. Air dilution
   C. Expiratory time
   D. Nebulization-inspiration
   E. Nebulization-expiration
   F. Negative pressure
   G. Sensitivity
   H. Terminal flow
   I. Peak flow
   J. Control pressure
   K. System pressure

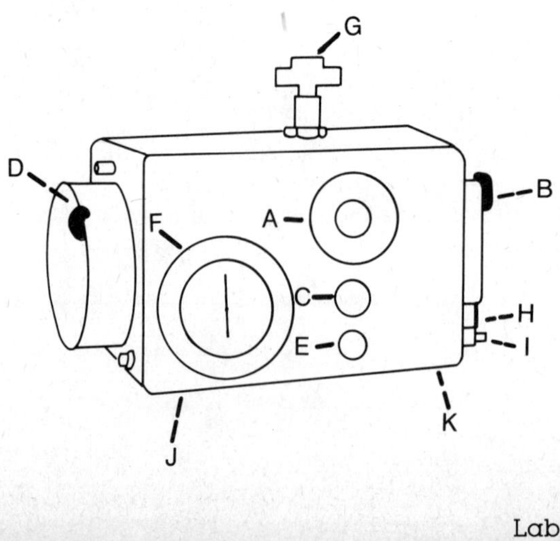

Fig. 15-1. Bird Mark 7 ventilator.

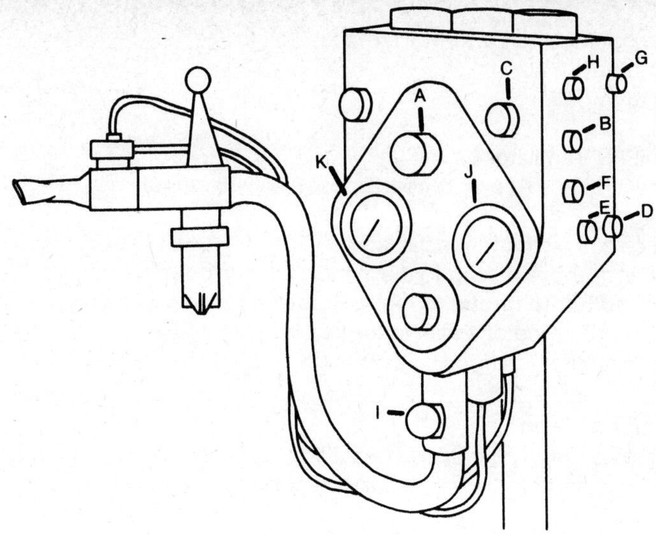

Fig. 15-2. Bennett PR-2.

Exercise B: Assembly of IPPB Breathing Circuit

1. Obtain a disposible or reusable IPPB ventilator circuit.
2. Identify the following IPPB ventilator circuit components:
   Mouthpiece or mask
   Medication nebulizer

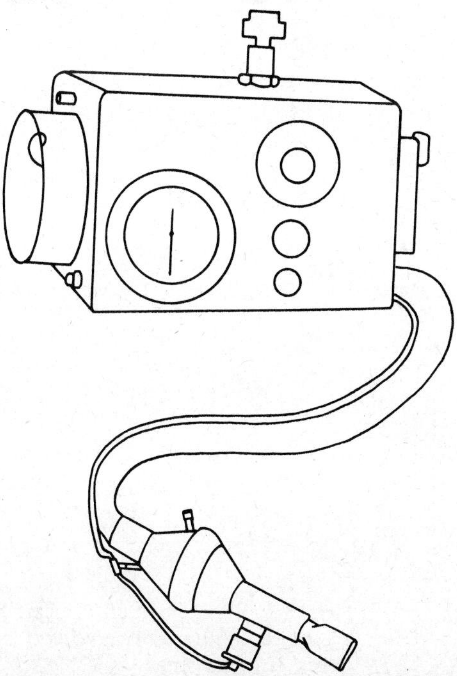

Fig. 15-3. Components of an IPPB breathing circuit.

Exhalation valve
Nebulizer and exhalation valve drive lines
Mainstream tubing
Exhalation valve outlet

Assembly of an IPPB Ventilator Circuit

1. Obtain either a disposable or a nondisposable IPPB circuit.
2. Wash your hands.
3. Remove the circuit from the plastic bag.
4. Connect the large-bore tubing to the ventilator gas outlet.
5. Connect the small-bore tubing to the exhalation valve gas outlet.
6. Connect the mouthpiece or mask to the circuit (Fig. 15-3).
7. Connect the ventilator to a gas source or plug in electrical cord.

Exercise C: Medication Injection

An IPPB treatment frequently includes the delivery of prescribed medication. When no medication is prescribed, sterile saline may be nebulized to provide some humidification of the inspired gas.

1. Obtain a single-dose of sterile H_2O medication.
2. Unscrew the nebulizer cup from the ventilator circuit.
3. Remove the top from the single dose medication.
4. Aseptically inject the sterile medication into the nebulizer cup.
5. Reconnect the nebulizer cup to the circuit.

Exercise D: Verification of Equipment Function

1. After assembling the ventilator circuit and injecting the medication, cycle the ventilator on with the hand-cycling mechanism.
2. The nebulized medication should be visible while the ventilator is in the inspiratory mode (Fig. 15-4).
   Note: Be certain to position the nebulizer properly in order to produce an aerosol.
3. Occlude the mouthpiece with sterile gauze or the plastic storage bag for the circuit.

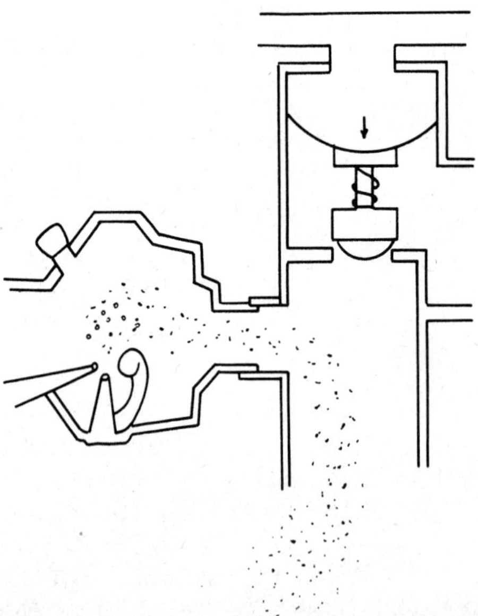

Fig. 15-4. Verification of nebulizer function by visualizing aerosol. *(Modified from Bird Corp. Palm Springs, CA)*

4. The ventilator should cycle off when the mouthpiece is occluded and at the preset pressure limit (Fig. 15-5).
Note: If the ventilator will not cycle off, a leak probably exists in the system. If an aerosol is not visible, then the medication is not in the medication chamber or the jet has become obstructed.

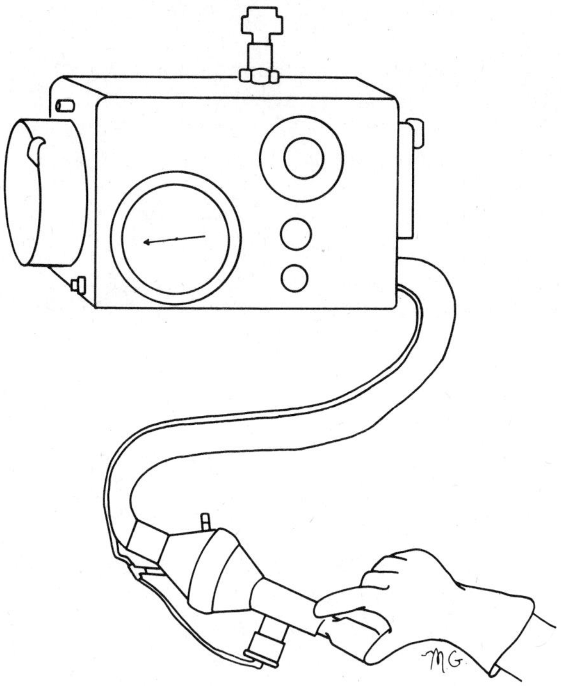

Fig. 15-5. Verification of cycling mechanism and accuracy check of pressure limit setting before IPPB administration.

Exercise E: Adjustment of Ventilator Controls

Administer IPPB to a laboratory partner. Before administration of a practice "treatment," review the following guidelines for adjustment of the ventilator controls.

- Pressure Limit and Tidal Volume. The delivered volume may be adjusted by regulating the pressure limit control. Initially, begin with a low pressure limit (5–10 cm H_2O) until the patient becomes accustomed to the sensation of positive pressure breathing. After several breaths, the pressure limit may be adjusted until the desired tidal volume is delivered. Typically, pressure limits between 5 and 25 cm H_2O are used. Observe the manometer when adjusting the pressure limit. The tidal volume must be measured.
- I:E Ratios. The inspiratory to expiratory time ratio (I:E ratio) is dependent on the delivered tidal volume (pressure limit), the gas flowrate, the cycling rate, and lung properties of resistance and compliance. After adjusting the tidal volume by means of the pressure limit control, adjust the flowrate to regulate the inspiratory time.
- Cycling Rate. Excessive rates (number of positive pressure breaths per minute) may cause alveolar hyperventilation, resulting in dizziness and paresthesia. To prevent excessive rates, provide proper instruction and monitoring. Also, adjust the sensitivity control to regulate the negative force required to turn the machine on. Observe

the manometer when adjusting the sensitivity. Typically, the sensitivity is set at -2 or -3 cm H_2O.

- Oxygen Concentration. Air may be used to power the ventilator unless oxygen is indicated for the treatment (or prevention) of hypoxia.

Administration of IPPB to a Laboratory Partner

1. Confirm the order for therapy.
2. Identify the patient and introduce yourself.
3. Explain the procedure to the patient and confirm patient understanding.
4. Wash hands. Obtain baseline pulse and breath sounds.
5. Assemble equipment.
6. Adjust the ventilator to deliver the following:
   VT of 10 ml/kg body weight
   I:E ratio of 1:2
   FI_{O_2} of 40% to 50%
7. Inject sterile H_2O medication.
8. Verify proper equipment function before applying it to the patient.
9. Allow the patient to take a few breaths from the machine. Explain that a tight seal is necessary if using a mouthpiece. Noseclips may be needed to obtain an effective seal.
10. Provide the following instructions:
    A. Obtain a tight seal around the mouthpiece.
    B. Inhale through the mouthpiece to turn the machine on.
    C. After triggering the machine on, inhale passively. Let the machine do the work of breathing.
    D. Keep a tight seal around the mouthpiece until the ventilator turns off.
    E. Exhale normally through mouthpiece.
    F. Remove the mouthpiece, and rest when needed.
11. Allow the patient to reach a stable ventilatory pattern before measuring the exhaled tidal volume.
12. Attach a spirometer to the exhalation port on the IPPB ventilator circuit (Fig. 15-6).
13. After the patient has reached a stable ventilatory pattern, measure the exhaled tidal volume. Adjust the pressure limit to deliver a minimum tidal volume of 10 ml/kg body weight.
14. Auscultate the lobes of the lungs to determine the effectiveness of therapy. Check the pulse during and after treatment.
15. Terminate the therapy when the medication has been delivered or if the pulse changes by

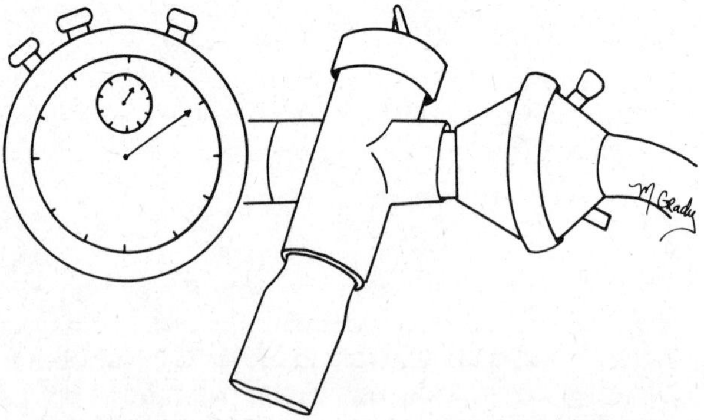

Fig. 15-6. Measurement of exhaled tidal volume during IPPB by attachment of a spirometer to the exhalation port.

A. increasing or decreasing more than 20 beats/minute from baseline; by
B. exceeding 140 beats/minute in an adult.

16. Remove any condensate from the nebulizer, and place the ventilator circuit in a clean plastic bag for storage.
17. Request a cough from the patient.
18. Document the performance of the procedure and any results of sputum production on the laboratory report. Be certain to record the following:
    A. Pressure limit
    B. Flowrate
    C. Sensitivity
    D. Tidal volume delivered
    E. Partner's body weight (in kg)

Optional: Administration of IPPB to a Laboratory Mannequin

1. Your instructor will provide you with a mannequin that may have an artificial airway in place.
2. Examine the methods that may be used to obtain an effective seal during IPPB administration (Fig. 15-7).
3. Assemble the equipment.
4. Connect a face mask to the ventilator circuit.
5. Explain the procedure to the patient and confirm patient understanding.
6. Adjust the ventilator controls to obtain the following:
   Tidal volume of 10 ml/kg body weight (peak pressure)
   I:E of 1:2 (flowrate)
   FI_{O_2} of 50%
7. Measure the exhaled tidal volume. Adjust the ventilator to deliver the desired tidal volume.

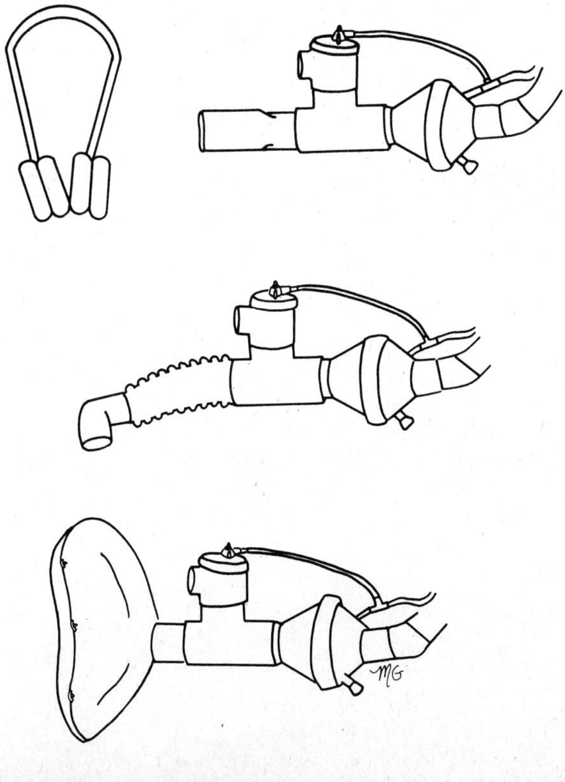

Fig. 15-7. Apparatus used during IPPB administration including a mouthpiece, noseclips, mask, or a flex tube 15.0 mm adapter for connection to a tracheostomy or endotracheal tube.

RECOMMENDED READING

Burton GG, Hodgkin JE: Respiratory Care. A Guide to Clinical Practice, 2nd ed. Philadelphia, JB Lippincott, 1984

Kacmarek RM, Dimas S, Mack C: Essentials of Respiratory Therapy, 2nd ed. Chicago, Year Book Medical Publishers, 1985

McPherson SP, Spearman CB: Respiratory Therapy Equipment, 3rd ed. St Louis, CV Mosby, 1985

Shapiro BA, Harrison RA, Kacmarek RM, Cane RD: Clinical Applications of Respiratory Care, 3rd ed. Chicago, Year Book Medical Publishers, 1985

Spearman CB, Sheldon RL: Egan's Fundamentals of Respiratory Therapy, 4th ed. St. Louis, CV Mosby, 1982

Laboratory Performance Evaluation (#15)

Topic: Intermittent Positive Pressure Breathing

Student ______________________ Course ______________________

Date ______________________ Section ______________________

Performance Elements	Acceptable	Unacceptable	Not Applicable	Comments
1. Verifies physician's order				
2. Selects appropriate equipment				
3. Washes hands				
4. Assembles and verifies proper equipment function				
5. Identifies simulated patient				
6. Introduces himself to simulated patient				
7. Instructs patient in method of performing procedure				
8. Confirms patient understanding				
9. Monitors simulated patient's pulse and breath sounds				
10. Implements therapy (assures a minimum tidal volume of 10 ml/kg body weight)				
11. Again monitors the pulse and breath sounds				
12. Modifies therapy, when indicated				

Performance Elements	Acceptable	Unacceptable	Not Applicable	Comments
13. Measures exhaled tidal volume				
14. Encourages patient to breathe deeply and cough				
15. Disassembles equipment				
16. Documents appropriate results				

Knowledge of Procedure

☐ Good; student is knowledgeable about rationale and theory related to procedure

☐ Fair; student has adequate understanding of rationale and theory related to procedure

☐ Poor; student has inadequate understanding of rationale and theory related to procedure

Performance Deficiencies (check those that apply)

☐ Excessive time needed to complete procedure

☐ Broke aseptic or sterile technique

☐ Gross inaccuracy noted

☐ Technique may be harmful to patient

☐ Incorrect dosage or gas concentration

☐ Incorrect equipment assembly/use

☐ Unable to answer questions correctly about rationale and/or theory related to procedure

☐ Other ______________________________

Evaluation Summary

☐ Satisfactory performance

☐ Unsatisfactory performance

Recommendations of Evaluator
☐ Skills may be applied/observed in clinical setting ☐ Specific evaluation deficiencies require correction ☐ Complete re-evaluation required ☐ Additional laboratory practice required

Signatures:

Evaluator ______________________ Date ______________________

Student ______________________ Date ______________________

Laboratory Report

Student ______________________ Acceptable ______________________

Date ______________________ Unacceptable ______________________

Course ______________________

Topic: Intermittent Positive Pressure Breathing

Data and Measurements

Estimated body weight (kg) ______________________

Delivered tidal volume (ml) ______________________

Pressure limit (cm H_2O)

Set ______________________

Measured ______________________

Sensitivity (cm H_2O)

Set ______________________

Measured ______________________

Flowrate setting ______________________

Scenario: You are a staff therapist assigned to a general medical ward in a medium-sized community hospital. Three of your patients are receiving IPPB every 4 hours while awake. One of the patients, Mr. Jones, has been diagnosed as suffering from emphysema. Another patient, Mr. Smith, suffers from chronic bronchitis, while the third patient, Ms. Williams, has been diagnosed as suffering from a lobar pneumonia. Please answer the following questions pertinent to your administration of IPPB to these patients.

1. How might you increase the volume of gas being delivered to Mr. Smith?

2. What ventilator control would you adjust when you hear the machine "chatter" and Ms. Williams cannot make it stop coming on?
   A. Pressure limit control
   B. Flowrate control
   C. Sensitivity control

3. In all probability, what is the cause when Mr. Jones complains, "I get a headache every time I use that thing"?

4. If the cause of Mr. Jones' headache is hyperventilation, what advice would you give him that might prevent the headache?

5. When administering IPPB therapy, which ventilator control adjusts

   A. tidal volume? ____________________

   B. I:E ratio? ____________________

   C. patient effort to initiate inspiration? ____________________

   D. FI_{O_2}? ____________________

6. Measurement of exhaled tidal volume during IPPB is made with a ____________________.
7. What is meant by the ventilatory pattern?

8. Which adjustments can be made with the ventilator for a patient who rapidly cycles the ventilator?

9. If a Bird ventilator remains "on" in the inspiratory phase, what is the most likely cause?

10. What is the function of the
   A. sensitivity?

   B. pressure limit?

   C. manometer?

chapter 16

Medication administration

INTRODUCTION

One of the most potentially dangerous activities in respiratory care is medication or drug administration. Since many pharmacologic agents used to treat cardiopulmonary disorders may produce serious side-effects, mistakes in medication administration may be harmful (or fatal) to critically ill patients. It is therefore essential to become thoroughly familiar with the medications commonly administered and to follow established guidelines for the mixing and administering of drugs. In addition, because each patient is unique, it is extremely important to monitor closely the physiologic response to drugs given. In this chapter, you are introduced to the guidelines and techniques for medication administration.

OBJECTIVES

After completing this chapter, you should be able to do the following:

1. *Prepare and administer medications for inhalation.*
2. *Administer medications for inhalation by intermittent nebulized aerosol therapy or intermittent positive pressure breathing.*
3. *Assemble a nebulizer for administering medications.*
4. *Identify the breathing pattern used for maximum aerosol deposition.*
5. *Evaluate the cardiovascular response to the inhalation of sympathomimetic drugs.*

EQUIPMENT NEEDED

- ☐ IPPB circuit
- ☐ Medication nebulizer
- ☐ Tuberculin syringe

- ☐ 3.0 ml syringe
- ☐ Unit dose vials of sterile water or saline
- ☐ Pharmacologic agents

Racemic epinephrine	2.25%
Isoetharine	1.0%
Isoproproterenol	0.5%
Acetylcysteine	20.0%
Ethyl alcohol	20.0%

ACTIVITIES

Exercise A: Verification of Physician Orders for Medication

In clinical practice, medications must be prescribed by a licensed physician. Prescriptions for respiratory care frequently are located in the patient's chart under "Physician's Orders" or the "Treatment and Medications" record. Prescriptions for medication must be written and signed by a physician before the medication is administered to the patient. Exceptions to this rule include the following:

- Acceptance of verbal orders by qualified therapists
- Respiratory care consultations by qualified therapists
- Emergency situations

In these cases, an order should be written and signed by a physician as soon as possible after the administration of therapy. If there is any doubt about an order, consult the physician for clarification. A therapist may not independently change or alter the physician's order in any way. If an order is incorrect, consult the physician and obtain a new order.

Review the following rules for medication administration recommended by Fields and colleagues.

RULES FOR MEDICATION ADMINISTRATION

1. The label on the medication is read
   before drawing medication into the syringe; after drawing medication into the syringe; and when placing the medication bottle in storage.
2. Use a syringe to measure medication.
3. When measuring medication, concentrate only on the medication quantity. *Never* talk to someone while drawing up medication.
4. Hold the syringe at eye level when measuring medication volume.
5. Give the right medication to the right patient at the proper time.
6. Thoroughly review the chart before administering medication to a new patient.
7. Know the maximum dose, contraindications, hazards, and side-effects of all medications administered. When in doubt, consult a *Physicians' Desk Reference* (PDR).
8. Check the expiration date on the label. Do *not* use outdated medication.

Exercise B: Preparation and Mixing of Medication

1. Obtain a syringe.
2. Examine the units of measure on the barrel of the syringe. Identify the milliliter unit of measure and other parts of the syringe (Fig. 16-1).
3. Identify the following components of a syringe:
   A. Needle
   B. Barrel
   C. Plunger
4. Measure the solute with the syringe. *Note:* Vials of saline or sterile water sealed with a rubber cap may require injection of a small volume of air into the vial in order to

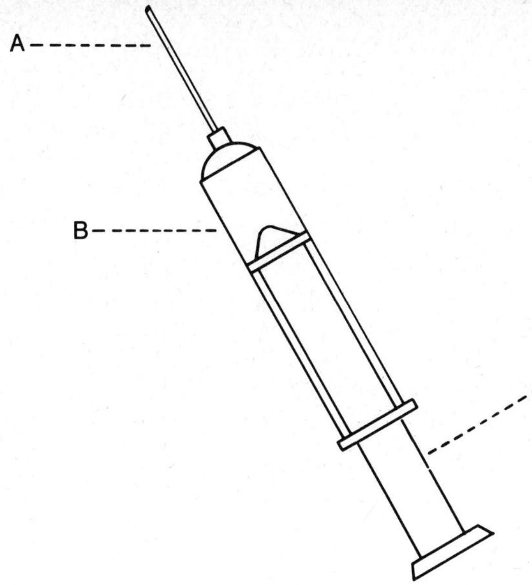

Fig. 16-1. Components of a syringe for measuring medications.

pressurize the container. When drawing medication from a sealed vial, invert the vial. After pressurization, hold the vial at eye level when withdrawing the desired volume of solution.

5. Aseptically prepare the following sample solutions by measuring the solute with the syringe and mixing the solute with solvent (H_2O or saline).
   - **A.** 0.5 ml Isoetharine
     + 2.5 ml H_2O
     3.0 ml total solution
   - **B.** 0.5 ml isoetharine
     2.0 ml acetylcysteine
     + 2.0 ml H_2O
     4.5 ml total solution
   - **C.** 0.25 ml racemic epinephrine
     + 2.5 ml H_2O
     2.75 ml total solution
   - **D.** 0.5 ml isoproterenol
     + 2.5 ml H_2O
     3.0 ml total solution
   - **E.** 5.0 ml of 20% ethyl alcohol
   - **F.** 5.0 ml of 0.9% saline
6. Your instructor may elect to add different colors of food dye to the medication vials in order to check your measurements. Have your instructor check the measured solutions.
7. After assembling the IPPB circuit or medication nebulizer, inject the solution into the nebulizer chamber.

Exercise C: Assembly of a Medication Nebulizer

1. Assemble a medication nebulizer by connecting one end of small-bore oxygen tubing to a flowmeter.
2. Connect the other end of a small-bore tubing to the medication nebulizer.
3. Attach an aerosol mask to the nebulizer.
4. Instill the premixed medication into the nebulizer.

5. Adjust the flowmeter to a flowrate of 6 to 10 liters/minute.
6. Instruct the patient to take slow, deep breaths through the mouth with a slight pause at the end of inspiration.
7. Apply the aerosol mask and medication nebulizer to the patient (Fig. 16-2).
   Note: Only sterile saline should be inhaled by a laboratory partner. If a mannequin is used to simulate a patient, tap water may be used.

EVALUATION OF TREATMENT RESPONSE

8. When administering sympathomimetic drugs, check the pulse before, during, and after treatment.
9. *Note:* Immediately stop the treatment and notify the physician if the heart rate exceeds 140 beats/minute (160–180 beats/minute in healthy, young adults) or if arrhythmias occur.
10. After the treatment, request a deep breath and a cough.
11. Evaluate sputum if the cough is productive.
12. Evaluate breath sounds.

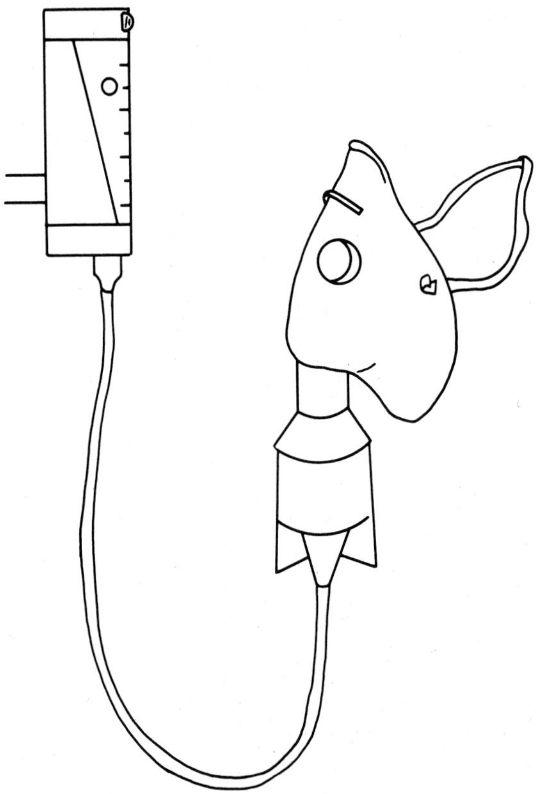

Fig. 16-2. Assembled medication nebulizer and aerosol mask.

Exercise D: Methods of Optimizing Topical Aerosol Deposition

1. For a spontaneously breathing patient using a mask and medication nebulizer, instruct the patient to inhale slowly through the mouth as deeply as possible with a slight pause at the end of inspiration.
2. Assemble a medication nebulizer connected to an incentive spirometer (Fig. 16-3).
3. Deep breathing required for optimal aerosol deposition may be induced by using an incentive spirometer during medication aerosolization.

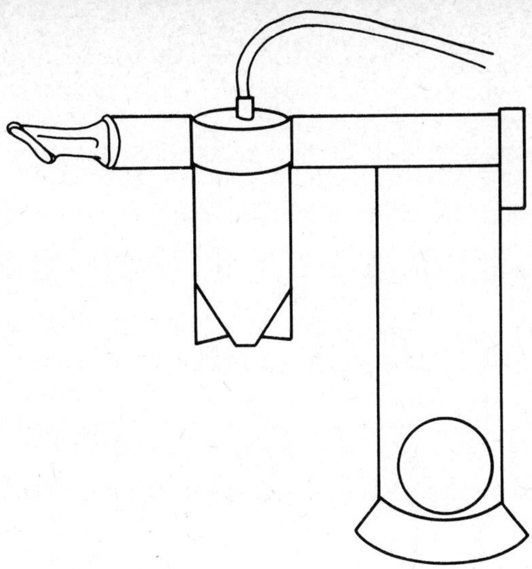

Fig. 16-3. Medication nebulizer with incentive spirometry.

4. Assemble a medication nebulizer used in a mechanical ventilator breathing circuit (Fig. 16-4).
5. During continuous ventilation, medication may be delivered by operation of the medication nebulizer. *Note:* during continuous ventilation, avoid prolonged interruptions when injecting the medication into the nebulizer. It is often desirable to premix the medication solution before creating a "leak" in the system by injecting the medication into the nebulizer.

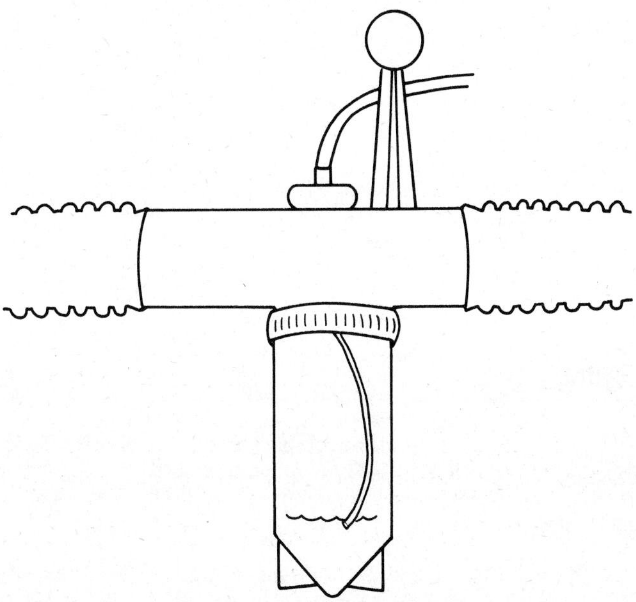

Fig. 16-4. Medication nebulizer in mechanical ventilator breathing circuit.

Exercise E: Metered Dose Medication Administration

1. Your instructor will provide you with a metered dose cartridge and mouthpiece for medication administration.
2. Assemble the metered dose device according to manufacturer's recommendations (Fig. 16-5).
3. Provide the following instructions as you would to a patient:
   A. Assemble the canister by removing any protective cover and connecting the mouthpiece to the dispensing canister.
   B. Shake the unit well.
   C. Place the mouthpiece in the mouth. Be certain that the tongue is kept beneath the mouthpiece and avoids contact with the aerosol.
   D. Exhale through the nose to residual volume.
   E. Activate the aerosol by depressing the canister while slowly inhaling at the same time. Hold your breath for a few seconds.
   F. Use only the prescribed number of puffs. If multiple puffs are prescribed, wait a few minutes between puffs.
   G. Replace the protective cover and keep the mouthpiece clean.

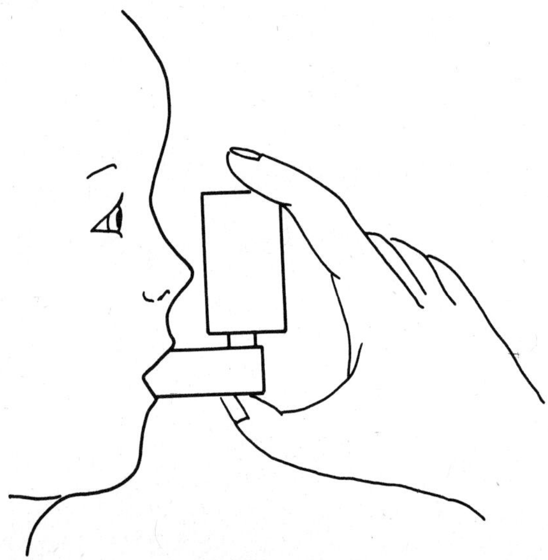

Fig. 16-5. Metered-dose inhaler.

RECOMMENDED READING

Fields LJ, Williams TJ, Garavaglia MM: Pharmacologic Review for Intensive Cardiopulmonary Therapy, 2nd ed. Chicago, Year Book Medical Publishers, 1978

Kacmarek RM, Dimas S, Mack C: Essentials of Respiratory Therapy, 2d ed. Chicago, Year Book Medical Publishers, 1985

Lehnert BE, Schacter EN: The Pharmacology of Respiratory Care. St Louis, CV Mosby, 1980

Shapiro BA, Harrison RA, Kacmarek RM, Cane RD: Clinical Applications of Respiratory Care, 3rd ed. Chicago, Year Book Medical Publishers, 1985

Ziment I: Respiratory Pharmacology and Therapeutics. Philadelphia, WB Saunders, 1978

Laboratory Performance Evaluation (#16)

Topic: Medication Administration

Student ______________________ Course ______________________

Date ______________________ Section ______________________

Performance Elements	Acceptable	Unacceptable	Not Applicable	Comments
1. Verifies medication order				
2. Washes hands				
3. Prepares aseptically and accurately the prescribed medication				
4. Assembles medication delivery device (nebulizer or IPPB equipment)				
5. Places prescribed dose of medication into appropriate device				
6. Checks equipment function				
7. Confirms simulated patient's understanding of therapy				
8. Instructs simulated patient in desired ventilatory pattern				
9. Monitors pulse before, during, and after treatment				
10. Monitors breath sounds				
11. Encourages cough				
12. Documents effects of therapy				

Knowledge of Procedure

☐ Good; student is knowledgeable about rationale and theory related to procedure

☐ Fair; student has adequate understanding of rationale and theory related to procedure

☐ Poor; student has inadequate understanding of rationale and theory related to procedure

Performance Deficiencies (check those that apply)

☐ Excessive time needed to complete procedure

☐ Broke aseptic or sterile technique

☐ Gross inaccuracy noted

☐ Technique may be harmful to patient

☐ Incorrect dosage or gas concentration

☐ Incorrect equipment assembly/use

☐ Unable to answer questions correctly about rationale and/or theory related to procedure

☐ Other ______________________________

Evaluation Summary

☐ Satisfactory performance

☐ Unsatisfactory performance

Recommendations of Evaluator

☐ Skills may be applied/observed in clinical setting

☐ Specific evaluation deficiencies require correction

☐ Complete re-evaluation required

☐ Additional laboratory practice required

Signatures:

Evaluator ______________________ Date ______________________

Student ______________________ Date ______________________

Laboratory Report

Student ____________________ Acceptable ____________________

Date ____________________ Unacceptable ____________________

Course ____________________

Topic: Medication Administration

Scenario: Mr. Strouse, a middle-aged man who suffers from chronic bronchitis and asthma, has arrived in the emergency room dyspneic, wheezing audibly, and using accessory muscles of ventilation. You have been asked to administer an aerosol treatment to him containing 0.5 ml isoetharine with 4.0 ml of normal saline. Please answer the following questions about this situation:

1. (T or F) A registered respiratory therapist may independently prescribe medication for therapeutic purposes.
2. Describe briefly what you would do if a physician prescribed 5.0 ml of isoproterenol for inhalation.
3. Medication nebulizers should be operated between flowrates of __________ liters/minute.
4. What breathing pattern is used for optimal deposition of aerosolized medication?
5. What are the major cardiovascular side-effects of sympathomimetics?
6. What procedure is used if an adult patient demonstrates marked tachycardia (greater than 140/minute) while inhaling a sympathomimetic?
7. List five "rules" for the safe administration of medications.

8. When you began administering the solution of isoproterenol and saline, Mr. Strouse's pulse rate was 88 beats/minute. Now, a few minutes later, his pulse rate is 110 beats/minute. Describe your response to this change in pulse rate.

9. Other than a medication nebulizer, how may drugs be administered as aerosols?

chapter 17

Sputum induction

INTRODUCTION

Many techniques may be used to obtain sputum samples from the tracheobronchial tree. The simplest and easiest way to obtain a sample is to request a cough. In the clinical environment, sputum samples are frequently obtained in the morning before meals. Patients should be instructed to brush their teeth and rinse out their mouths before expectorating a sample. Sputum produced from the tracheobronchial tree should not be kept in the mouth but should be expectorated immediately.

Another technique used for sputum induction is aerosol administration. Aerosols are frequently administered to patients with a nonproductive cough. Normal, hypotonic, or hypertonic saline may be administered in order to stimulate mucokinesis. Nebulized sterile water, which is quite irritating, may be used to stimulate a cough. The aerosolized solutions may be given by medication, jet, or ultrasonic nebulizer. The administration of a super-heated aerosol with hypertonic saline may induce bronchorhea for a relatively prolonged period (24–48 hours).

All of the aforementioned techniques may be used to induce sputum samples when a cooperative patient can cough adequately. When the cough is inadequate, a sputum sample can be obtained by nasotracheal aspiration.

Nasotracheal aspiration of a sputum sample is never a routine or benign procedure. It is important to realize that the technique of nasotracheal suction may be associated with dangerous complications and has occasionally resulted in sudden death. Regardless of the method used to obtain a sputum sample, the labeled specimen must be transported to the laboratory and analyzed while warm and fresh. In this chapter, you are introduced to the techniques used to obtain tracheobronchial sputum specimens.

OBJECTIVES

After completing this chapter, you should be able to do the following:

1. *Understand the procedures used for sputum inductions.*
2. *Identify the pharmacologic agents that are aerosolized to induce sputum.*

3. *Analyze the physical properties of an expectorated sputum sample.*
4. *Compare and contrast "spit" with sputum.*
5. *Describe the breathing pattern used for optimal aerosol deposition.*
6. *Describe the method of preparing the sample for laboratory analysis.*

EQUIPMENT NEEDED

- ☐ Gas source, flowmeter, nipple adapter
- ☐ Medication nebulizer
- ☐ Aerosol mask
- ☐ Aerosol tubing
- ☐ Sputum trap (Leuken's tube)
- ☐ Large reservoir or ultrasonic nebulizer
- ☐ Suction catheter kit (gloves, catheter, sterile specimen cup)
- ☐ Oxygen source, flowmeter, connecting tubing
- ☐ Partial rebreathing mask
- ☐ Lubricant
- ☐ Vacuum source and suction bottle
- ☐ Induction agents
  - Sterile saline (normal and hypertonic)
  - Sterile H_2O
  - Acetylcysteine

ACTIVITIES

Exercise A: Identification and Selection of Sputum Induction Agents

1. Your instructor will provide you with pharmacologic agents used for sputum induction. Identify the following agents:
   A. Sterile water
   B. Sterile isotonic (0.9%) saline
   C. Sterile hypotonic (0.45%) saline
   D. Sterile hypertonic (1.0–15.0%) saline
   E. Acetylcysteine
2. Note the concentration and expiration date of the pharmacologic agents provided.

Exercise B: Aerosol Administration

1. Request that the patient brush his teeth and rinse his mouth. Assemble a medication nebulizer by connecting one end of small-bore oxygen tubing to a flowmeter.
2. Connect the other end of small-bore tubing to the medication nebulizer.
3. Attach an aerosol mask to the nebulizer.
4. Instill 5.0 ml of 0.9% sterile saline into the medication nebulizer.
5. Adjust the flowmeter to a flowrate of 8 liters/minute.
6. Instruct the patient to take slow, deep breaths through the mouth with a slight pause at the end of inspiration.
7. Apply the aerosol mask and medication nebulizer to the simulated patient (Fig. 17-1).
8. After the saline has been nebulized, request a deep breath and a forceful cough.
9. If sputum is produced, have the patient put it in a sterile container or cup. *Note:* When requesting a cough, ask the simulated patient to turn away from you and to cover the mouth while coughing.

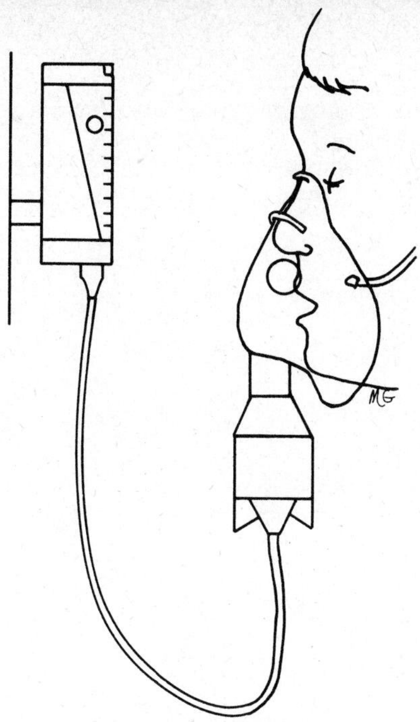

Fig. 17-1. Administration of aerosol by medication nebulizer.

Exercise C: Super-Heated Aerosol Administration

1. Obtain a large reservoir (jet) nebulizer with an immersion heater.
2. Assemble the nebulizer (see previous laboratory exercise on aerosol therapy).
3. Pour sterile, hypertonic saline (10%) into the nebulizer.
4. Adjust the nebulizer heater to obtain a temperature between 140° and 185°F.
5. Apply the aerosol delivery device to the patient (Fig. 17-2).
6. Allow the aerosol to be delivered for about 30 minutes.
7. Request a deep breath and a cough.
8. If the cough is productive, obtain the sample in a sterile sputum cup.
9. Label the specimen. Include the patient's name, the date, and the time the sample was obtained.

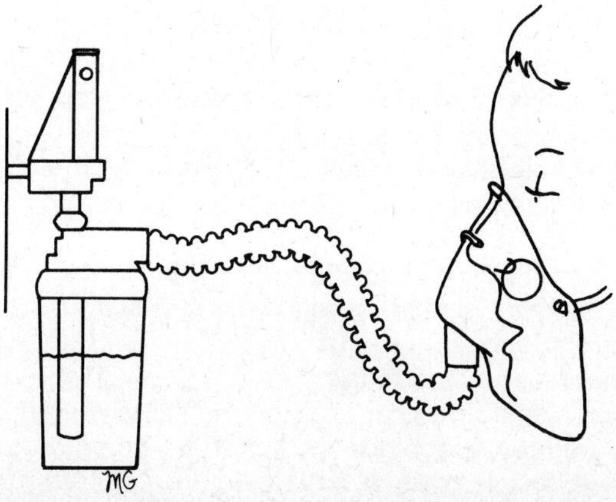

Fig. 17-2. Administration of super-heated aerosol.

Exercise D: Ultrasonic Generated Aerosols

1. Obtain an ultrasonic nebulizer.
2. Assemble the nebulizer (see previous laboratory exercise on aerosol generators).
3. Verify that water is present in the couplant.
4. Pour sterile saline into the medication chamber.
5. Adjust the amplitude control to regulate the aerosol density.
6. Apply an aerosol delivery device to the aerosol tubing that is connected to the ultrasonic nebulizer (Fig. 17-3).
7. Allow the aerosol to be delivered for several minutes.
8. Request a deep breath and a cough.
9. Obtain the sputum sample in a sterile cup.

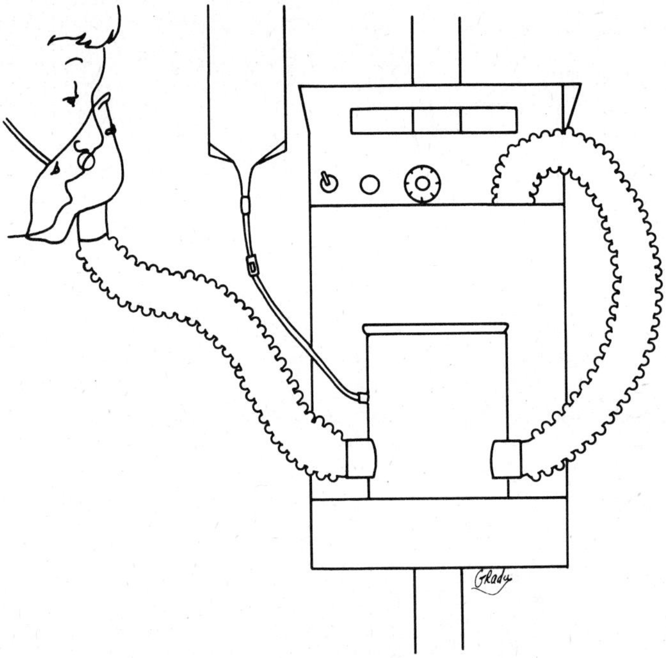

Fig. 17-3. Ultrasonic nebulizer used for sputum induction.

Exercise E: Nasotracheal Aspiration of a Sputum Sample

1. Your instructor will provide you with a sterile suction catheter kit or supplies containing the catheter, gloves, sterile specimen container (sputum trap), and rinse cup.
2. You will also be provided with a mannequin, which you may assume is a simulated patient.
3. Identify yourself and your department.
4. Inform the patient of the procedure. Wash your hands with antimicrobial solution.
5. Place the patient in the Fowler's (sniffing) position. Be certain that the nose, chin, and thyroid cartilage are midline.
6. Assemble a partial or nonrebreathing mask.
7. Administer 100% oxygen while you prepare your suctioning equipment. (The oxygen mask may be adjusted to provide access to the external nares during suction (Fig. 17-4).

8. Obtain a baseline pulse and heart rhythm (if applicable).
9. Check the suction pressure and function of the suction apparatus by occluding the suction tubing and adjusting the negative pressure (Fig. 17-5).
10. Connect the sputum trap to the suction tubing.
11. Using aseptic technique, open the suction catheter and sterile glove package. Put on the sterile glove and grasp the catheter with the sterile glove (Fig. 17-6).
12. Using aseptic technique, lubricate the catheter with sterile lubricant.
13. Advance the catheter slowly through the nares to just above the vocal cords while administering oxygen.
14. Listen for sounds of air flow at the proximal end of the catheter.
15. When respiratory air flow sounds are loudest, advance the catheter during *inspiration*.
16. If the catheter enters the trachea, the patient will cough violently. If the catheter enters the esophagus, no breath sounds will be heard and the patient may swallow. Quickly connect the catheter to the sputum trap and suction tubing (Fig. 17-7).
17. Briefly apply suction (15 seconds maximum) (Fig. 17-8).
18. Remove the catheter.
19. Administer oxygen and check vital signs.
20. Disassemble the sputum trap and label the specimen.
    Note: Nasotracheal sputum samples are not recommended for anaerobic cultures.

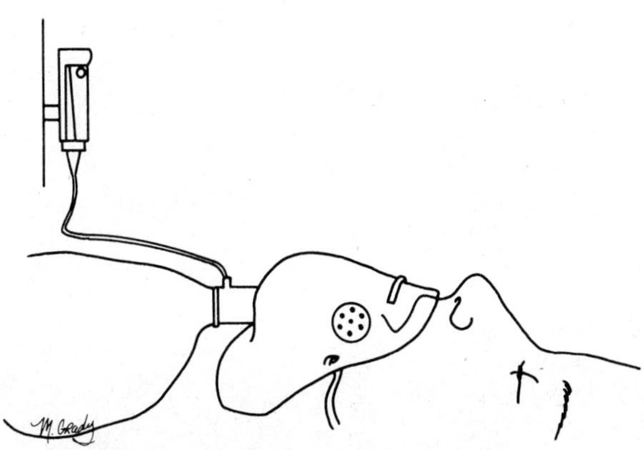

Fig. 17-4. Administration of 100% oxygen during nasotracheal suction.

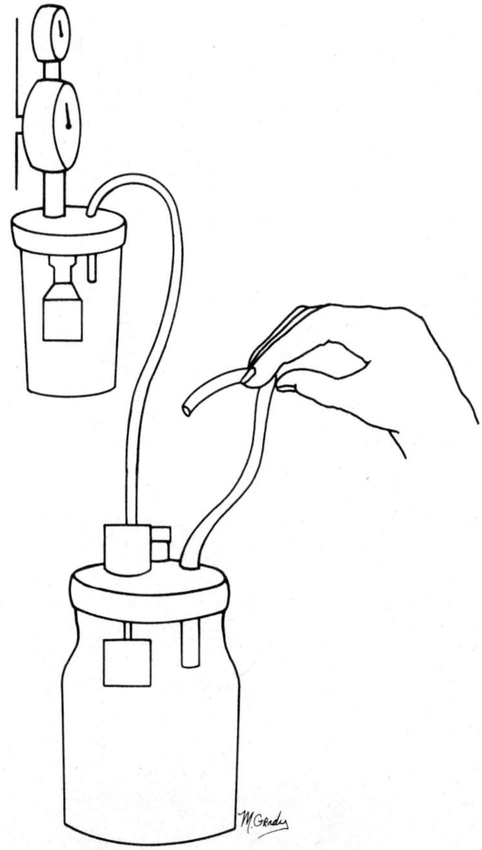

Fig. 17-5. Occlusion of suction tubing to check or adjust suction pressure.

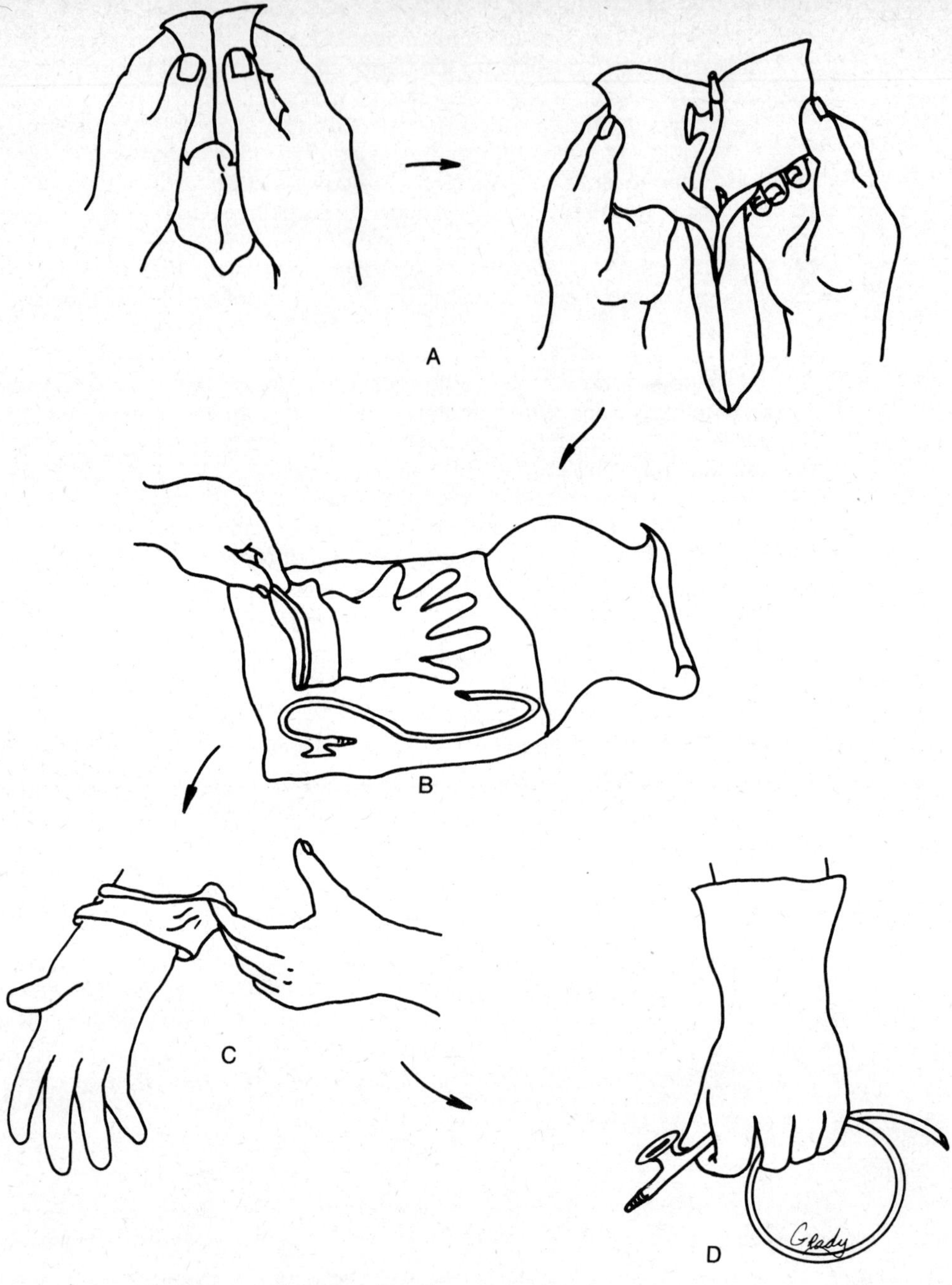

Fig. 17-6. Aseptic technique for nasotracheal suction.
A. Opening sterile catheter package.
B. Maintenance of sterile field.
C. Aseptic application of sterile glove.
D. Grasping sterile catheter with sterile glove.

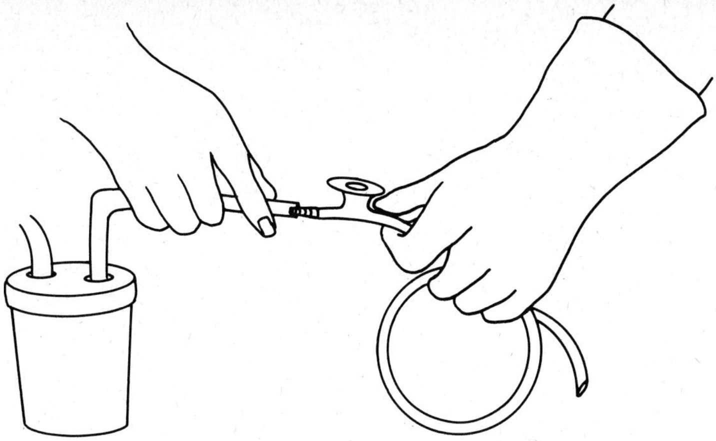

Fig. 17-7. Connection of sputum trap.

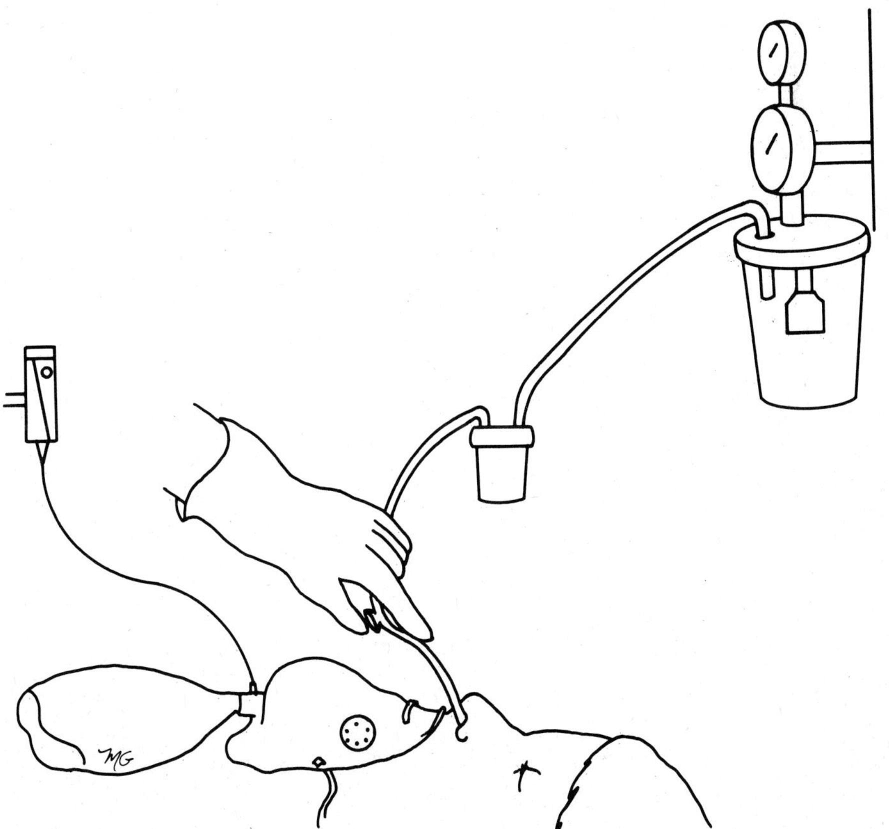

Fig. 17-8. Nasotracheal suction. Note the continuous administration of oxygen during suctioning to minimize hypoxemia.

Exercise F: Preparation of a Sputum Sample for Analysis

1. Obtain a sputum sample.
2. Note the color, odor, amount, viscosity, consistency, and time of expectoration.
3. Note the temperature of the sample.
4. Label the specimen with the name, date, and time obtained.

   Note: Bacteriostatic or preservative agents should not be present in normal saline used to "wash" sputum samples.

RECOMMENDED READING

Burton GG, Hodgkin JE: Respiratory Care. A Guide to Clinical Practice, 2nd ed. Philadelphia, JB Lippincott, 1984

Shapiro BA, Harrison RA, Kacmarek RM, Cane RD: Clinical Applications of Respiratory Care, 3rd ed. Chicago, Year Book Medical Publishers, 1985

Spearman CB, Sheldon RL: Egan's Fundamentals of Respiratory Therapy, 4th ed. St Louis, CV Mosby, 1982

Laboratory Performance Evaluation (#17)

Topic: Sputum Induction and Nasotracheal Aspiration

Student ______________________ Course ______________________

Date ______________________ Section ______________________

Performance Elements	Acceptable	Unacceptable	Not Applicable	Comments
1. Assembles necessary equipment for sputum induction: A. Medication nebulizer B. Jet nebulizer C. Nasotracheal suctioning equipment and supplies				
2. Obtains nasotracheal sputum sample: A. Washes hands B. Explains procedure to simulated patient C. Confirms patient understanding of procedure D. Positions head and neck E. Preoxygenates with 100% O_2 F. Lubricates catheter G. Maintains supplemental O_2 throughout suctioning procedure H. Maintains sterile technique throughout procedure I. Limits suction time to 15 seconds J. Evaluates pulse after suctioning K. Obtains sputum sample L. Prepares obtained specimen for analysis (labels and so forth)				
3. Documents procedure				

Knowledge of Procedure
☐ Good; student is knowledgeable about rationale and theory related to procedure
☐ Fair; student has adequate understanding of rationale and theory related to procedure
☐ Poor; student has inadequate understanding of rationale and theory related to procedure

Performance Deficiencies (check those that apply)
☐ Excessive time needed to complete procedure
☐ Broke aseptic or sterile technique
☐ Gross inaccuracy noted
☐ Technique may be harmful to patient
☐ Incorrect dosage or gas concentration
☐ Incorrect equipment assembly/use
☐ Unable to answer questions correctly about rationale and/or theory related to procedure
☐ Other ______________________________

Evaluation Summary
☐ Satisfactory performance
☐ Unsatisfactory performance

Recommendations of Evaluator
☐ Skills may be applied/observed in clinical setting
☐ Specific evaluation deficiencies require correction
☐ Complete re-evaluation required
☐ Additional laboratory practice required

Signatures:

Evaluator ______________________ Date ______________________

Student ______________________ Date ______________________

Laboratory Report

Student ______________________ Acceptable ______________________

Date ______________________ Unacceptable ______________________

Course ______________________

Topic: Sputum Induction

Scenario: Today, you have been assigned sputum inductions, which includes the following: clinic patients referred to the laboratory, bedridden patients on the wards, and patients in the critical care units—in other words, any patient from whom a sputum sample needs to be obtained. Please answer the following questions:

1. Mr Woodley, who has a feeble or weak cough at best, has been scheduled for a sputum induction. What would be the method of choice for obtaining an adequate sample from him?

2. What information should be contained on the label of the container of the sputum sample?

3. What pharmacologic agents may be used for sputum induction? Why?

4. Why is a super-heated aerosol used to induce expectoration?

5. Suction should not be applied in the trachea longer than __________.
6. List three complications of nasotracheal suctioning.

7. How will a sputum sample be affected if suction pressure is applied to a catheter while the catheter is withdrawn through the oropharynx or nasopharynx?

8. When using a super-heated aerosol for sputum induction, what is the suggested temperature range for the aerosol?

chapter 18

History and physical examination for respiratory care

INTRODUCTION

An organized, systematic approach to the physical examination of the chest is an essential skill for the clinical application of respiratory care. The initial phase of the examination process may consist of the history, in which symptoms and related subjective information are solicited from the patient. The history should also include the primary reason that medical attention has been sought or the "chief complaint." The history may be obtained before or during the physical examination process.

An organized physical examination of the chest comprises four steps: inspection, palpation, percussion, and auscultation. Inspection consists of the systematic observation of the chest and breathing pattern. Palpation involves the tactile sense of touch to detect physical abnormalities. Percussion is the step in which the chest is struck in order to create vibrations that may audibly indicate abnormalities. The final step in the examination of the chest is auscultation, or listening to lung sounds. The purpose of this chapter is to introduce you to the history and physical examination process for respiratory care.

OBJECTIVES

After completing this chapter, you should be able to do the following:

1. *Obtain a history relevant to respiratory care.*
2. *Evaluate the cardiopulmonary system using the techniques of inspection, palpation, percussion, and auscultation.*
3. *Identify normal and abnormal breath sounds.*
4. *Document the results of the chest examination.*

EQUIPMENT NEEDED

- ☐ Binaural stethoscope
- ☐ Watch with a second hand

- ☐ Tape recorder (cassette)
- ☐ Cassette tape of breath sounds

ACTIVITIES

Exercise A: Respiratory History

1. Assure that the environment is conducive to obtaining a history and performing a physical examination. Be certain that a private room or area is available and that both the temperature and noise level are acceptable. *Note:* In the laboratory, a man should perform the physical examination of a woman *only* with the permission of your instructor.
2. After introducing yourself and identifying your department, an excellent way to begin an interview of a simulated patient is to ask, "How are you feeling today?"
3. The interview should be used to ascertain the following general information:
   A. Speech pattern—severe shortness of breath may result after only one or two spoken words before "catching the breath"
   B. Sensorium—awareness of orientation to time and place
   C. Emotional status
   D. Ability to comply with directions
   E. Presence of shortness of breath
   F. Patient's subjective account of respiratory status
4. Obtain the following additional information:
   A. Chief complaint or reason for seeking medical assistance (if applicable)
   B. Previous cardiopulmonary disease(s)
   C. Family history of cardiopulmonary disease
   D. Social exposure to cardiopulmonary disease
   E. Occupational exposure to dusts such as asbestos, silica, cotton, or coal dust
   F. Residential exposure to agents of pulmonary disease (Ohio or Mississippi River Valley, San Joaquin Valley in California, or southeastern United States)
   G. Chest surgery
   H. Chest injuries
   I. Smoking history—quantify the smoking history in terms of pack years (1 pack year is equivalent to smoking 1 pack of cigarettes per day for a full year)
   J. Current medications
5. Inquire about the following primary symptoms of pulmonary disease:
   A. Cough—suggests an abnormality when present
   B. Expectoration—sputum or mucus production
   C. Dyspnea—difficulty breathing
   D. Chest pain—requires differential diagnosis
   E. Hemoptysis—coughing up blood
6. Pursue a positive response to the aforementioned symptoms by obtaining as much quantitative detail as possible:
   A. Cough (dry or productive of sputum?)
      1) Type
      2) Frequency
      3) Time of occurrence
   B. Expectoration of sputum
      1) Sputum color
      2) Odor
      3) Volume produced
      4) Consistency
      5) Time produced

C. Dyspnea
   1) Specify activity or degree of exertion that causes dyspnea
D. Chest pain
   1) Localized or general
   2) Type of pain
   3) Association with breathing phases
   4) Associated with shortness of breath
   5) Associated with local tenderness
   6) Related to coughing, sneezing, or straining
E. Hemoptysis
   1) Associated with cough
   2) Color (brown versus bright red)
   3) History of nasal bleeding or gastrointestinal disorder

Exercise B: Inspection

1. Make the following general observations:
   A. Overall appearance
   B. Age
   C. Sex
   D. Weight
2. Observe the basic body positioning (Fig. 18-1).

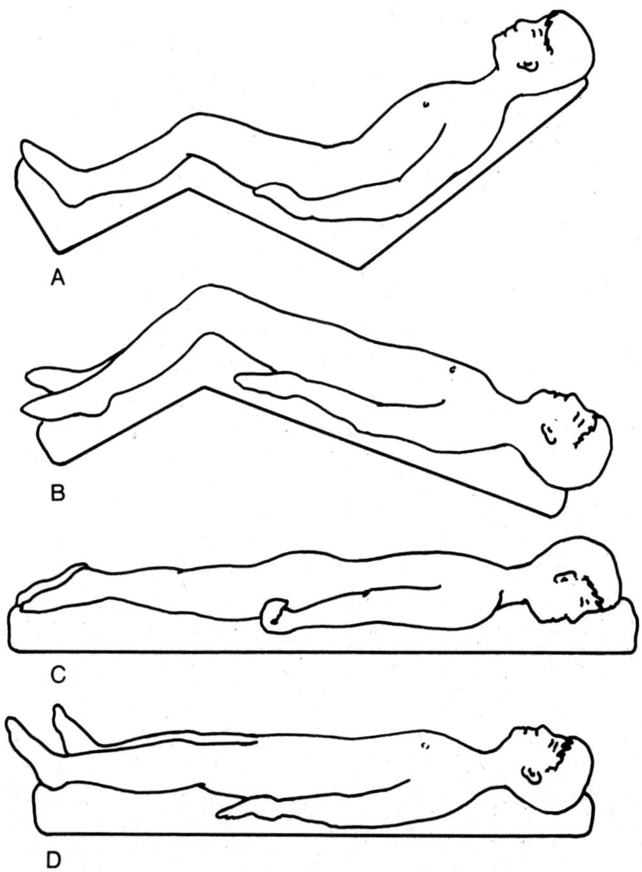

Fig. 18-1. Common body positions.

3. Common positions assumed by patients in the clinical setting include the following:
   A. Fowler's
   B. Trendelenburg
   C. Prone
   D. Supine

   Orthopnea is a term used to describe breathing difficulty that may be relieved in the sitting position.
4. Inspect the shape of the chest (Fig. 18-2).
5. Examine the shape of the chest for the following abnormalities:
   A. Pectus carinatum (pigeon chest)
   B. Pectus excavatum (funnel chest)
   C. Kyphosis
   D. Scoliosis
   E. Barrel chest
6. Observe the movement of the chest during breathing. Compare the excursion of the right side of the chest with that of the left side.

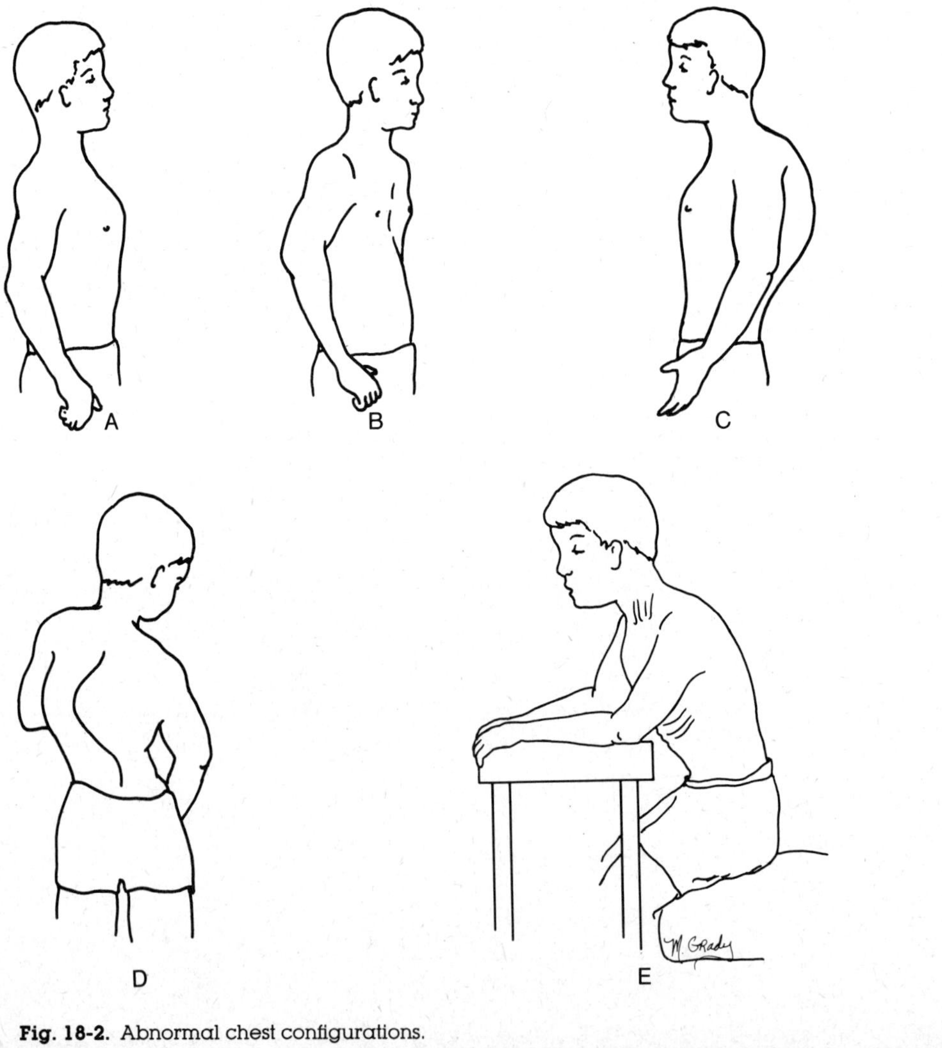

Fig. 18-2. Abnormal chest configurations.

7. Determine the muscles that are active during both inspiration and expiration (Fig. 18-3).
8. Observe the epigastric area for a slight protrusion during inspiration to evaluate the diaphragmatic activity.
9. Evaluate the fingers for the presence of tobacco stains (in chronic cigarette abuse) and digital clubbing (Fig. 18-4).
10. Evaluate the sternal, intercostal, and supraclavicular regions for retractions of the chest or a pulling inward of the chest wall during inspiration (Fig. 18-5).
11. Observe the neck for distension or bulging of the jugular veins.
12. Examine the chest for the presence of old or recent surgical scars.
13. Observe the skin for the presence of cyanosis, pallor, flushing, diaphoresis, or lesions.
14. Evaluate the wrists and ankles for the presence of swelling due to fluid or peripheral edema.
15. Observe large muscle groups for muscle wasting or atrophy.
16. Examine the position of the trachea.
17. Look for obvious nodes or masses on the chest.
18. Observe the breathing pattern by noting the rate and depth of breathing.
19. Observe the intercostal region for "paradoxical" breathing in which the chest wall moves inward (rather than outward) during inspiration.

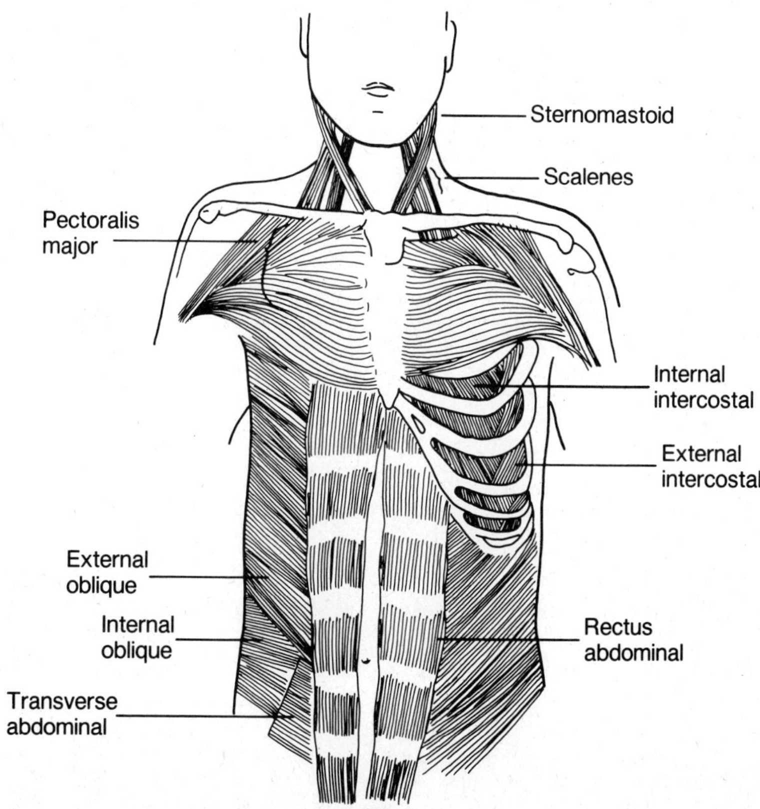

Fig. 18-3. Muscles of ventilation. *(Redrawn from Spearman CB, Sheldon RL: Egan's Fundamentals of Respiratory Therapy, 4th ed. St Louis, CV Mosby, 1982)*

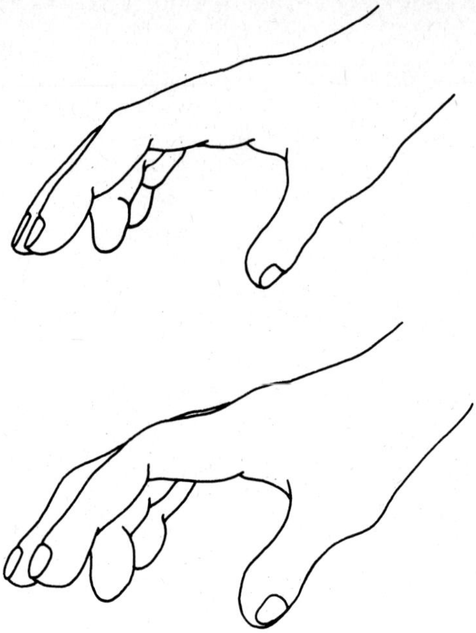

Fig. 18-4. Normal fingers and digital clubbing.

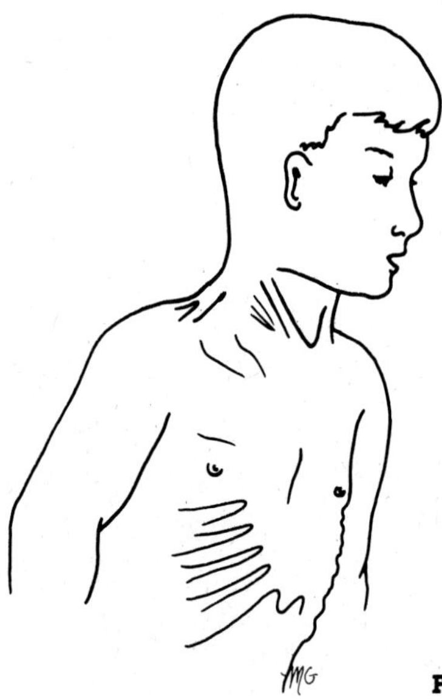

Fig. 18-5. Chest wall retractions during inspiration.

20. Evaluate the ability to cough by requesting that the simulated patient
  A. inhale deeply.
  B. turn his face away from your face.
  C. coughing.

21. Note any sputum produced.

22. If applicable, note the odor of the breath.

23. Observe the ankles and wrists for enlargement or osteoarthropathy.

24. Some practitioners systematically inspect the chest by proceeding from the top of the chest (at the neck) to the base of the chest wall.

Exercise C: Palpation

1. Palpate the chest wall while the patient says "ninety-nine" to detect abnormal vibrations or tactile fremitus. The fingertips, palm of the hand, or side of the hand may be used to detect tactile fremitus (Fig. 18-6).
2. The hands may be placed on each side of the chest to detect symmetrical chest movement. After placing the hands at the upper, midchest, or lower chest, request a deep inhalation to observe hand motion. The hands should move an equal distance in symmetrical chest movement (Fig. 18-7).
3. The capillary refill time may reflect peripheral perfusion. Evaluate capillary refill by alternately compressing and releasing the nail bed of a finger (Fig. 18-8).
4. The position of the trachea may be palpated by inserting a finger into the space superior to the manubrium (Fig. 18-9).
5. The trachea is normally positioned midline.
6. Using the side of the hand, palpate the point of maximal cardiac impulse (PMI). The PMI is normally located proximal to the fifth intercostal space at the junction of the midclavicular line (Fig. 18-10).
7. Evaluate the wrist or ankle for the presence of pitting edema by compressing the area with a finger. In the presence of significant edematous fluid, an indentation may remain in the compressed area (Fig. 18-11).
8. The presence of pitting edema, jugular vein distention, and hepatomegaly (enlargement of the liver) may be associated with right heart failure.
9. Palpate the skin for crepitation, which may be associated with a benign condition called subcutaneous emphysema.

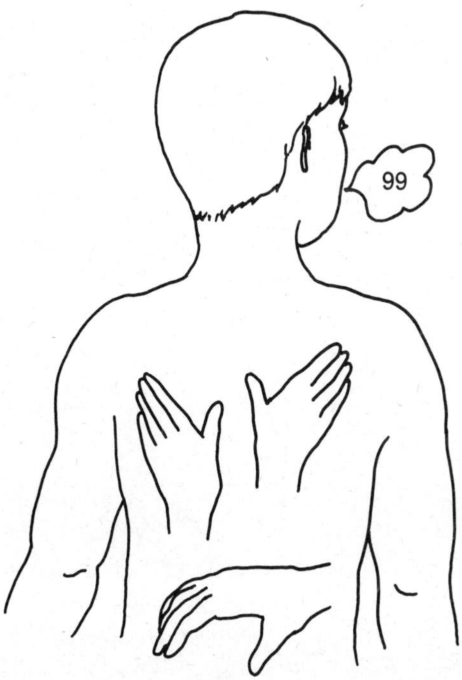

Fig. 18-6. Palpation of chest for tactile fremitus. *(Modified from Frownfelter D: Chest Physical Therapy and Pulmonary Rehabilitation: An Interdisciplinary Approach. Chicago, Year Book Medical Publishers, 1978)*

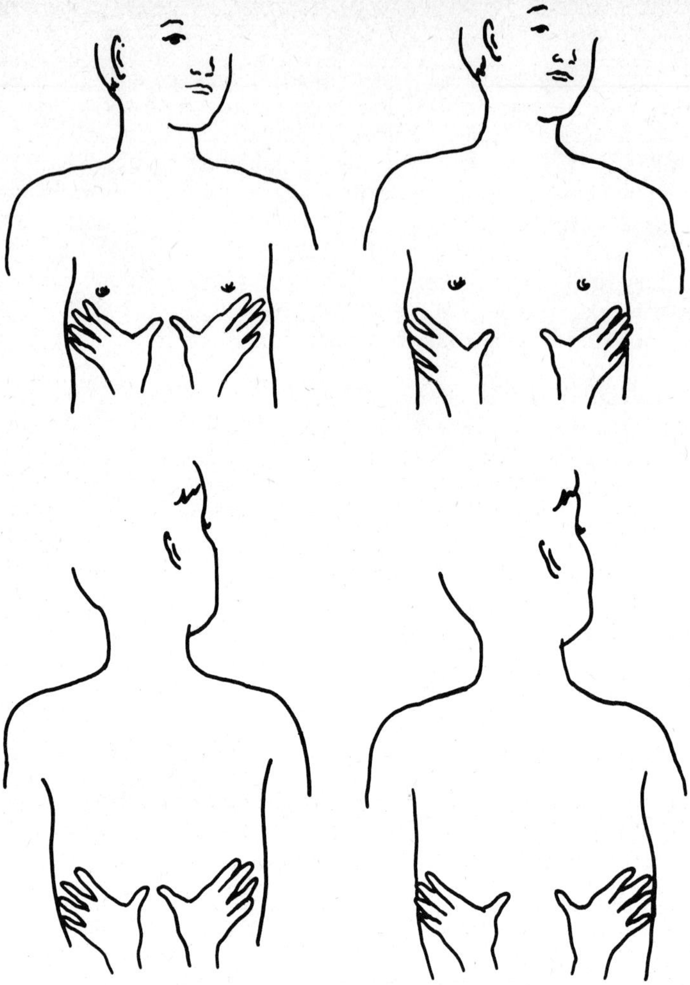

Fig. 18-7. Palpation for symmetrical chest excursion.

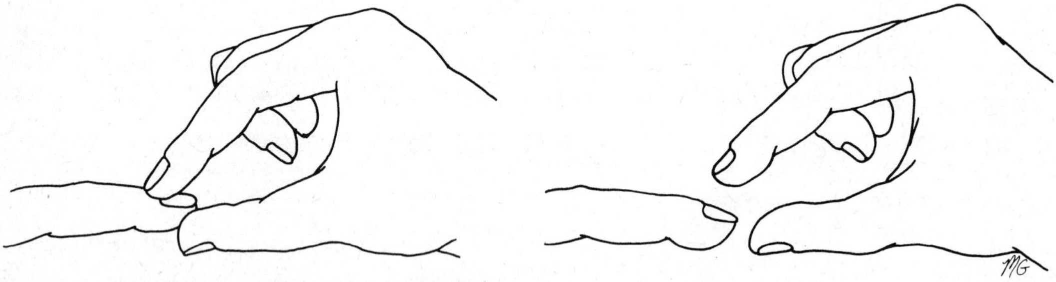

Fig. 18-8. Determination of capillary refill.

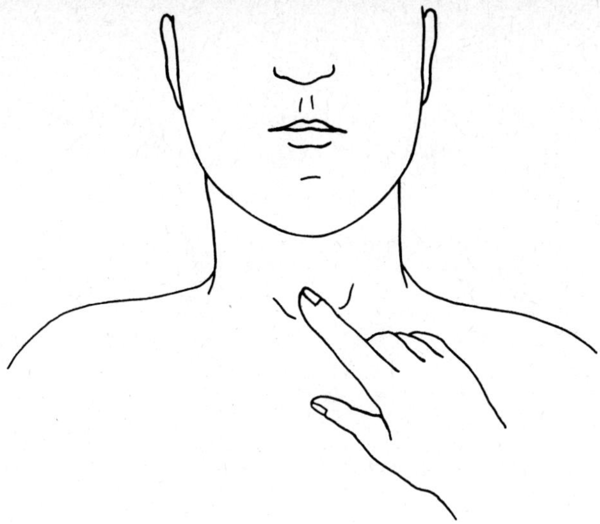

Fig. 18-9. Palpation of tracheal position.

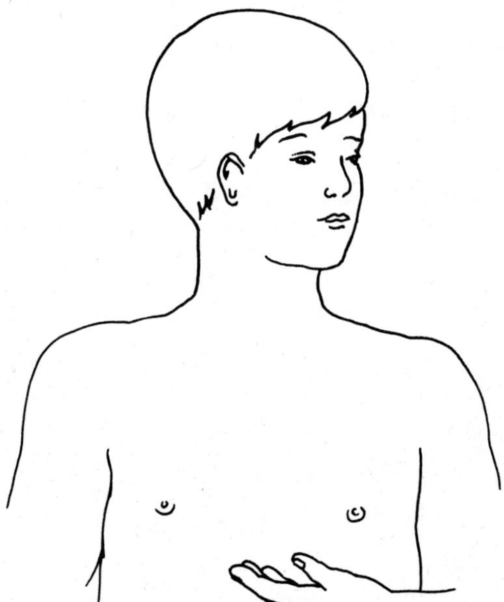

Fig. 18-10. Palpation of point of maximal impulse (cardiac PMI).

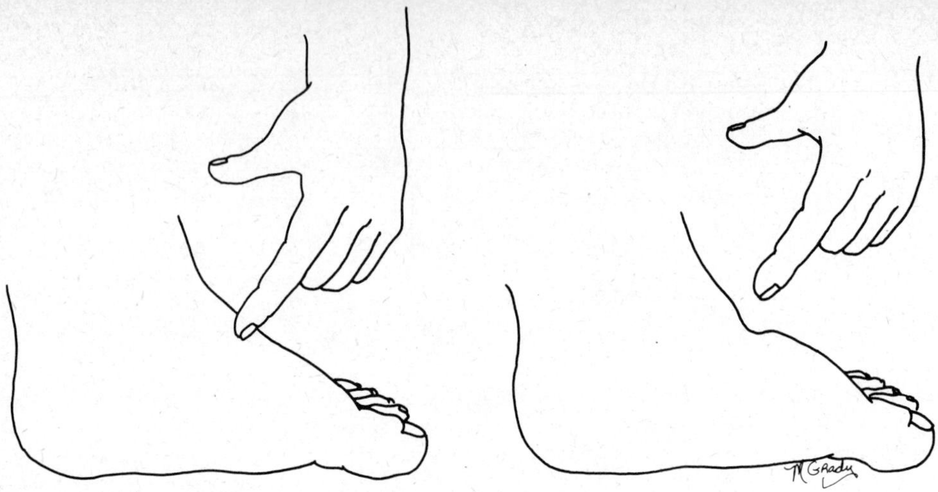

Fig. 18-11. Pitting edema.

Exercise D: Percussion

1. Percussion of the chest may be performed by directly striking the chest wall with a finger (immediate percussion) or by striking a finger placed against the chest wall (mediate percussion). Mediate percussion of the chest is performed by placing the finger of one hand flat against the chest wall in between the ribs. The finger of the other hand is used to tap or percuss the finger against the chest wall (Fig. 18-12).
2. After creating a percussion note, determine the quality, intensity, and duration of the note produced. The note produced over healthy, aerated lung tissue is termed a resonant note. With hyperinflation or with a pneumothorax, a tympanic note may be detected. In the presence of consolidated (solidified) lung tissue or abnormal fluid such as blood, pus, or chyle present in the pleural space, a dull (flat) note may be present.
3. Percuss the area over the heart or liver to create a dull note.
4. Compare the quality, intensity, and duration of a dull note to the sound created when percussing over healthy, aerated lung tissue.

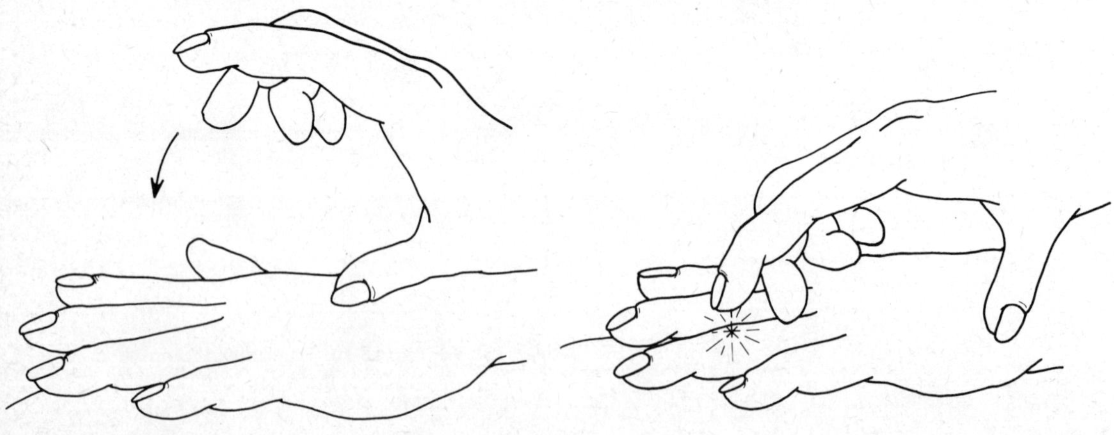

Fig. 18-12. Percussion technique.

5. Compare percussion notes between the right and left lung. A recommended path for percussion notes is shown in the following diagram (Fig. 18-13).
6. Make additional comparisons between anterior and posterior surfaces of the chest and over right and left apices.
7. Percussion may also be used to determine the extent of diaphragmatic excursion. Owing to the availability of fluorosscopy in the clinical setting, however, percussion is rarely used for this purpose.

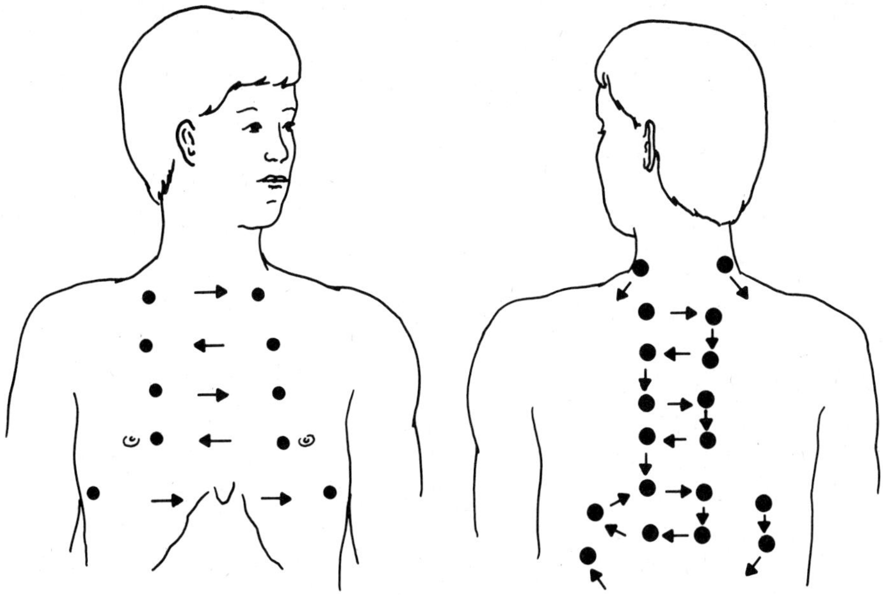

Fig. 18-13. Path of percussion. *(Modified from Des Jardins T: Clinical Manifestations of Respiratory Disease. Chicago, Year Book Medical Publishers, 1984)*

Exercise E: Auscultation of the Chest

1. Examine a stethoscope. Identify the bell, diaphragm, and ear tips (Fig. 18-14).
2. Auscultation of lung sounds is frequently performed with the diaphragm, whereas heart sounds are frequently heard with the bell of the stethoscope.
3. Insert the ear tips into your ears. The ear tips should be facing anteriorly when viewed from the side. Gently tap the diaphragm to determine whether the diaphragm is functioning. If the bell portion is functioning, rotate the bell and diaphragm assembly until the diaphragm fuctions.
4. Review the topographic locations of the lung lobes in relation to the chest (Fig. 18-15).
5. Identify the following lobes of the right lung in the anterior, posterior, and lateral views:
   A. Upper lobe
   B. Middle lobe
   C. Lower lobe
6. Identify the lobes of the left lung in the anterior, posterior, and lateral views:
   D. Upper lobe (includes the lingula)
   E. Lower lobe
7. After ensuring a private, quiet environment, instruct your laboratory partner to assume a sitting position and disrobe to the waist.

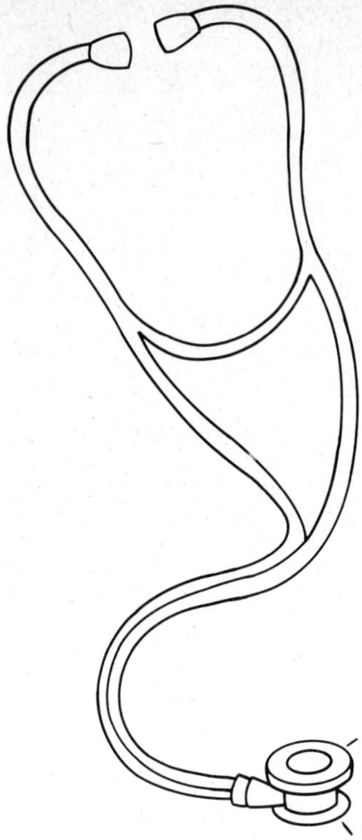

Fig. 18-14. Components of a stethoscope.

8. Using a stethoscope, auscultate the chest. Prepare the "patient" by requesting slow, deep breathing through the mouth. Place the diaphragm of the stethoscope flat against the chest. Auscultate the lobes of both lungs.
9. A recommended path of chest auscultation is shown in the following diagram (Fig. 18-16).
10. During auscultation, it is essential to determine
    - A. the existence of bilateral breath sounds.
    - B. whether sounds are increased, decreased, or absent.
    - C. abnormal sounds such as the following:
        1) Absent—no sound heard over the affected area
        2) Amphoric—cavernous sound similar to blowing air over an open bottle, usually due to air contacting a cavity in the lung
        3) Stridor—high-pitched crowing sound heard during inspiration; may be associated with partial airway obstruction
        4) Rales (crackles)—discontinuous sound frequently associated with fluid (edema) or sudden opening of terminal airways
        5) Rhonchi—continuous sound frequently associated with secretions in the airways
        6) Rubs—sound similar to creaking shoe leather usually due to abnormalities of the pleura
        7) Wheeze—musical pulmonary sound frequently associated with spasm of bronchial smooth muscle or obstruction of airway's lumen
11. Obtain a respiratory history and perform a complete chest examination on a laboratory partner. Record the results on the laboratory report for one complete examination.

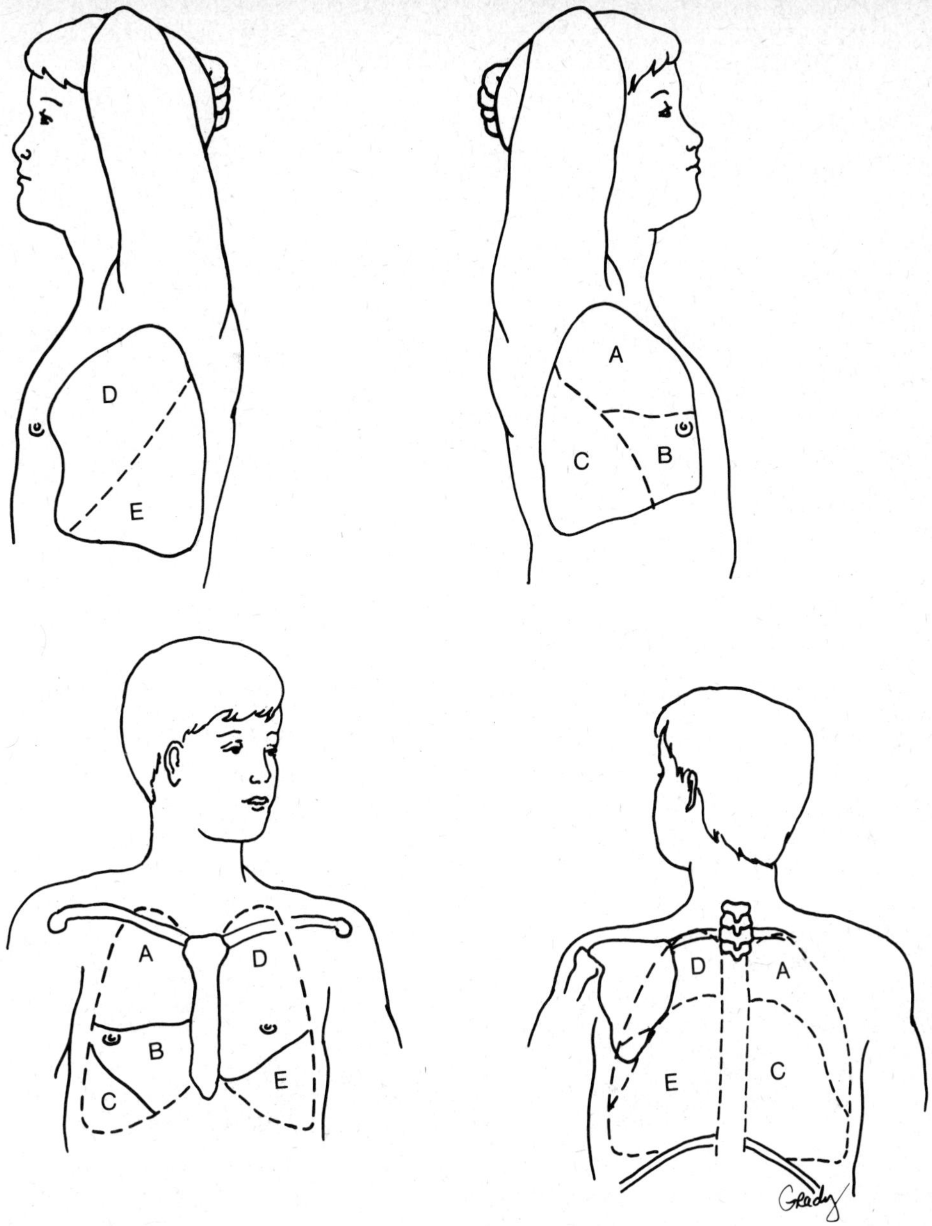

Fig. 18-15. Topographic location of lung lobes.

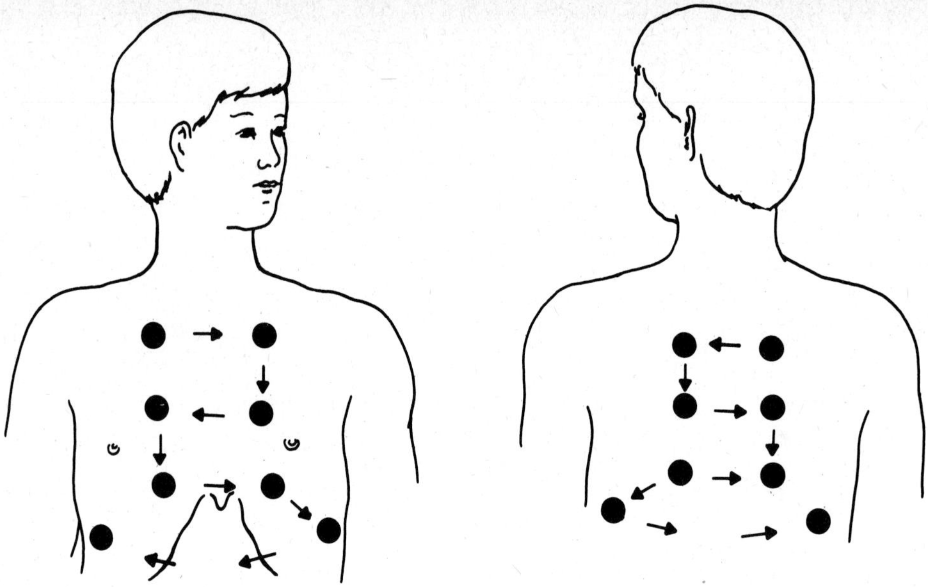

Fig. 18-16. Path for anterior and posterior chest auscultation. *(Modified from Des Jardins T: Clinical Manifestations of Respiratory Disease. Chicago, Year Book Medical Publishers, 1984)*

Exercise F: Determination of "Unknown"

1. Your laboratory instructor will provide you with a tape recording of breath sounds. Identify the "unknown" sounds on the laboratory report.

RECOMMENDED READING

Bates BA: A Guide to Physical Examination. Philadelphia, JB Lippincott, 1974

Burton GG, Hodgkin JE: Respiratory Care. A Guide to Clinical Practice, 2nd ed. Philadelphia, JB Lippincott, 1984

Fraser RG, Pare JAP: Diagnosis of Diseases of the Chest, volume I, 2nd ed. Philadelphia, WB Saunders, 1978

Hinshaw C, Murray JF: Diseases of the Chest, 4th ed. Philadelphia, WB Saunders, 1980

Lehrer S: Understanding Lung Sounds. Philadelphia, WB Saunders, 1984

Shapiro BA, Harrison RA, Kacmarek RM, Cane RD: Clinical Application of Respiratory Care, 3rd ed. Chicago, Year Book Medical Publishers, 1985

Laboratory Performance Evaluation (#18)

Topic: History and Physical Examination for Respiratory Care

Student ______________________ Course ______________________

Date ______________________ Section ______________________

Performance Elements	Acceptable	Unacceptable	Not Applicable	Comments
1. Obtains a respiratory history				
2. Inspects the chest				
3. Palpates the chest: **A.** Position of trachea **B.** Point of maximal impulse **C.** Fremitus **D.** Rhonchi **E.** Chest expansion **F.** Capillary refill **G.** Pitting edema				
4. Percusses the chest: **A.** Percusses each lobe				
5. Auscultates the chest: **A.** Auscultates each lobe **B.** Identifies normal sounds				

Knowledge of Procedure

☐ Good; student is knowledgeable about rationale and theory related to procedure

☐ Fair; student has adequate understanding of rationale and theory related to procedure

☐ Poor; student has inadequate understanding of rationale and theory related to procedure

Performance Deficiencies (check those that apply)

☐ Excessive time needed to complete procedure

☐ Broke aseptic or sterile technique

☐ Gross inaccuracy noted

☐ Technique may be harmful to patient

☐ Incorrect dosage or gas concentration

☐ Incorrect equipment assembly/use

☐ Unable to answer questions correctly about rationale and/or theory related to procedure

☐ Other ______________________________

Evaluation Summary

☐ Satisfactory performance

☐ Unsatisfactory performance

Recommendations of Evaluator

☐ Skills may be applied/observed in clinical setting

☐ Specific evaluation deficiencies require correction

☐ Complete re-evaluation required

☐ Additional laboratory practice required

Signatures:

Evaluator ______________________ Date ______________________

Student ______________________ Date ______________________

Laboratory Report

Student ______________________ Acceptable ______________________

Date ______________________ Unacceptable ______________________

Course ______________________

Topic: History and Physical Examination for Respiratory Care

Data or Measurements

"Unknown" Breath Sounds

1. ______________________

2. ______________________

3. ______________________

4. ______________________

5. ______________________

6. ______________________

Results of Complete Chest Examination:

General Information

Age ________ Sex ________ Body Weight (g) ________

Position (check one)

Sitting ________ Supine ________ Prone ________ Reclining ________

Right or Left Side Dependent ________ Orthopnea ________

History

Cough ________ Dyspnea ________ Chest Pain ________

Cough Effort (check) None ________ Poor ________ Adequate ________

Strong ________

Expectoration Time Produced ________ Amount ________

Consistency ________

Expectorant Color (check)

Clear ______ White ______ Yellow ______ Green ______

Brown ______ Bloody ______

Smoking History Packs Per Day ______ Number of Years ______

Pack Years ______

Previous Cardiopulmonary Disease ______

Personal/Family History of Lung Disease ______

Occuptional Exposure to Irritants ______

Current Medication ______

Inspection

Respiratory Rate ______ Diaphoresis ______

Pheripheral (Pitting) Edema ______ Cyanosis ______

Digital Clubbing ______

Intercostal or Sternal Retractions ______

Asymmetrical Chest Movement ______

Accessory Muscle Activity ______ Venous Distension ______

Thoracic Shape (check)

Normal ______ Barrel Chest ______ Kyphoscoliosis ______

Pectus Excavatum ______ Pectus Carinatum ______

Flail ______

Pursed Lip Breathing ______ Other ______

Palpation

Pulse Rate ______ Nodes ______

Symmetrical Chest Movement ______

Vocal Fremitus ______ Tactile Fremitus ______

Tracheal Deviation ______ Point of Maximal Impulse ______

Percussion (Check, note, and cite location)

Flat ________ Dull ________ Resonant ________ Hyperesonant ________

Location ________

Auscultation (check)

Normal Bilateral Sounds ________

Decreased, Absent, or Unequal Sounds ________

Rhonchi ________ Wheezing ________ Rub ________

Crackles (Rales) ________ Stridor ________

Location of Abnormal Sounds (Diagram and Shade Lung Lobes):

Scenario: You have been asked to perform a respiratory care consult on the patient in Room 206 of Ward 8A. Your review of the chart produces the following: Mr. Harris, an elderly white man, was found earlier this morning huddled beneath an empty shipping carton at a nearby warehouse. The security guard who found him stated that he was delirious and carried no identification. On admission, his temperature was 102°F, pulse 102/minute, and respiratory rate 25 breaths/minute.

Your initial impression: He is an emaciated and unkempt elderly man, with an obvious barrel chest and hypertrophied accessory muscles. He is receiving oxygen at 4 liters/minute by means of nasal cannula. He is diaphoretic and mildly tachypneic. You also notice that the index and middle fingers of his right hand are heavily stained with nicotine. The ER note beneath diagnosis states "COPD, CVA, and possible pneumonia." Please answer the following questions pertinent to Mr. Harris.

1. In addition to the barrel chest, what other *inspection* findings may indicate chest wall abnormalities?
   A.
   B.
   C.
2. What are three additional points noted during inspection?
   A.
   B.
   C.
3. Where would the point of maximal impulse be in a healthy person?

4. Palpation might reveal the following for a consolidated pneumonia:
   A.
   B.
   C.
5. If Mr. Harris has a right lower lobe consolidation, what sort of percussion note would be
   A. on the left posterior thorax?

   B. on the right posterior thorax?

6. Describe the auscultation findings most commonly associated with abnormal breath sounds.

chapter 19

Pulmonary mechanics (bedside pulmonary functions)

INTRODUCTION

Pulmonary mechanics testing provides valuable data that may be used in several ways. In conjunction with clinical assessment and other diagnostic tests, the pulmonary mechanics data may be used to determine the feasibility of weaning or initiating continuous mechanical ventilation and the effectiveness of therapeutic techniques. In addition, pulmonary mechanics may be useful in detecting the ability to breathe deeply and cough effectively, which is essential in the maintenance of bronchial hygiene.

Pulmonary mechanics, or bedside pulmonary functions, usually consist of the following tests:

- ☐ Tidal volume (V_T)
- ☐ Minute volume (V_E)
- ☐ Vital capacity(VC)
- ☐ Peak expiratory flowrate (PEFR)
- ☐ Negative inspiratory force (NIF)
- ☐ Positive expiratory force (PEF)

Tidal volume is the average volume of gas inhaled and exhaled during resting breathing. Minute volume is the total volume of gas exhaled during resting breathing for an interval of 1 minute. Vital capacity is the maximum volume of gas that can be forcefully exhaled after a maximum inhalation. Forced vital capacity is an index of the ability to breathe deeply and cough effectively. Peak expiratory flowrate is the maximum gas flowrate at which the vital capacity is exhaled. The PEFR may be used to evaluate the response to bronchodilator therapy. The negative inspiratory force measurement may be used to evaluate improvement or deterioration of the respiratory system in neuromuscular disease. The negative inspiratory force and positive expiratory force measurements are indicative of respiratory muscular strength and may also reflect the ability to breathe deeply and cough effectively. The purpose of this chapter is to introduce you to the measurement of pulmonary mechanics.

OBJECTIVES

After completing this chapter, you should be able to do the following:

1. *Identify the apparatus needed to measure the mechanics test.*
2. *Prepare a patient for the measurement of pulmonary mechanics.*
3. *Assemble the apparatus needed for measuring pulmonary mechanics.*
4. *Measure and record pulmonary mechanics on four spontaneously breathing classmates.*
5. *Measure and record pulmonary mechanics on an intubated adult mannequin.*

EQUIPMENT NEEDED

- ☐ Manometer
- ☐ Spirometer
- ☐ Pneumotachometer
- ☐ Face mask or mouthpieces and noseclips
- ☐ T-tube and one-way valve system

ACTIVITIES

PREPARATION OF A SIMULATED PATIENT FOR PULMONARY MECHANICS

1. Request that the patient assume an upright sitting position (if possible).
2. Explain the following before performing each test:
   - The tests are painless.
   - Maximum effort should be exerted for each test, and rest will be allowed between tests.
   - The patient will be unable to breathe any air during the negative force test.
3. Determine the body weight in kilograms.

Exercises A and B: Measurement of Minute Volume and Average Tidal Volume

1. Obtain a portable spirometer (Fig. 19-1).
2. Identify the (a) on/off switch; (b) reset button and volume increments. *Note:* The small hand indicates volume in tenths of a liter; the large hand indicates the volume in liters.
3. Connect a face mask to a portable spirometer.
4. Explain the procedure and reassure the subject. Request normal breathing from the subject.
5. Cover the subject's mouth and nose with a mask and spirometer (Fig. 19-2).
6. Turn the spirometer "on" for 60 seconds.
7. While measuring the exhaled volume, count the respiratory rate for 60 seconds.
8. After 60 seconds, turn the spirometer "off."
9. Read and record minute volume. Record respiratory rate.
10. Calculate the average tidal volume according to the following equation:

$$V_T = \frac{V_E}{RR}, \text{ where}$$

V_T = tidal volume (ml)
V_E = minute volume (ml/minute)
RR = respiratory rate.

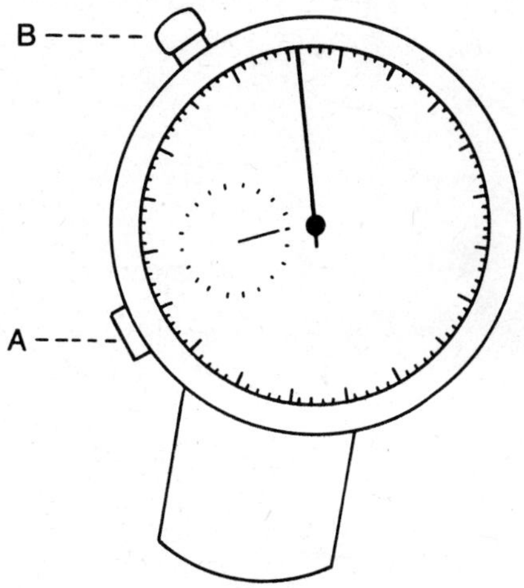

Fig. 19-1. Portable spirometer.

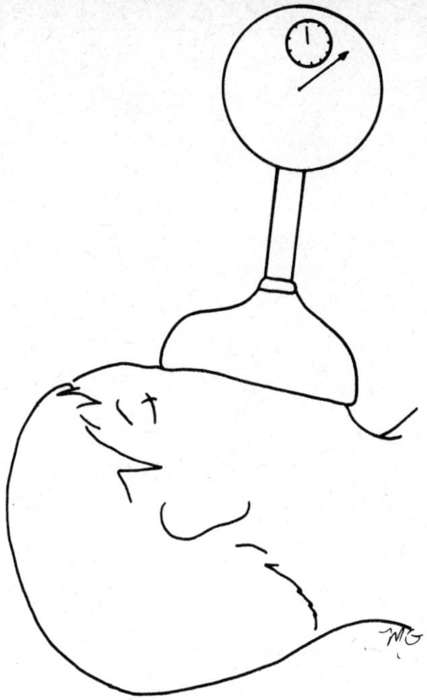

Fig. 19-2. Face mask and portable spirometer for measurement of gas volumes.

Exercise C: Measurement of Vital Capacity

1. Explain the procedure.
2. Occlude the mouth and nose with a face mask and spirometer.
3. Request a maximal inhalation and exhalation.
4. Repeat two or three times.
5. Read and record the best vital capacity. *Note:* Do *not* forcefully exhale into a Wright's spirometer.

Exercise D: Measurement of Peak Expiratory Flowrate

1. Obtain a pneumotachometer (Fig. 19-3).
2. Connect a mouthpiece to the pneumotachometer.
3. Explain the procedure and reassure the subject.
4. Request a maximal inspiration and both a *forceful* and a *complete* expiration.
5. Read and record the expiratory flowrate.

Exercise E: Measurement of Inspiratory and Expiratory Pressure

1. Connect a face mask to a manometer (Fig. 19-4).
2. Explain the procedure and reassure the subject by stating that the patient will be unable to breathe for one breath during the test. *Note:* In the laboratory, the student should not perform a maximal inhalation because of the potential of inner ear discomfort.
3. Cover the subject's mouth and nose with a mask and manometer.
4. Occlude the thumb port in the manometer connection.
5. Request a deep inspiration from the subject.
6. Read and record negative inspiratory pressure.

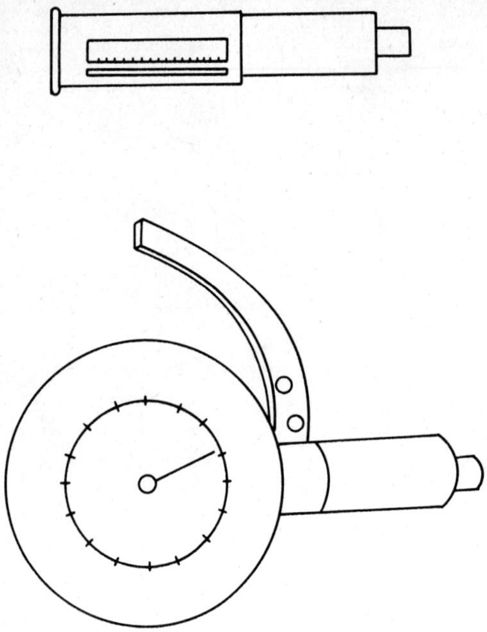

Fig. 19-3. Pneumotachometer.

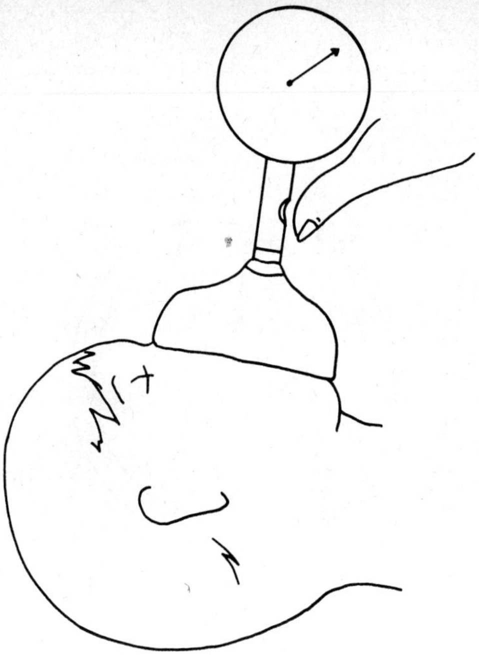

Fig. 19-4. Face mask and manometer for inspiratory force measurement.

7. Allow normal breathing through the thumb port.
8. Occlude the thumb port.
9. Request a maximal expiration from subject.
10. Read and record the expiratory pressure.
11. Measure and record the following test results from four laboratory partners on the laboratory report.
    - Minute volume
    - Respiratory rate
    - Tidal volume
    - Forced vital capacity
    - Negative inspiratory force

Exercise F: Determination of "Unknown"

MEASUREMENT OF PULMONARY MECHANICS IN AN INTUBATED ADULT PATIENT

1. Your laboratory instructor will provide you with an intubated mannequin.* You may assume that the mannequin is breathing spontaneously through the endotracheal tube.
2. The technique for measuring pulmonary mechanics is essentially the same with some important differences:
   A. An intubated patient must be reconnected immediately to any therapeutic apparatus (i.e., a T-tube or ventilator) after performing each individual test.
   B. Intubated patients as well as any patient in borderline respiratory failure must be allowed to rest in-between individual tests for optimal performance.

* Note to instructor: An intubated mannequin may be modified to provide known values for pulmonary mechanics "unknown" determinations by students. To modify an intubated mannequin, see the steps outlined above.

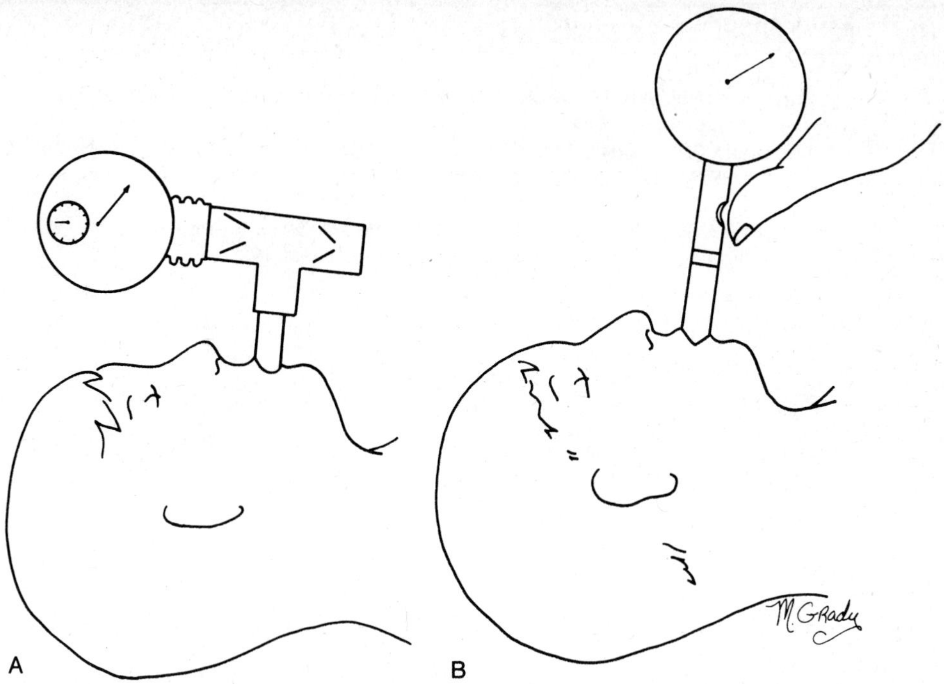

Fig. 19-5. Apparatus required to measure pulmonary mechanics by connection to an artificial airway using (A) a spirometer and (B) a manometer.

3. Assemble the apparatus by applying one-way valves or adapters for connection to the endotracheal tube as shown in Figure 19-5.
4. Measure and record the unknown values for
   A. V_T
   B. V_E
   C. RR
   D. FVC
   E. NIFM

MODIFICATION OF AN INTUBATED MANNEQUIN

1. Orally intubate the mannequin with a No. 8 mm ID endotracheal tube.
2. Insert the No. 8 tube down into the right main stem bronchus.
3. Remove the right lung from the right main stem bronchus.
4. Insert the cuff of a No. 5 mm ID endotracheal tube into the right main stem bronchus within the No. 8 tube.
5. Inflate the cuffs on both the No. 8 and No. 5 tubes.
6. Assemble a volume ventilator breathing circuit.
7. Attach the breathing circuit to the No. 5 endotracheal tube adapter.
8. Turn the ventilator on and adjust the desired settings for the tidal volume, rate, and minute volume.
9. The manual breath or sigh may provide an FVC.
10. Connect a syringe to the No. 5 tube and aspirate for the negative force measurement.

RECOMMENDED READING

Burton GG, Hodgkin JE: Respiratory Care. A Guide to Clinical Practice, 2nd ed. Philadelphia, JB Lippincott, 1984

Kacmarek RM, Dimas S, Mack C: Essentials of Respiratory Therapy, 2nd ed. Chicago, Year Book Medical Publishers, 1985

Ruppel G: Manual of Pulmonary Function Testing, 2nd ed. St Louis, CV Mosby, 1979

Shapiro BA, Harrison RA, Kacmarek RM, Cane RD: Clinical Application of Respiratory Care, 3rd ed. Chicago, Year Book Medical Publishers, 1985

Laboratory Performance Evaluation (#19)

Topic: Pulmonary Mechanics

Student ______________________ Course ______________________

Date ______________________ Section ______________________

Performance Elements	Acceptable	Unacceptable	Not Applicable	Comments
1. Obtains necessary equipment				
2. Washes hands				
3. Assembles equipment properly: A. Spirometer B. Manometer C. Pneumotachometer				
4. Explains procedure to simulated patient				
5. Disconnects patient from CMV system				
6. Measures the following correctly: A. Tidal volume (VT) B. Minute volume (V) C. Ventilatory frequency (f) D. Negative inspiratory force E. Vital capacity				
7. Reconnects simulated patient to premeasurement systems				
8. Interprets measured results properly				
9. Records results				

Knowledge of Procedure

- ☐ Good; student is knowledgeable about rationale and theory related to procedure
- ☐ Fair; student has adequate understanding of rationale and theory related to procedure
- ☐ Poor; student has inadequate understanding of rationale and theory related to procedure

Performance Deficiencies (check those that apply)

- ☐ Excessive time needed to complete procedure
- ☐ Broke aseptic or sterile technique
- ☐ Gross inaccuracy noted
- ☐ Technique may be harmful to patient
- ☐ Incorrect dosage or gas concentration
- ☐ Incorrect equipment assembly/use
- ☐ Unable to answer questions correctly about rationale and/or theory related to procedure
- ☐ Other ______________________________

Evaluation Summary

- ☐ Satisfactory performance
- ☐ Unsatisfactory performance

Recommendations of Evaluator

- ☐ Skills may be applied/observed in clinical setting
- ☐ Specific evaluation deficiencies require correction
- ☐ Complete re-evaluation required
- ☐ Additional laboratory practice required

Signatures:

Evaluator ______________________ Date ______________________

Student ______________________ Date ______________________

Laboratory Report

Student ______________________ Acceptable ______________________

Date ______________________ Unacceptable ______________________

Course ______________________

Topic: Pulmonary Mechanics

Data or Measurements

A. Results of pulmonary mechanics measurements from four classmates

	1	2	3	4	Average
Name					
Body Weight (kg)					
Tidal Volume					
Respiratory Rate					
Vital Capacity					
Negative Force					
Positive Force					

B. Results of pulmonary mechanics "unknown" measurement from intubated adult

Tidal Volume ______________________

Minute Volume ______________________

Respiratory Rate ______________________

Vital Capacity ______________________

Negative Force ______________________

Scenario: Mr. Harris, you recall, was the unfortunate who had been found during a recent cold snap huddled beneath shipping cartons. Your physical examination reinforced earlier pulmonary findings of emphysema and pneumonia. Upon consultation, you had recommended an increase in supplemental oxygen, bedside PFTs, and, most importantly, *vigorous* bronchial hygiene. It has been 48 hours since your recommendations were implemented, and you are going to obtain follow-up bedside pulmonary mechanics.

Please answer the following questions.

1. Specifically, which pulmonary function tests will you use at Mr. Harris' bedside?
A.

B.

C.

D.

E.

F.

2. Improvement in which of the above would indicate the effectiveness of bronchial hygiene?

3. In a healthy, resting adult, what is the range of normal values for

A. tidal volume? ____________

B. minute volume? ____________

C. respiratory rate? ____________

D. vital capacity? ____________

E. negative inspiratory force? ____________

4. Which pulmonary mechanics tests are the most dependent on patient effort?

5. What is the significance of a markedly decreased vital capacity?

6. Which pulmonary mechanics test(s) may indicate
   A. the ability to breathe deeply and cough effectively?

   B. muscular power of the respiratory muscles?

7. What apparatus is needed to measure

   A. V_T? ______________________________

   B. V_E? ______________________________

   C. FVC? ______________________________

   D. NIFM? ______________________________

   E. PEFR? ______________________________

chapter 20

Arterial puncture

INTRODUCTION

Puncture of an artery is performed to obtain an anaerobic sample of arterial blood. After the procedure, the sample is analyzed to measure *p*H, the partial pressure of carbon dioxide, and the partial pressure of oxygen. The measurement of arterial blood gases is a cornerstone test used in the diagnosis of hypoxemia and ventilatory failure.

It is important to review several anatomical points concerning arteries before performing a puncture. Arteries comprise three tissue layers: From within the lumen to the outside of an artery, these layers include the tunica intima, the tunica media, and the tunica adventitia. Because of the relatively thick layers of elastic connective tissue and smooth muscle, the diameter of arteries is usually smaller than that of neighboring veins. In addition, arteries lie deeper beneath the skin than do the more superficial veins. In the adult, the most common sites used for puncture include the radial, brachial, and femoral arteries. In the neonate, the temporal and radial arteries are commonly used.

In a healthy person, several differences exist between arterial and venous blood. Arterial blood is transported under much higher pressure (mean = 100 mmHg) than venous blood (mean = 1 - 10 mm Hg). Because of the pressure gradient between arterial blood and ambient pressure, blood will usually pulsate and fill a syringe during arterial puncture. The color of arterial blood is bright red (because of oxyhemoglobin), compared to the dark blue color of venous blood.

Another important difference between arterial and venous blood is the blood gas values. After analysis, the typical blood gas values for arterial and venous blood in a young, healthy adult are as follows:

	Arterial	Venous
*p*H	7.40	7.36
Pa_{CO_2} (mm Hg)	40	46
Pa_{O_2} (mm Hg)	100	40

Since visualization of the vessel is impossible during a pucture, these differences may allow the differentiation between an arterial and a venous sample.

Performance of an arterial puncture is not without the risk of significant complications. Extreme caution should be exercised in the presence of

- low platelet count (normal, 180, 000–300, 000 mm^3)
- prolonged clotting time
- bleeding diathesis
- history of multiple punctures
- anticoagulant therapy (heparin, protamine, or warfarin sodium)
- hemophilia
- acquired immune deficiency syndrome (AIDS)

The aforementioned conditions may require consultation with a physician or modification of the procedure.

In this chapter, you are introduced to the technique of arterial puncture and preparation of a blood sample for analysis.

OBJECTIVES

After completing this chapter, you should be able to do the following:

1. *Identify drugs and physiologic disorders that may affect the procedure of arterial puncture.*
2. *Select a site for arterial puncture.*
3. *Differentiate between an arterial and venous blood sample.*
4. *Assemble the equipment needed for blood sampling.*
5. *Explain the procedure to the patient.*
6. *Perform the Allen's test for collateral circulation.*
7. *Prepare the puncture site.*
8. *Aseptically puncture the artery.*
9. *Apply pressure to the puncture site, and verify the cessation of bleeding.*
10. *Prepare the anaeraobic sample for transportation to the blood gas analyzer.*

EQUIPMENT NEEDED

- ☐ Syringe (preheparinized or unheparinized)
- ☐ 22-gauge needle (for adults)
- ☐ Sterile swabs
- ☐ Sterile cotton
- ☐ Iodine disinfectant swab
- ☐ Ice
- ☐ Heparin (1000 U/ml or dry)
- ☐ Band-Aid
- ☐ Arterial puncture simulator

ACTIVITIES

Exercise A: Preliminary Steps

Your laboratory instructor may provide you with an arterial simulator. You may simulate the procedure of arterial puncture in the clinical environment by interacting with a laboratory partner acting as a "patient." *Note:* Do *not* perform the actual puncture on a laboratory partner without sterile equipment and instructor permission.

1. Review the patient's chart and evaluate the following:
   - **A.** Physician order (or enter a verbal order)
   - **B.** Patient history and current status (clotting disorders)

C. Medications (anticoagulants)
D. Previous blood samples
E. Prescribed FI_{O_2}

2. Identify the patient by name and by checking the wrist band.
3. Introduce yourself and identify your department.
4. Explain the procedure to the patient.
5. Wash your hands.

Exercise B: Equipment Preparation

1. Aseptically prepare the equipment for arterial puncture.
   A. Attach needle to syringe.
   B. If using a syringe that is not preheparinized, withdraw 0.5 ml of sodium heparin (1000 U/ml).
   C. Lubricate the barrel of the syringe.
   D. Expel the sodium heparin and any air bubbles.
2. *Note:* Excessive heparin may affect the accuracy of the blood gas and *p*H values. A volume of heparin of 0.05 ml per 1.0 ml of blood is recommended.

Exercise C: Site Preparation

1. Select the puncture site (Fig. 20-1). Commonly used sites in the adult include the
   A. radial artery.
   B. brachial artery.
   C. femoral artery.
2. If the radial artery is selected as the puncture site, perform the Allen's test for collateral circulation (Fig. 20-2).
   A. Palpate the radial and ulnar arteries.
   B. Request that the patient make a tight fist.
   C. Occlude both the radial and ulnar arteries.
   D. Release the ulnar artery and verify a rapid color return to the blanched area of the hand. The color should return within 10 to 15 seconds.
3. Disinfect the selected puncture site with isopropyl alcohol and iodine solutions.
4. Disinfect your fingers that will palpate the artery with the alcohol and iodine solution.
5. Place both the patient and yourself in comfortable positions. The equipment should be easily retrievable.

Exercise D: Performing the Puncture

1. Before puncturing the artery, 1.0 ml of 2% lidocaine may be injected as a skin wheal. This is an optional procedure and is indicated when the puncture must be repeated or is difficult to perform.
2. Palpate the arterial puncture site. Attempt to visualize the location of the artery by palpating several points in a straight line.
3. Stabilize the artery to prevent it from moving during insertion of the needle.
4. Hold the syringe at a 45° angle to the arm, with the bevel of the needle facing up (Fig. 20-3).
5. Inform the patient of a "stick" and insert the needle through the skin.
6. While palpating the artery, advance the needle slightly until blood pulsates in the syringe barrel. While performing the puncture, avoid
   A. repeated punctures (sewing machine punctures).
   B. deep punctures of the radial artery.
   C. pulling on the plunger of the syringe to withdraw blood "quicker."

7. After obtaining an appropriate volume of blood (adults, 1.5–2.0 ml), smoothly withdraw the needle and immediately apply pressure to the site for a minimum of 5 minutes with sterile cotton gauze.
8. After 5 minutes, verify that bleeding has stopped. Apply a Band-Aid or sterile gauze to the site. When anticoagulant therapy is being administered, pressure may be required for longer periods of time to stop bleeding.
9. If bleeding continues, apply firm pressure to the site, elevate the wrist above the head, and notify a physician.

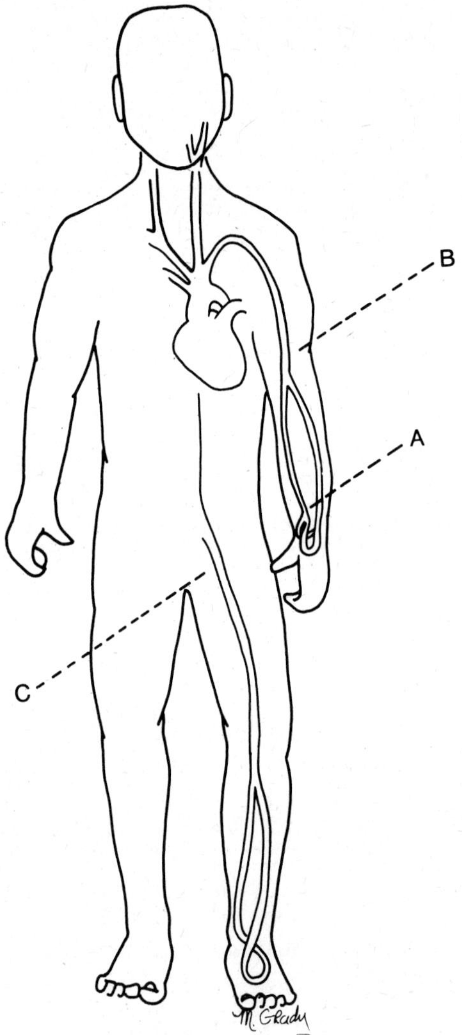

Fig. 20-1. Location of radial, brachial, and femoral arteries.

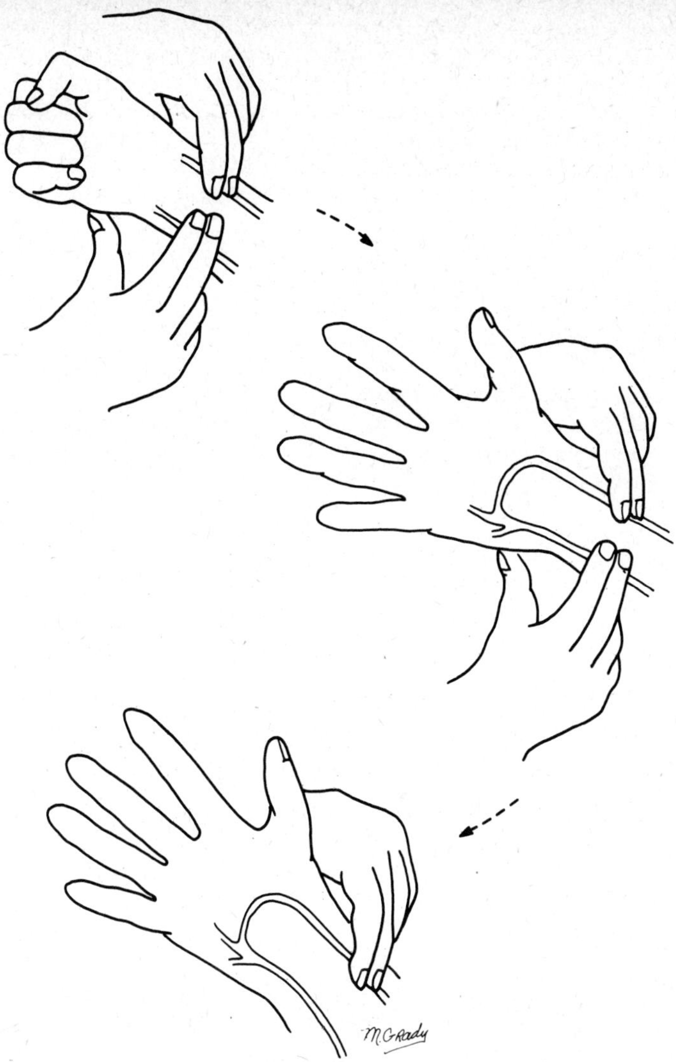

Fig. 20-2. Allen's test for collateral circulation of the hand.

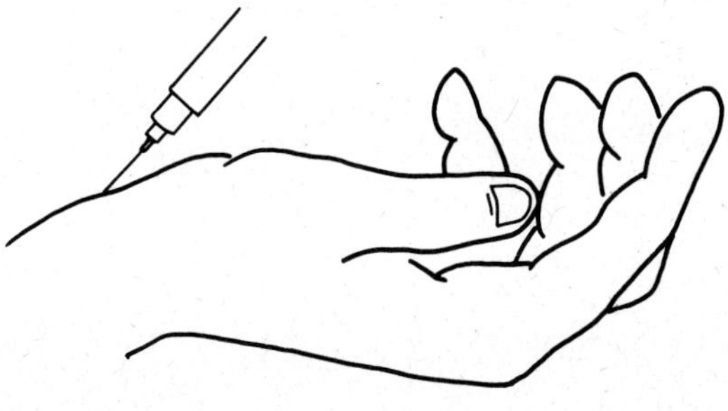

Fig. 20-3. Puncture of radial artery.

Exercise E: Sample Preparation for Analysis

1. Prepare the blood sample for transport to the analyzer.
   A. Remove air bubbles by holding the needle upright, tapping gently, and depressing the plunger.
   B. Place a cap or rubber stopper on the syringe.
   C. Label the syringe with the patient name and time drawn.
   D. Place the syringe in an ice slush. The optimal temperature for storage of a sample is 4°C
   E. Note the FI_{O_2}.

Exercise F: Neonatal Arterial Puncture

1. Puncture of a neonate's radial artery is similar to that of an adult's with the following important differences:
   A. A 25-gauge butterfly needle is used.
   B. The 25-gauge butterfly needle is connected to a tuberculin syringe.
   C. A small volume of blood is obtained (0.2–0.3 ml), compared to the volume usually obtained for adult samples (2.0–3.0 ml).
2. Heparinize the syringe and butterfly needle.
3. Palpate the radial artery.
4. Cleanse the skin with iodine and alcohol.
5. With the bevel of the butterfly needle up, puncture the skin at a 35° to 45° angle (Fig. 20-4).
6. Gently insert the needle until a pulsatile flow of blood enters the butterfly tubing.
7. Connect the 1.0 ml syringe and obtain a 0.3 ml sample of blood
8. Remove the needle and apply pressure to the site for a minimum of 5 minutes.
9. Prepare the sample for analysis in a manner similar to that for an adult sample.

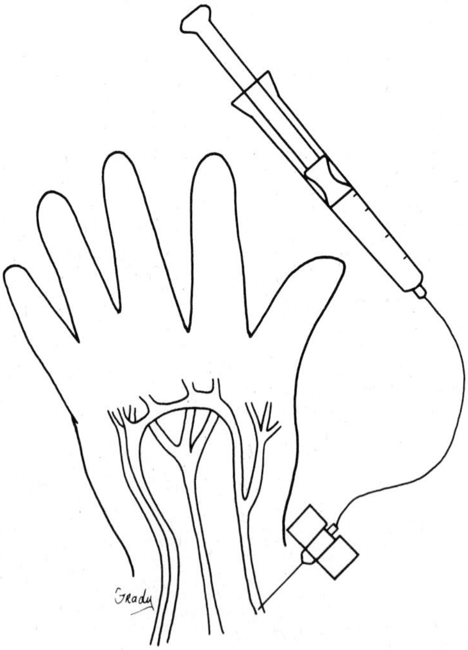

Fig. 20-4. Puncture of the radial artery in a neonate with a 25-gauge "butterfly" needle.

RECOMMENDED READING

Burgess WR, Chernick V: Respiratory Therapy in Newborn Infants and Children. New York, Thieme-Stratton, 1982

Burton GG, Hodgkin JE: Respiratory Care. A Guide to Clinical Practice, 2nd ed. Philadelphia, JB Lippincott, 1984

Lough MD, Williams TJ, Rawson JE: Newborn Respiratory Care. Chicago, Year Book Medical Publishers, 1979

Shapiro BA, Harrison RA, Walton JR: Clinical Application of Blood Gases, 3rd ed. Chicago, Year Book Medical Publishers, 1982

Laboratory Performance Evaluation (#20)

Topic: Arterial Puncture

Student ______________________ Course ______________________

Date ______________________ Section ______________________

Performance Elements	Acceptable	Unacceptable	Not Applicable	Comments
1. Verifies the order				
2. Inspects chart for anticoagulant drug therapy or clotting disorders				
3. Washes hands				
4. Obtains necessary and appropriate equipment				
5. Prepares aseptically and efficiently the arterial puncture equipment				
6. Identifies simulated patient properly				
7. Introduces self to simulated patient and explains procedure				
8. Prepares aseptically and thoroughly the puncture site				
9. Performs an Allen test				
10. Penetrates artery, using sterile technique and accepted method				
11. Obtains simulated arterial blood sample				

Performance Elements	Acceptable	Unacceptable	Not Applicable	Comments
12. Applies pressure to puncture site for appropriate amount of time				
13. Checks for adverse side-effects or complications				
14. Reassures the patient				
15. Prepares the obtained sample properly: **A.** Removes air bubbles **B.** Places on syringe rubber stopper or alternative occluding device **C.** Labels correctly the blood gas sample **D.** Places sample in container of ice water slush				

Knowledge of Procedure

☐ Good; student is knowledgeable about rationale and theory related to procedure

☐ Fair; student has adequate understanding of rationale and theory related to procedure

☐ Poor; student has inadequate understanding of rationale and theory related to procedure

Performance Deficiencies (check those that apply)

☐ Excessive time needed to complete procedure

☐ Broke aseptic or sterile technique

☐ Gross inaccuracy noted

☐ Technique may be harmful to patient

☐ Incorrect dosage or gas concentration

☐ Incorrect equipment assembly/use

☐ Unable to answer questions correctly about rationale and/or theory related to procedure

☐ Other ______________________________

Evaluation Summary
☐ Satisfactory performance ☐ Unsatisfactory performance

Recommendations of Evaluator
☐ Skills may be applied/observed in clinical setting ☐ Specific evaluation deficiencies require correction ☐ Complete re-evaluation required ☐ Additional laboratory practice required

Signatures:

Evaluator ____________________ Date ____________________

Student ____________________ Date ____________________

Laboratory Report

Student ______________________ Acceptable ______________________

Date ______________________ Unacceptable ______________________

Course ______________________

Topic: Arterial Puncture

Scenario: Mr. Baldwin, an elderly man well known to the department for his hospitalizations caused by exacerbations of his COPD, is again residing on Ward 4B. His admitting arterial blood gas values on room air were as follows: $Pa_{O_2} = 40$ mm Hg, $Pa_{CO_2} = 55$ mm Hg, and a pH of 7.32. He currently is receiving an FI_{O_2} of 0.35 from Venturi Mask. The physician has ordered an arterial blood gas sample to evaluate the effectiveness of 0.35 FI_{O_2}.

Please respond to the following questions:

1. Please describe the manner in which you prepare a site for arterial puncture.

2. What type of antiseptic agent is preferred for preparation of an arterial puncture site?

3. Why is the obtained sample immersed in a container of ice water?

4. Specifically, what information should be placed on the label of the arterial blood sample?

5. Briefly state the purpose of the Allen's test.

6. List two physiologic disorders in which arterial puncture may be dangerous.

7. As a therapist, what should be done if the skin does not resume its color after an Allen's test?

8. How may a sample be verified to be arterial blood?

9. List the three most common sites of arterial puncture in an adult.

chapter 21

Indwelling arterial line sampling

INTRODUCTION

Intermittent or occasional arterial blood samples are usually obtained by arterial puncture. In the critically ill or unstable patient, frequent or multiple arterial blood samples may necessitate the insertion of an indwelling arterial catheter. In addition to blood sampling, the catheter may allow the continuous measurement of arterial blood pressure.

In the adult, the catheter is usually inserted into the radial or brachial artery. In the neonate, a catheter may be inserted into an umbillical artery. Because the blood within an indwelling catheter exists under pressure, a sterile, pressurized solution of diluted anticoagulant counterbalances the force of arterial blood pressure. Since the pressure of the anticoagulant solution is usually maintained higher than that of arterial blood, the anticoagulant solution may be infused or "flushed" through the catheter to prevent the formation of blood clots.

The use of an arterial catheter for blood sampling is not without risk. Poor aseptic technique may result in the introduction of microbes directly into the vasculature, causing infection. Carelessness in the adjustment of the stopcock valve or accidental tubing disconnection may result in massive blood loss. Inattention to the maintenance of catheter patency may cause thrombus formation and dysfunction of the system. The purpose of this chapter is to introduce you to the technique of indwelling arterial blood sampling.

OBJECTIVES

After completing this chapter, you should be able to do the following:

1. *Understand the functions of an arterial line catheter.*
2. *Obtain an arterial blood sample from an arterial line.*
3. *Flush an arterial line with a heparin solution.*
4. *Trace the flow of blood and fluid through an arterial line.*

EQUIPMENT NEEDED

- ☐ Syringes (preheparinized or unheparinized)
- ☐ Sterile alcohol swabs
- ☐ Sterile cotton gauze
- ☐ Iodine disinfectant swab
- ☐ Ice
- ☐ Heparin 1000 U/ml
- ☐ Arterial puncture simulator
- ☐ Controlled infusion device
- ☐ Three-way stopcocks
- ☐ Arterial catheter
- ☐ Pressure transducer
- ☐ Pressure monitor
- ☐ Fluid pressure infusion setup

ACTIVITIES

Exercise A: Identification of Arterial Line System Components

1. Examine an arterial line. (Your laboratory instructor will provide you with a simulated human arm with an arterial catheter in place—Figure 21-1).
2. Identify the following components:
   - A. Arterial catheter
   - B. Three-way stopcock and protective cap
   - C. Intraflow device
   - D. Intravenous tubing
   - E. Pressure gauge
3. Identify the remaining components of the system (Fig. 21-2).
   - A. Pressure transducer
   - B. Transducer cable

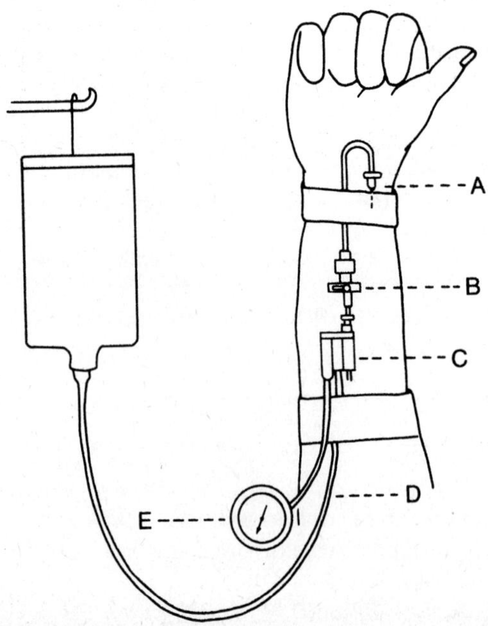

Fig. 21-1. Arterial catheter. *(Modified from Schroeder JS, Daily Ek: Techniques in Bedside Hemodynamic Monitoring. St Louis, CV Mosby, 1976)*

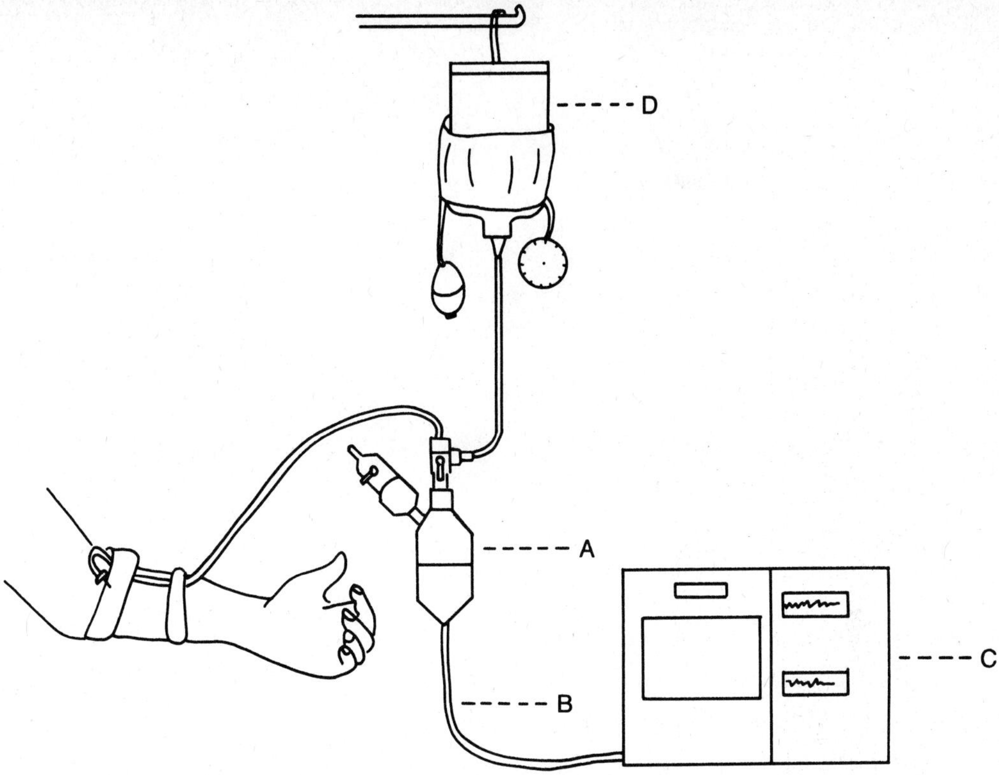

Fig. 21-2. Arterial line system. *(Modified from Schroeder JS, Daily EK: Techniques in Bedside Hemodynamic Monitoring. St Louis, CV Mosby, 1976)*

C. Pressure monitor
D. Intravenous fluid (pressurized bag)

4. Examine a three-way stopcock (Fig. 21-3). It is essential to understand flow through a stopcock in order to use an arterial line safely. *Note:* The stopcock handle (or lever) is always over the closed port, and flow occurs through the remaining ports.
5. Closely examine a controlled infusion (intraflow) device located near the arterial catheter (Fig. 21-4).
6. Identify the components:
   A. Valve stem
   B. Transducer connection
   C. Catheter connection
   D. Fluid source luer connector
   E. Protective caps
7. Trace the flow of "flush" solution as the valve stem is displaced.

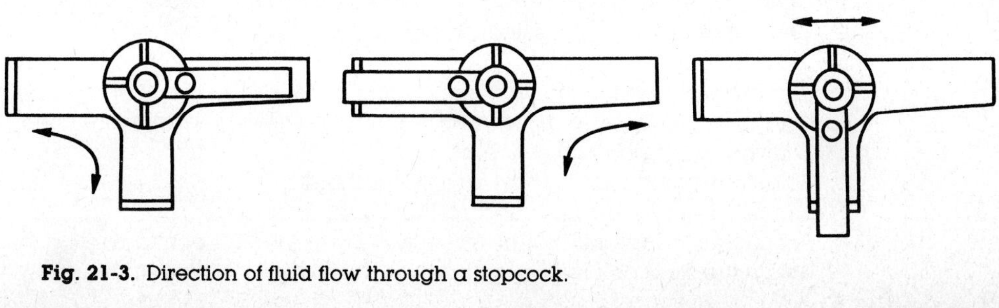

Fig. 21-3. Direction of fluid flow through a stopcock.

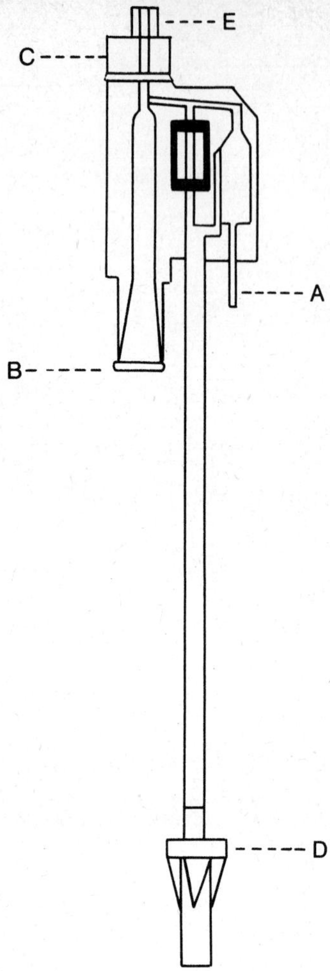

Fig. 21-4. Controlled infusion device. *(Redrawn from Burton GG, Gee GG, Hodgkin JE: Respiratory Care. A Guide to Clinical Practice. Philadelphia, JB Lippincott, 1977)*

Exercise B: Equipment Preparation

1. Obtain two 10.0 ml syringes.
2. Preheparinize one of the syringes using aseptic technique.
3. Label the heparinized syringe.
4. Obtain an alcohol swab.

Exercise C: Obtaining a Blood Sample from an Arterial Line

1. Obtain two 10.0 ml syringes.
2. Verify that one syringe is preheparinized.
3. Using asseptic technique, remove the protective cap and attach a nonheparinized syringe to the three-way stopcock (Fig. 21-5).
4. Rotate the stopcock lever toward the intraflow device and connecting tubing.
5. Withdraw about 5.0 ml of blood.
6. Rotate the stopcock lever toward the catheter.
7. Remove the syringe and discard the 5.0 ml of blood.
8. Aseptically attach the heparinized syringe to the luer connector.
9. Rotate the stopcock lever toward the intraflow device and connecting tubing.

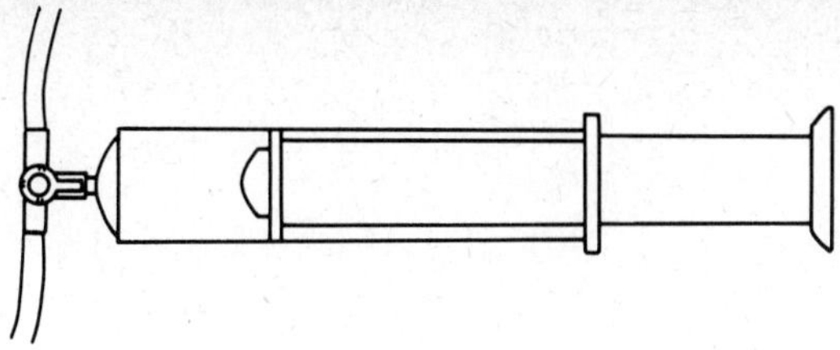

Fig. 21-5. Connection of a syringe to a stopcock.

10. Withdraw 2 or 3 ml of blood.
11. Rotate the stopcock lever toward the catheter.
12. Remove the syringe.

Exercise D: Maintenance of Arterial Line Patency

1. After removal of the syringe, the stopcock lever should still be rotated toward the catheter.
2. Place the sterile gauze beneath the stopcock.
3. Displace the valve stem two or three times to flush the tubing
4. Rotate the stopcock lever toward the protective cap; swab the luer connector on the stopcock with alcohol. Replace the protective cap. Displace the valve stem two or three times. Verify adequate flushing. Blood remaining within the tubing should appear to be flushed into the catheter.

Exercise E: Sample Preparation

1. Remove any air bubbles in the sample.
2. Cap the blood sample.
3. Roll the syringe several times between your hands to mix the blood sample adequately with heparin.
4. Label the sample and place the syringe in an ice slush.
5. Clean and replace all equipment. If the arterial arm simulator will not be in use for a prolonged period, adjust the valve to prevent blood flow into the arm.

RECOMMENDED READING

Blodgett D: Manual of Respiratory Care Procedures. Philadelphia, JB Lippincott, 1980

Schroeder JS, Daily EK: Techniques in Bedside Hemodynamic Monitoring. St. Louis, CV Mosby, 1976

Laboratory Performance Evaluation (#21)

Topic: Indwelling Arterial Line Sampling

Student ______________________ Course ______________________

Date ______________________ Section ______________________

Performance Elements	Acceptable	Unacceptable	Not Applicable	Comments
1. Verifies order				
2. Obtains appropriate equipment				
3. Washes hands				
4. Prepares a heparinized syringe properly				
5. Attaches syringes aseptically				
6. Operates appropriate stopcock correctly				
7. Obtains an initial sample				
8. Discards initial sample				
9. Obtains arterial blood sample for analysis				
10. "Flushes" the arterial line properly				
11. Returns stopcock to proper positions				
12. Prepares the obtained sample properly: A. Removes air bubbles B. Labels the sample appropriately C. Place sample in a container of ice water slush				

Knowledge of Procedure

- ☐ Good; student is knowledgeable about rationale and theory related to procedure
- ☐ Fair; student has adequate understanding of rationale and theory related to procedure
- ☐ Poor; student has inadequate understanding of rationale and theory related to procedure

Performance Deficiencies (check those that apply)

- ☐ Excessive time needed to complete procedure
- ☐ Broke aseptic or sterile technique
- ☐ Gross inaccuracy noted
- ☐ Technique may be harmful to patient
- ☐ Incorrect dosage or gas concentration
- ☐ Incorrect equipment assembly/use
- ☐ Unable to answer questions correctly about rationale and/or theory related to procedure
- ☐ Other ______________________________

Evaluation Summary

- ☐ Satisfactory performance
- ☐ Unsatisfactory performance

Recommendations of Evaluator

- ☐ Skills may be applied/observed in clinical setting
- ☐ Specific evaluation deficiencies require correction
- ☐ Complete re-evaluation required
- ☐ Additional laboratory practice required

Signatures:

Evaluator ______________________ Date ______________________

Student ______________________ Date ______________________

Laboratory Report

Student ______________________ Acceptable ______________________

Date ______________________ Unacceptable ______________________

Course ______________________

Topic: Indwelling Arterial Line Sampling

Scenario: Over the weekend, Mr. Kalb, a patient who had shown marked improvement, has deteriorated. In Report this morning, you learn that he has been reintubated and transferred to the medical intensive care unit. He is being ventilated with a volume ventilator. A Swan-Ganz catheter and indwelling arterial line are in place.

Also during Report, you are informed that arterial samples obtained from Mr. Kalb's line by the night nurse have been unreliable. Your shift supervisor has suggested that the erroneous results are probably due to the technique used to obtain the sample. Your first order of business for the a.m. is to obtain a reliable arterial blood sample from Mr. Kalb's line. Please describe in detail the following:

1. Equipment necessary before drawing the sample.

2. Technique used to obtain the sample from the line.

3. Why is the arterial line "flushed" occasionally?

4. Name three complications associated with indwelling arterial lines:
   A.

   B.

   C.

5. Describe the manner in which you will prepare your obtained sample for analysis.

6. Diagram and label the parts in an arterial line system.
   A. Arterial catheter
   B. Three-way stopcock
   C. Connecting tubing
   D. Intravenous fluid (pressurized)
   E. Pressure transducer
   F. Transducer cable
   G. Valve stem
   H. Intraflow device
   I. Luer connectors
7. In which direction will blood flow if the catheter stopcock lever is rotated:
   A. toward the catheter?
   B. toward the syringe?
   C. toward the intraflow device?
8. What is the function of a valve stem in an arterial line?

9. Why must a pressurized heparin solution be used to maintain patency in an artificial line?

10. Immediately after withdrawing a blood sample from an arterial line, you need to take what steps to

A. prevent blood clots from forming?

B. prevent the transmission of microbes?

chapter 22

Blood gas analysis

INTRODUCTION

Blood gas analysis consists of exposing a blood sample to special electrodes that measure the *p*H, partial pressure of carbon dioxide (P_{CO_2}), and partial pressure of oxygen (P_{O_2}) in blood. The *p*H is potentiometrically measured with a Sanz electrode. A modification of the Sanz *p*H electrode, the Severinghaus electrode, is used in the potentiometric measurement of P_{CO_2}. The P_{O_2} of blood is amperometrically measured with a Clark electrode.

Before the introduction of a blood sample into the analyzer, the electrodes should be calibrated to improve the accuracy of the measurement. Calibration involves the exposure of the electrodes to known values or standards and subsequent adjustment of the analyzer electronics to indicate the known value. One or two-point calibration may be performed before the analysis. The calibration of the *p*H electrode involves a solution of buffer containing a known *p*H, whereas the Severinghaus and Clark electrodes are usually exposed to special mixtures of calibration gases in which the P_{CO_2} and P_{O_2} may be determined. By convention, the electrodes are usually maintained at 37° C and calibrated under conditions of body temperature and pressure saturated (BTPS). When extreme precision is required, however, the electrode temperature may be adjusted to that at which the blood sample was obtained.

In recent years, blood gas analyzers have evolved into highly sophisticated, computerized instruments that have simplified the calibration and analysis procedures; however, the student may benefit from learning to manually calibrate and operate a blood gas analyzer. In this chapter, you are introduced to the technique of blood gas analysis.

OBJECTIVES

After completing this chapter, you should be able to do the following:

1. *Understand the procedure of blood gas and pH analysis.*
2. *Calculate the P_{CO_2} and P_{O_2} calibration points given the barometric pressure and concentration of calibration gases.*

3. *Understand the functions of the Sanz, Severinghaus, and Clark electrodes.*
4. *Identify common sources of error in blood gas analysis.*

EQUIPMENT NEEDED

☐ Blood gas analyzer and calibration gases
☐ High and low pH buffer solutions (7.384 and 6.840)
☐ pH electrode flush solution
☐ Tonometered blood samples, an arterial blood sample, or calibration fluid controls

ACTIVITIES

Exercise A: Identification of Blood Gas Analyzer Components and Controls

1. The laboratory instructor will provide you with a blood gas analyzer. Identify the typical controls of a blood gas analyzer (Fig. 22-1)
   - **A.** pH display
   - **B.** P_{CO_2} display
   - **C.** P_{O_2} display
   - **D.** pH balance control
   - **E.** P_{CO_2} balance control
   - **F.** P_{O_2} balance control
   - **G.** Mode selector
   - **H.** pH slope control
   - **I.** P_{CO_2} slope control
   - **J.** P_{O_2} slope control
   - **K.** Temperature selector switches
   - **L.** Power light
   - **M.** On/off switch
   - **N.** Sample inlet valve

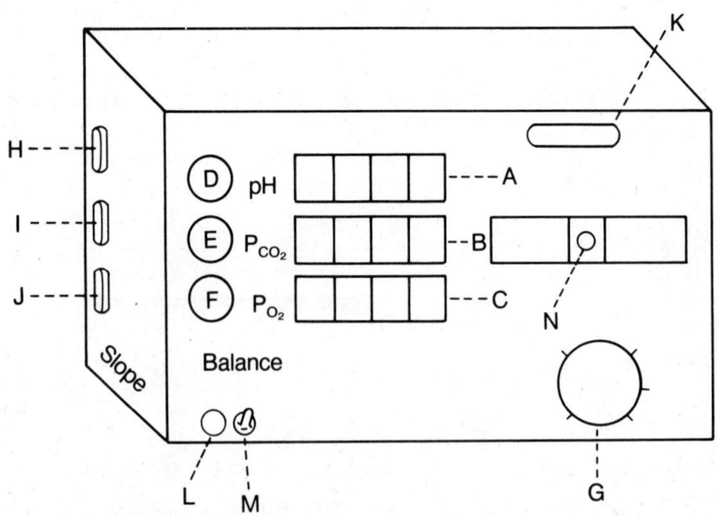

Fig. 22-1. Components of a blood gas analyzer.

Exercise B: Preparation of Analyzer for Analysis

Each student is expected to calibrate the blood gas analyzer and simulate the actual analysis of a blood sample. At no time is a student to practice the calibration or analysis of a sample without the supervision of the instructor.

Warm-up. To function accurately, the heater, sample chamber, and all electrodes must have reached a stable temperature of 37°C (or the temperature selected by the operator). In addition, the flow rate bubble chambers must be equilibrated with the calibrating gases. Allow 20 minutes for warm-up.

Calculations. Analyzed gases of known carbon dioxide and oxygen contents are used as calibration standards for the P_{CO_2} and P_{O_2} electrodes. Calculations should be determined as follows:

1. Determine the ambient barometric pressure of the day in millimeters of mercury by reading a mercury barometer. *Note:* When reading a mercury barometer, read the scale that corresponds to the mercury level (Fig. 22-2).
2. Subtract the water vapor pressure (47 mm Hg at a temperature of 37°C).
3. Multiply the remainder, the pressure of the gas alone, by the decimal fraction of the carbon dioxide and the oxygen of each of the calibration gas mixtures to obtain the partial pressure for these gases.

Example 1

PB = 760 mm Hg
pH_2O = 47 mm Hg
Low calibration gas = 0.05 CO_2
X = Partial pressure of CO_2(P_{CO_2} low calibration point)
X = $(pB - PH_20) \times$ percent gas
$= (760 - 47) \times 0.05$
$= 713 \times 0.05$
P_{CO_2} low calibration point = 35.7 mm Hg

Example 2

PB = 755 mm Hg
PH_2O = 47 mm Hg
High calibration gas = 0.12 CO_2
X = P_{CO_2} (high calibration point)

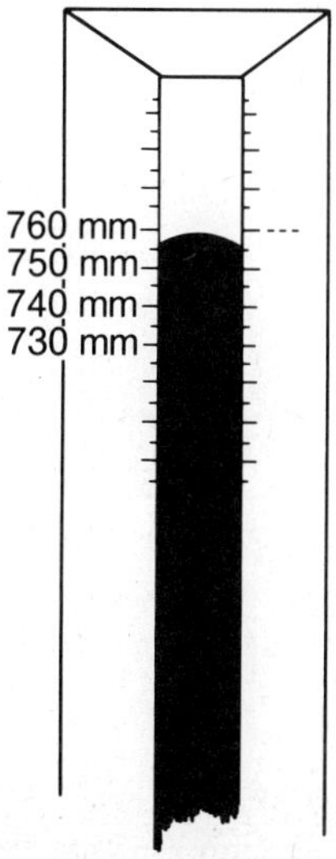

Fig. 22-2. Example of mercury barometer reading.

$$X = (PB = PH_2O \times \text{percent gas}$$
$$= (755 - 47) \times 0.12$$
$$= 708 \times 0.12$$

P_{CO_2} high calibration point = 84.96 mm Hg

Therefore, in example one, the P_{CO_2} balance control is adjusted to 35.7 mm Hg after exposing the electrode to the calibration gas.

Exercise C: Analyzer Calibration

Two-Point Calibration: A two-point calibration is usually performed after prolonged periods of analyzer inactivity. The specific calibration procedure may vary according to individual instruments. Consult your laboratory instructor or the operator's manual for the specific sequence of steps required for the analyzer you are using. A two-point calibration usually involves the following steps:

pH

- Introduce low pH buffer solution (6.840) into the pH electrode
- Adjust the pH balance control to 6.840
- Flush the pH electrode
- Introduce high pH buffer solution (7.384) into the pH electrode
- Adjust the pH slope control to 7.384

P_{CO_2} AND P_{O_2} ELECTRODES

- Determine the high and low calibration points for P_{CO_2} from the percentage concentration of the calibration gases and the observed barometric pressure.
- Expose the P_{CO_2} and P_{O_2} electrodes to the low calibration gas.
- Adjust the P_{CO_2} balance control to the low calibration point.
- Expose the P_{CO_2} and P_{O_2} electrodes to the high calibration gas.
- Adjust the P_{CO_2} slope control to the high calibration point.
- Adjust the P_{O_2} slope control to zero.
- Re-expose the P_{CO_2} and P_{O_2} electrodes to the low calibration gas.
- Check the P_{CO_2} reading. If necessary, adjust the P_{CO_2} with the balance control.
- Adjust the P_{O_2} balance control to the appropriate calibration point.

Exercise D: Sample Analysis

1. Before analysis of a sample, a one-point calibration of the analyzer is needed. The following steps are usually involved in a manual one-point calibration.

   One-Point Calibration

   - Flush the pH electrode.
   - Expose the pH electrode to high buffer (7.384).
   - Adjust the balance control to 7.384.
   - Expose the P_{CO_2} and P_{O_2} electrodes to the low calibration gas.
   - Adjust the P_{CO_2} and P_{O_2} balance controls to the appropriate calibration points.
2. An example of a one-point calibration at a barometric pressure of 760 mm Hg and using calibration gas containing 12% O_2 and 5% CO_2 follows (Fig. 22-3).
3. Adjust the analyzer mode selector to the sample position.
4. Mix the blood sample by rolling the syringe between your hands or by shaking the sample. (Fig. 22-4).
5. Remove the cap to the sample.
6. Slowly inject the blood sample into the sample chamber. Be certain that no air bubbles are introduced (Fig. 22-5).

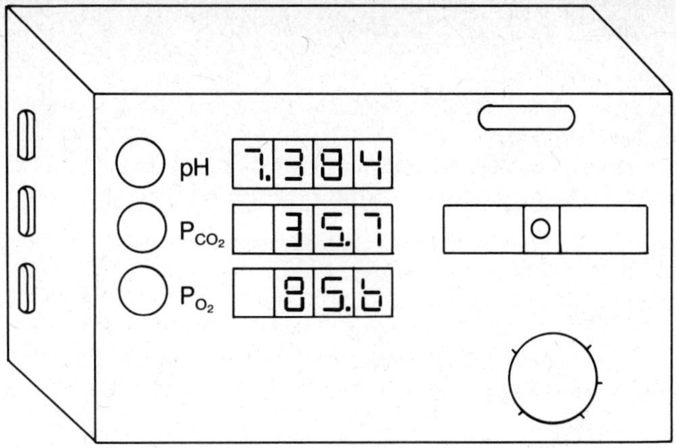

Fig. 22-3. One-point calibration of a blood gas analyzer using the balance controls.

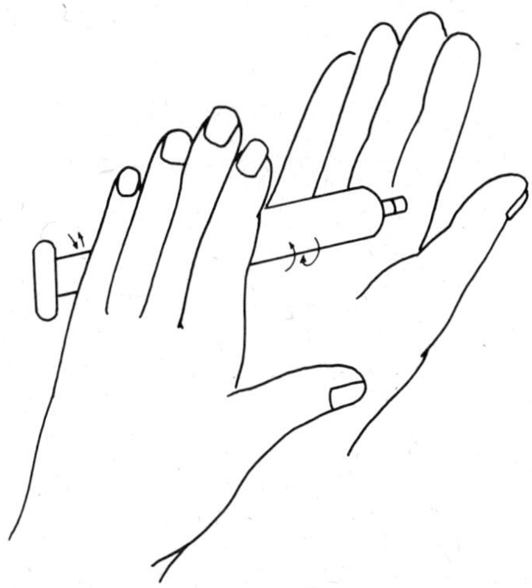

Fig. 22-4. Mixing of blood sample before injection in order to mix blood with heparin.

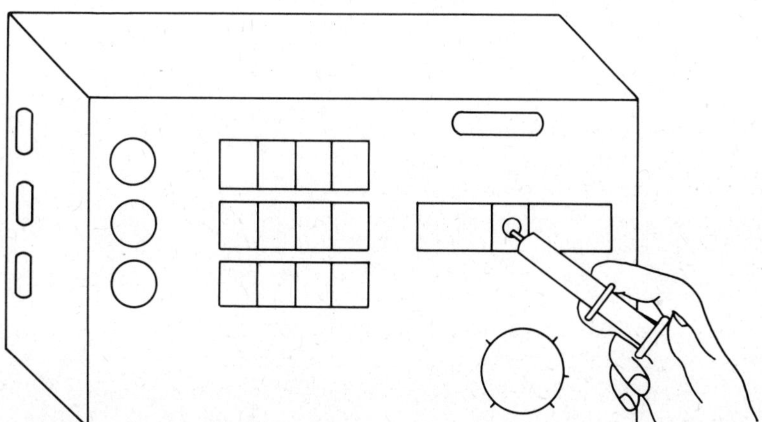

Fig. 22-5. Injection of a blood sample into the sampling inlet of a blood gas analyzer.

Exercise E: Preparation of Analyzer for Standby Mode

1. Flush the sample chamber with saline.
2. Allow saline to soak the P_{CO_2} and P_{O_2} electrodes by leaving a saline-filled syringe attached to the sample inlet.
3. Aspirate fresh 7.384 buffer into the *p*H measuring electrode.
4. Turn the electrometer mode selector to the standby position.

Exercise F: Determination of "Unknown"

Your laboratory instructor will provide you with an "unknown" sample for analysis. Analyze the sample after performing a one-point calibration. Record the results of the analysis (*p*H, P_{CO_2}, and P_{O_2}) on the laboratory report. *Note to the instructor:* An "unknown" sample may consist of tonometric blood or commercially available quality control fluids.

RECOMMENDED READING

Burton GG, Hodgkin JE: Respiratory Care. A guide to Clinical Practice, 2nd ed. Philadelphia, JB Lippincott, 1984

Kacmarek RM, Dimas S, Mack C: Essentials of Respiratory Therapy, 2nd ed. Chicago, Year Book Medical Publishers, 1985

Ruppel G: Manual of Pulmonary Functon Testing, 2nd ed. St Louis, CV Mosby, 1979

Shapiro BA, Harrison RA, Walton JR: Clinical Application of Blood Gases, 3rd ed. Chicago, Year Book Medical Publishers, 1982

Laboratory Performance Evaluation (#22)

Topic: Blood Gas Analysis

Student ______________________ Course ______________________

Date ______________________ Section ______________________

Performance Elements	Acceptable	Unacceptable	Not Applicable	Comments
1. Allows machine adequate warm-up time				
2. Performs a one-point calibration: **A.** Flushes sample chamber **B.** Adjusts *p*H balance control				
3. Determines P_{CO_2} and P_{O_2} calibration points **A.** Adjusts P_{CO_2} balance control **B.** Adjusts P_{O_2} balance control				
4. Mixes blood sample				
5. Injects blood sample into analyzer				
6. Reads and records results				
7. Flushes sample chamber				
8. Sets/returns analyzer to "standyby" mode				

Knowledge of Procedure

- ☐ Good; student is knowledgeable about rationale and theory related to procedure
- ☐ Fair; student has adequate understanding of rationale and theory related to procedure
- ☐ Poor; student has inadequate understanding of rationale and theory related to procedure

Performance Deficiencies (check those that apply)

- ☐ Excessive time needed to complete procedure
- ☐ Broke aseptic or sterile technique
- ☐ Gross inaccuracy noted
- ☐ Technique may be harmful to patient
- ☐ Incorrect dosage or gas concentration
- ☐ Incorrect equipment assembly/use
- ☐ Unable to answer questions correctly about rationale and/or theory related to procedure
- ☐ Other ______________________________

Evaluation Summary

- ☐ Satisfactory performance
- ☐ Unsatisfactory performance

Recommendations of Evaluator

- ☐ Skills may be applied/observed in clinical setting
- ☐ Specific evaluation deficiencies require correction
- ☐ Complete re-evaluation required
- ☐ Additional laboratory practice required

Signatures:

Evaluator ______________________ Date ______________________

Student ______________________ Date ______________________

Laboratory Report

Student ______________________ Acceptable ______________________

Date ______________________ Unacceptable ______________________

Course ______________________

Topic: Blood Gas Analysis

Data and/or Measurements

Unknown Sample Results

*p*H ______________________

P_{CO_2} ______________________

P_{O_2} ______________________

Scenario: For the past week, you have been working the evening shift in the blood gas laboratory. About halfway through the shift, your main analyzer become inoperable. The laboratory's standby analyzer is one of the older models, but you will need it to analyze arterial blood samples by performing a single-point calibration.

1. List in the sequence that you would perform them, the steps for performing a single-point calibration.

   A.

   B.

   C.

   D.

   E.

2. What are three common causes of inaccuracy of results obtained from arterial blood gas analysis?

   A.

   B.

   C.

3. When should a two-point calibration be performed on an analyzer?

4. When or how often should a single-point calibration be performed on a blood gas analyzer?

5. At what temperature is the water bath of a blood gas analyzer maintained?

6. Given the barometric pressure is 762 mm Hg and the low calibration gas contains 5% O_2 with 83% N_2 and 12% CO_2, what is the

P_{CO_2} calibration point? ________________________________

P_{O_2} calibration point? ________________________________

7. Briefly describe the function of
the Sanz electrode:

the Clark electrode:

the Severinghaus electrode:

chapter 23

Transcutaneous gas analysis

INTRODUCTION

The measurement of respiratory gases that have diffused from arterial blood through skin is known as transcutaneous gas analysis. The partial pressure of oxygen and carbon dioxide may be measured by the application of specially modified electrodes to the skin. Transcutaneous oxygen tension may be polarographically measured by means of a modified Clark electrode. The use of a modified Severinghaus electrode allows for the potentiometric measurement of transcutaneous carbon dioxide tension. When the modified electrodes are heated and applied to the skin, hyperemia or "arterialization" of skin blood flow may occur. Although transcutaneous gases are physiologically different from arterial blood gases, the values may be similar when local perfusion, skin thickness, blood pressure, and cardiac index are adequate. In the clinical setting, transcutaneous gas analysis may be used as a dynamic reflection of arterial blood gas milieu. The purpose of this chapter is to introduce you to transcutaneous gas analysis.

OBJECTIVES

After completing this chapter you should be able to do the following:

1. *Identify the typical components of a transcutaneous gas analyzer.*
2. *Prepare an electrode for application to the skin.*
3. *Perform a two-point calibration of a transcutaneous gas analyzer.*
4. *Measure the transcutaneous P_{O_2} during oxygen administration.*

EQUIPMENT NEEDED

- ☐ Transcutaneous analyzer
- ☐ Electrode preparation kit

- ☐ Calibration gases or zeroing solution
- ☐ Barometer
- ☐ Electrode contact gel and stablilizing ring
- ☐ Alcohol swab
- ☐ Tape
- ☐ Oxygen source
- ☐ Venturi mask

ACTIVITIES

Exercise A: Identification of Analyzer Components and Controls

1. Your instructor will provide you with a transcutaneous gas analyzer and the operator's manual or additional learning materials. Become thoroughly familiar with the operation of the analyzer before completing these exercises. In addition, assemble a Venturi mask near the transcutaneous monitor before beginning Exercise D.
2. Examine the transcutaneous analyzer and its electrode(s) (Fig. 23-1)
3. Identify the following typical controls and components:
   - A. P_{O_2} electrode
   - B. Zero calibration dial
   - C. High calibration dial
   - D. Temperature selection switch
   - E. Transcutaneous P_{O_2} display
   - F. Temperature display
   - G. System power switch
   - H. P_{O_2} high/low alarms
   - I. Temperature high/low alarms
   - J. Maximum electrode power
   - K. Electrode storage holder
   - L. Chart paper (if appplicable)
4. Prepare the unit for use by activating the power source and turning the system power switch on. A 15 to 20 minute warm-up period is typically needed for most units.

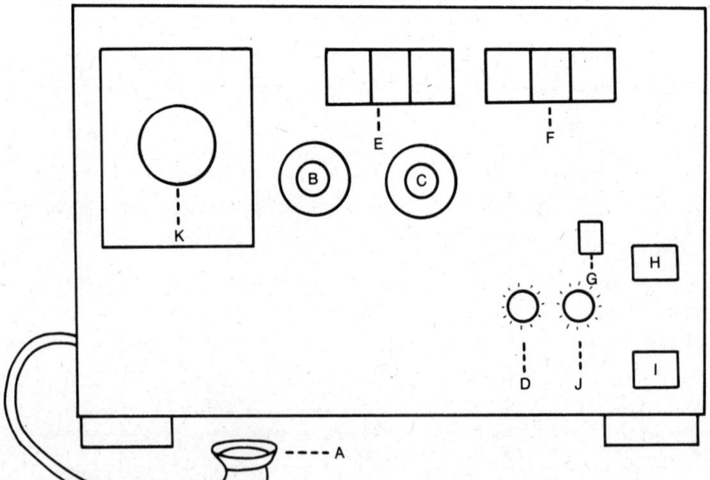

Fig. 23-1. Transcutaneous gas analyzer and electrode.

5. Silence any audible alerts or alarms.
6. Verify that the electrode has been plugged into the monitor inlet.

Exercise B: Preparation of Electrode

1. Prepare the transcutaneous oxygen electrode according to the manufacturer's recommendations. Preparation of the electrode usually involves the application of electrolyte and attachment of a disposable membrane to the electrode.
2. Verify that no air bubbles have been trapped within the membrane or electrolyte when the electrode was prepared. The presence of large air bubbles may be a source of inaccurate measurements.
3. Adjust the electrode temperature to the desired setting. Allow an adequate period for stabilization of the temperature. With normal cardiac index, blood pressure, local perfusion, and skin thickness, good correlations between transcutaneous and arterial P_{O_2} occur at the following temperatures:

Adult	44–45°C
Neonate	43–44°C

4. Be certain that the electrode has reached a stable temperature before attempting calibration of the electrode.
5. At any time, should the membrane become loose or leak electrolyte solution, the entire preparation procedure should be repeated.

Exercise C: Analyzer Calibration

1. Calibrate the analyzer according to manufacturer's recommendations. Frequently, a two-point calibration procedure is performed by exposing the electrode to both high and low P_{O_2} values and adjusting the analyzer accordingly.

Low Calibration

2. The two-point calibration may involve exposure of the electrode to a partial pressure of oxygen equal to zero. The calibration of the analyzer to a P_{O_2} of zero may be accomplished by exposing the electrode to calibration gas containing no oxygen or by use of a P_{O_2} zeroing solution.
3. Following electrode exposure to zero oxygen, adjust the zero calibration control to read zero on the transcutaneous P_{O_2} display. Allow an adequate period for stabilization to occur.

High Calibration

4. Remove the zeroing solution with gauze (or expose the electrode to the high calibration gas mixture).
5. Expose the electrode to ambient air (or to a high calibration gas). The barometric pressure and ambient temperature determine the partial pressure of oxygen to which the analyzer is adjusted. *Note:* At a barometric pressure of 760 mm Hg, relative humidity of 50%, and ambient temperature of 22° or 24°C, the partial pressure of oxygen in room air is equal to 157 mm Hg. For calibration conditions other than those listed, see your laboratory instructor for assistance.
6. Adjust the high calibration knob until the desired P_{O_2} value is indicated on the transcutaneous P_{O_2} display (Fig. 23-2).
7. Recalibrate the analyzer each time the electrode is removed from a sampling site.
8. After calibration of the electrode, the transcutaneous P_{O_2} reading should remain relatively stable. To observe responsiveness of the electrode, gently exhale air into the electrode. The electrode should measure a slight decrease in the P_{O_2} of air, and the reading should correspondingly decrease several millimeters of mercury for a few moments. After the momentary decrease, the reading should approach and stabilize near the high calibration point.

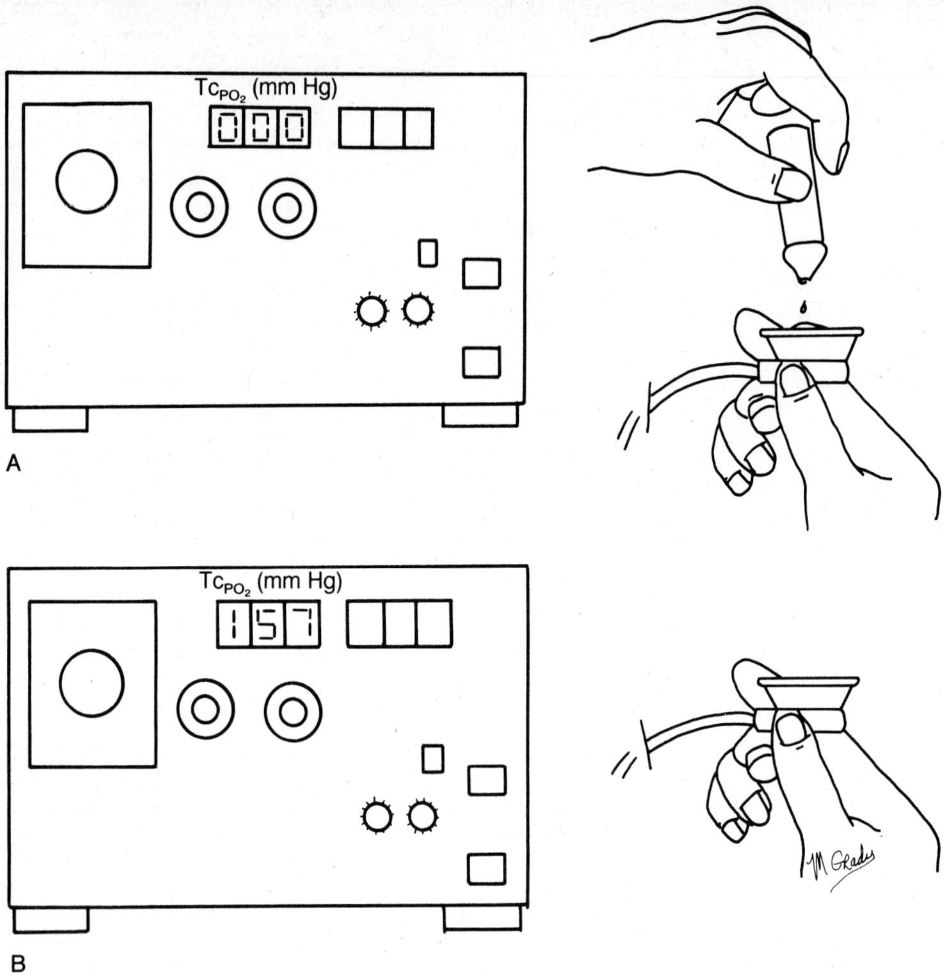

Fig. 23-2. Two-point calibration of oxygen electrode with *(A)* zeroing solution and *(B)* ambient air.

Exercise D: Site Preparation and Electrode Attachment

1. Select a site for attachment of the electrode. Criteria for adequate attachment sites include a flat surface, good perfusion, and normal skin thickness. Bony areas and locations with large fat deposits are to be avoided. For adults, the upper chest (beneath the clavicles) and abdomen are sites frequently used. In neonates, the upper chest, temporal region, abdomen, and inner thigh areas may be used (Fig. 23-3).
2. Degrease the site by swabbing the skin with alcohol. Allow the alcohol to dry.
3. Apply and remove a piece of cellophane tape to the area to remove dead skin.
4. If necessary, shave the area to allow an airtight fit between the electrode and the skin.
5. Attach an adhesive ring (if applicable) to the electrode.
6. Apply a drop of contact gel to the membrane of the electrode. Avoid contact between the contact gel and the adhesive ring.
7. Remove the protective layer of the adhesive ring, and firmly press the electrode against the skin (Fig. 23-4).

8. The transcutaneous P_{O_2} reading should show a large decrease until stabilization occurs. Allow the electrode to stabilize for 15 to 20 minutes. After stabilization of the transcutaneous P_{O_2} reading, monitor and record the transcutaneous P_{O_2} during breathing of ambient air ($F_{IO_2} = 0.21$).

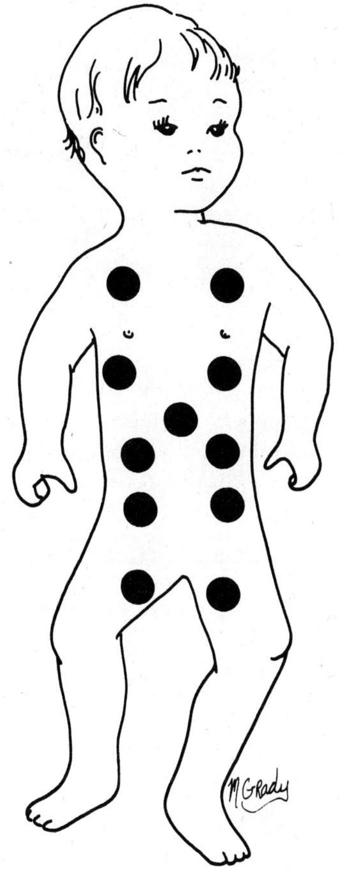

Fig. 23-3. Common sites for transcutaneous electrode placement on a neonate.

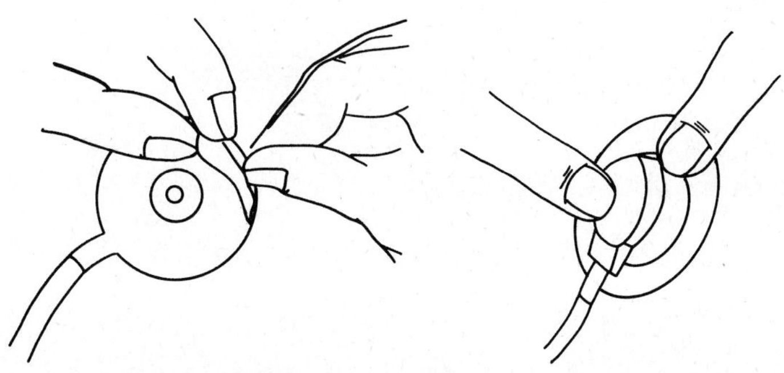

A B

Fig. 23-4. Preparation of the transcutaneous electrode for attachment to the skin by *(A)* removal of adhesive ring and *(B)* attachment to the skin. *(Modified from Novametrix Medical Systems, Wallingford, CT)*

Exercise E: Analysis of Transcutaneous Gas Tensions During Oxygen Inhalation

1. After stabilization of the transcutaneous P_{O_2} electrode, determine the effect of oxygen inhalation on the transcutaneous P_{O_2}.
2. Set up a Venturi mask to deliver the following oxygen concentrations:

   FI_{O_2}

   A. 0.21
   B. 0.24
   C. 0.28
   D. 0.40
   E. 0.50
3. After the application of a transcutaneous P_{O_2} electrode to either yourself or a laboratory partner, allow breathing of each of the indicated oxygen concentrations for 15 to 20 minutes or until a stabilized transcutaneous P_{O_2} value is indicated on the monitor.
4. Record the transcutaneous P_{O_2} value obtained after breathing each of the indicated oxygen concentrations on the laboratory report.
5. Disassemble all equipment. Remove the electrode and carefully place it in a protective container. Turn the power off to the monitor.
6. Evaluate the sampling site. Because transcutaneous electrodes apply heat to the skin, complications may occur, including blisters, erythema (diffuse redness), edema, and eschar (scab) formation. In clinical use, close monitoring of the sampling site and changing the location of the electrode at regular intervals (2–6 hours) may minimize complications.

RECOMMENDED READING

Blodgett D: Manual of Pediatric Respiratory Care Procedures. Philadelphia, JB Lippincott Company, 1982

Burgess WR, Chernick V: Respiratory Therapy in Newborn Infants and Children. New York, Thieme-Stratton, 1982

Lough MD, Williams TJ, Rawson JE: Newborn Respiratory Care. Chicago, Year Book Medical Publishers, 1979

McPherson SP, Spearman CB: Respiratory Therapy Equipment, 3rd ed. St Louis, CV Mosby, 1985

Ruppel G: Manual of Pulmonary Function Testing, 3rd ed. St Louis, CV Mosby, 1979

Laboratory Performance Evaluation (#23)

Topic: Transcutaneous Gas Analysis

Student ______________________ Course ______________________

Date ______________________ Section ______________________

Performance Elements	Acceptable	Unacceptable	Not Applicable	Comments
1. Obtains appropriate equipment				
2. Washes hands				
3. Prepares transcutaneous electrode(s) for use				
4. Adjusts electrode to desired temperature				
5. Calibrates transcutaneous gas analyzer: A. Zero calibration B. High calibration				
6. Prepares simulated sample site				
7. Attaches electrode to sample site				
8. Monitors electrode and analyzer function				
9. Evaluates condition of sample site				
10. Documents observations				

Knowledge of Procedure

☐ Good; student is knowledgeable about rationale and theory related to procedure

☐ Fair; student has adequate understanding of rationale and theory related to procedure

☐ Poor; student has inadequate understanding of rationale and theory related to procedure

Performance Deficiencies (check those that apply)

☐ Excessive time needed to complete procedure

☐ Broke aseptic or sterile technique

☐ Gross inaccuracy noted

☐ Technique may be harmful to patient

☐ Incorrect dosage or gas concentration

☐ Incorrect equipment assembly/use

☐ Unable to answer questions correctly about rationale and/or theory related to procedure

☐ Other ____________________

Evaluation Summary

☐ Satisfactory performance

☐ Unsatisfactory performance

Recommendations of Evaluator

☐ Skills may be applied/observed in clinical setting

☐ Specific evaluation deficiencies require correction

☐ Complete re-evaluation required

☐ Additional laboratory practice required

Signatures:

Evaluator ____________________ Date ____________________

Student ____________________ Date ____________________

Laboratory Report

Student ______________________ Acceptable ______________________

Date ______________________ Unacceptable ______________________

Course ______________________

Topic: Transcutaneous Gas Analysis

Data or Measurements

	FI_{O_2}	Stabilized Transcutaneous P_{O_2} (mm Hg)
A.	0.21	____________
B.	0.24	____________
C.	0.28	____________
D.	0.40	____________
E.	0.50	____________

Scenario: This week, for orientation purposes, you have been assigned to work in the intensive care nursery. The neonatologist in charge of the unit phones to inform you that the transport team will be arriving with a 1000 g premature infant. The estimated time of arrival is 30 minutes from now. You have been asked to prepare a transcutaneous gas analyzer for use on this patient. Please answer the following questions:

1. Assuming a barometric pressure of 757 mm Hg and a relative humidity of 50%, describe (in the order of their performance) the steps taken when performing a two-point calibration.
   A.

   B.

   C.

   D.

   E.

   F.

2. How often and when should the transcutaneous analyzer be recalibrated?

3. In this situation, the electrode should be maintained within what temperature range?

4. Describe the method used to prepare the electrode site.

5. Describe the method used to prepare the electrode.

6. How does the absence of an airtight seal between skin and electrode affect transcutaneous gas analysis?

7. What complications are associated with transcutaneous gas analysis?

8. List three accepted placement sites for transcutaneous electrodes on a neonate.

9. Compare and contrast advantages and disadvantages of arterial blood sampling and transcutaneous gas sampling.

chapter 24

Pulmonary function tests: spirometry

INTRODUCTION

Spirometry is a basic diagnostic tool used to detect and evaluate pulmonary disease. A specific quantity of gas that may be measured during a known point in the breathing cycle is a lung volume. The sum of two or more lung volumes may be defined as a lung capacity. An instrument used to measure lung volumes and capacities is a spirometer. The purpose of this chapter is to introduce you to the measurement of lung volumes and capacities using a water-sealed spirometer.

OBJECTIVES

After completing this chapter you should be able to do the following:

1. *Prepare a water-sealed spirometer for use.*
2. *Explain the breathing maneuver required for the measurement of the vital capacity.*
3. *Define the following volumes and capacities:*
   - A. *Tidal volume (VT)*
   - B. *Inspiratory reserve volume (IRV)*
   - C. *Expiratory reserve volume (ERV)*
   - D. *Residual volume (RV)*
   - E. *Inspiratory capacity (IC]*
   - F. *Functional residual capacity (FRC)*
   - G. *Vital capacity (VC)*
   - H. *Total lung capacity (TLC)*
4. *Measure the lung volumes and capacities on three laboratory partners.*
5. *Convert the measured volumes and capacities to body temperature.*

EQUIPMENT NEEDED

- ☐ Water-sealed spirometer
- ☐ Mouthpieces
- ☐ Noseclips
- ☐ Spirometer (kymograph) paper
- ☐ Disinfectant solution

ACTIVITIES

Exercise A: Spirometer Preparation

1. Examine the primary components of a water-sealed spirometer (Fig. 24-1).
2. Identify the following components:
   - **A.** Mouthpiece
   - **B.** Breathing valve
   - **C.** Kymograph
   - **D.** Pen
   - **E.** Thermometer
   - **F.** Kymograph speed switch
3. Prepare the spirometer for use according to the manufacturer's specifications or to the satisfaction of your laboratory instructor. Preparation may include the following steps:
   - **A.** Align the graph paper on the kymograph.
   - **B.** Stabilize the graph paper.

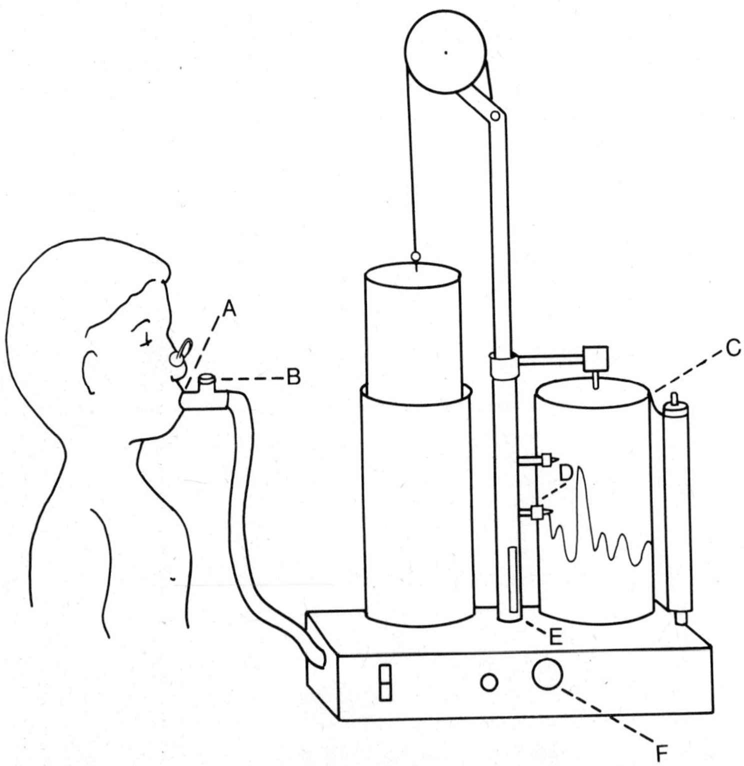

Fig. 24-1. Components of a water-sealed respirometer.

C. Adjust the kymograph speed switch to the slowest pattern.
D. Adjust the breathing valve to allow movement of the bell.
E. Lift the bell to position the pen at the lower third of the graph paper.
F. Turn the breathing valve to "lock" the bell and pen.
G. Apply a clean mouthpiece.

Exercise B: Subject Preparation

1. Request that a laboratory partner serve as a subject for measuring the lung volumes and capacities.
2. Prepare the subject for testing. Preparation should include the following steps:
   A. Inform the subject that the procedure is easy to do and is painless.
   B. Place noseclips on the subject.
   C. Request that the subject insert the mouthpiece. Explain the importance of a tight seal with the lips around the mouthpiece.
   D. Clearly give instructions to the subject to obtain a tidal volume. The subject should be told "to relax and breathe normally" (for 3–5 breaths).
   E. After the subject has become accustomed to breathing through the spirometer, turn the breathing valve on to allow the subject to breathe gas from within the bell. (The bell should move down during inhalation.)
   F. Turn the kymograph power on. The kymograph speed should be set at 160 mm/minute.
   G. Obtain a vital capacity by asking the subject to "inhale as deeply as possible and blow out all the air."
   H. Tell the subject to relax and then to remove the mouthpiece.
   I. Turn the kymograph power off.

Exercise C: Measurement of Lung Volumes and Capacities

1. Review the following definitions of the four lung volumes and four lung capacities:

   Lung Volumes

   A. Tidal volume (VT)—volume of air inhaled or exhaled during normal, resting breathing.
   B. Inspiratory reserve volume (IRV)—maximum volume of air that can be inhaled following a resting inhalation.
   C. Expiratory reserve volume (ERV)—maximum volume of air that can be exhaled following a normal, resting exhalation.
   D. Residual volume (RV)—volume of air remaining in the lungs after a complete exhalation; is not measured on a spirogram.

   Lung Capacities

   E. Inspiratory capacity (IC)—sum of the tidal volume and inspiratory reserve volume. The maximum volume of air that can be inhaled following a resting exhalation.
   F. Functional residual capacity (FRC)—the maximum volume of air in the lungs following a resting exhalation.
   G. Vital capacity (VC)—maximum amount of gas that can be exhaled following a maximum inhalation.
   H. Total lung capacity (TLC)—maximum volume of gas in the lungs after a maximum inhalation.
2. Using the following diagram, identify the lung volumes and capacities (Fig. 24–2).

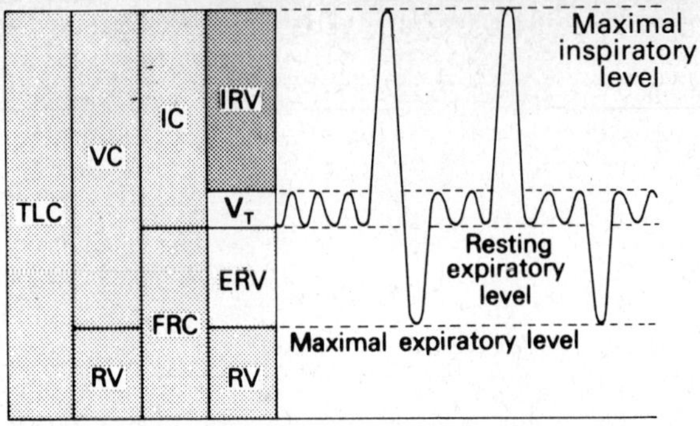

Fig. 24-2. Lung volumes and capacities. *(Adopted from Comroe JH Jr. et al: The Lung, 2nd ed. Chicago, Year Book Medical Publishers, 1962)*

3. Using the spirogram obtained from a laboratory partner, calculate the following lung volumes and capacities:
   IRV
   VT
   ERV
   VC
   IC
4. Record the calculated values on the laboratory report.
5. Obtain a spirogram tracing from two additional laboratory partners. Calculate the lung volumes and capacities and record the results on the laboratory report.

Exercise D: Temperature Conversion to BTPS

1. Since the spirometer measures the lung volumes under conditions of ambient temperature and pressure saturated (ATPS), the measured values must be converted to those which exist within the lung at body temperature and pressure saturated (BTPS). In other words, as the temperature of the exhaled gas decreases, the volume of exhaled gas deceases, as predicted by Charles' law.
2. Your laboratory instructor will provide you with a temperature conversion factor for the ambient temperature of the laboratory. Be certain to multiply the measured volumes and capacities by the temperature conversion factor. *Note:* Depending on the spirometer and system used, the results may require conversion by multiplication with a bell conversion factor. If necessary, your laboratory instructor will provide you with the appropriate conversion factor.

RECOMMENDED READING

Burton GG, Hodgkin JE: Respiratory Care. A guide to Clinical Practice, 2nd ed. Philadelphia, JB Lippincott, 1984

Kacmarek RM, Dimas S, Mack C: Essentials of Respiratory Therapy, 2nd ed. Chicago, Year Book Medical Publishers, 1985

Ruppel G: Manual of Pulmonary Functon Testing, 2nd ed. St Louis, CV Mosby, 1979

Spearman CB, Sheldon RL: Egan's Fundamentals of Respiratory Therapy, 4th ed. St Louis, CV Mosby, 1982

Laboratory Performance Evaluation (#24)

Topic: Pulmonary Function Tests: Spirometry

Student ______________________ Course ______________________

Date ______________________ Section ______________________

Performance Elements	Acceptable	Unacceptable	Not Applicable	Comments
1. Prepares spirometer				
2. Aligns paper on kymograph				
3. Adjusts kymograph speed				
4. Lifts bell so that pen is centered on graph				
5. Turns main valve to "lock" bell and pen				
6. Washes hands				
7. Instructs patient on proper method of performing procedure				
8. Places noseclips on subject				
9. Inserts mouthpiece into simulated patient				
10. Repeats the instructions to the patient: A. Relax and breathe normally B. Inhale as deeply as possible C. Exhale forcefully all air				
11. Runs kymograph as patient carries out instructions				
12. Turns kymograph off				
13. Records obtained results				

Knowledge of Procedure

☐ Good; student is knowledgeable about rationale and theory related to procedure

☐ Fair; student has adequate understanding of rationale and theory related to procedure

☐ Poor; student has inadequate understanding of rationale and theory related to procedure

Performance Deficiencies (check those that apply)

☐ Excessive time needed to complete procedure

☐ Broke aseptic or sterile technique

☐ Gross inaccuracy noted

☐ Technique may be harmful to patient

☐ Incorrect dosage or gas concentration

☐ Incorrect equipment assembly/use

☐ Unable to answer questions correctly about rationale and/or theory related to procedure

☐ Other ____________________

Evaluation Summary

☐ Satisfactory performance

☐ Unsatisfactory performance

Recommendations of Evaluator

☐ Skills may be applied/observed in clinical setting

☐ Specific evaluation deficiencies require correction

☐ Complete re-evaluation required

☐ Additional laboratory practice required

Signatures:

Evaluator ____________________ Date ____________________

Student ____________________ Date ____________________

Laboratory Report

Student ______________________ Acceptable ______________________

Date ______________________ Unacceptable ______________________

Course ______________________

Topic: Pulmonary Function Tests: Spirometry

Data and Measurements

Subj. No.	Name	Age	Sex	Wt. (kg)	IRV (BTPS)	V_T (BTPS)	ERV (BTPS)	IC (BTPS)	VC (BTPS)
1									
2									
3									
Average									

Review Questions

1. Why must expired gas volume measurements be corrected to BTPS?

2. What lung volumes must be measured in order to calculate

A. TLC?

B. VC?

C. IC?

3. List and define the four lung volumes.

4. List and define the four lung capacities.

5. Which lung volumes and capacities may not be measured with a water-sealed spirometer?

chapter 25

Pulmonary function tests: flowrates

INTRODUCTION

Flowrate measurements, or airflow volume tests, are dynamic tests that may be useful in detecting and evaluating airway obstruction. The flowrate measurements may be obtained from computerized, electronic pulmonary function apparatus or from the spirographic tracing obtained during a timed, forced vital capacity maneuver. In general, flowrates may be calculated by measuring the volume of gas exhaled during a specific time interval. The purpose of this chapter is to introduce you to the measurement of flowrates during pulmonary function testing.

OBJECTIVES

After completing this chapter, you should be able to do the following:

1. *Obtain a spirogram of a timed, forced vital capacity maneuver.*
2. *Determine the following flowrates from the spirogram:*
   A. *Forced expiratory volume (FEV_T)*
   B. *Forced vital capacity (FVC)*
   C. *Forced expiratory volume/forced vital capacity ratio ($FEV_T/FVC\%$)*
   D. *Forced expiratory flow $_{200-1200}$ ($FEF_{200-1200}$)*
   E. *Forced expiratory flow $_{25\%-75\%}$ ($FEF_{25\%-75\%}$)*
3. *Convert the measured flowrates to conditions of body temperature and pressure saturated (BTPS).*
4. *Compare the measured flowrates to the predicted flowrates by using a nomogram.*
5. *Calculate the percentage of predicted value for gas flowrates.*

EQUIPMENT NEEDED

- ☐ Water-sealed spirometer
- ☐ Mouthpiece

- ☐ Noseclips
- ☐ Spirometer kymograph paper
- ☐ Disinfectant solution
- ☐ CO_2 absorbent (soda lime)
- ☐ Straightedge
- ☐ Calculator

ACTIVITIES

Exercises A and B: Measurement of Forced Vital Capacity (FVC) and Forced Expiratory Volume (FEV_T)

1. Request that a laboratory partner serve as a subject for testing.
2. Prepare a water seal or other spirometer for use (see Chapter 24, Exercise A).
3. Prepare the subject for testing. Preparation for a forced vital capacity maneuver should include the following steps:
   A. Have the subject sit up straight in a comfortable position.
   B. Explain that the test is painless and easy to do.
   C. Place noseclips on the subject.
   D. Request that the subject insert the mouthpiece into his mouth. Explain the importance of a tight seal around the mouthpiece.
   E. Tell the subject to relax and breathe normally.
   F. After the subject has become accustomed to breathing through the spirometer, turn the breathing valve on to allow breathing of gas from within the spirometer bell (or activate the spirometer).
   G. Turn the kymograph power switch to the "on" position. The kymograph speed should be set at 160 mm/minute.
   H. Ask the subject to "inhale as much air as possible."
   I. Switch kymograph to high speed (1920 mm/minute).
   J. Ask the subject to completely blow out all air as quickly as possible.
   K. Tell the subject to resume normal breathing.
   L. Turn the kymograph power off.
4. Examine the FVC spirogram (Fig. 25-1).
5. Calculate the FVC.
   A. Measure the recorded FVC by determining the volume that corresponds to the highest and lowest point in the FVC.
   B. Subtract the lowest from the highest volume.
   C. Multiply the result by appropriate correction factors* and by the temperature conversion factor.
   D. Record the results on the laboratory report.

$$FVC_{(BTPS)} = \text{Calculated FVC} \times \text{temperature conversion factor} \times \text{(bell factor if applicable)}$$

$FEV_{1.0}$ and $FEV_{3.0}$

Calculate the forced expiratory volume in 1 second ($FEV_{1.0}$) and the forced expiratory volume in 3 seconds ($FEV_{3.0}$) (Figs. 25-2 and 25-3).

A. When referring to the examples in Figures 25-2 and 25-3, determine the point at which exhalation begins on the vital capacity curve of your spirogram. The

* *Note:* Depending on the spirometer system used, a bell correction factor may be required. Your laboratory instructor will inform you if this factor is necessary.

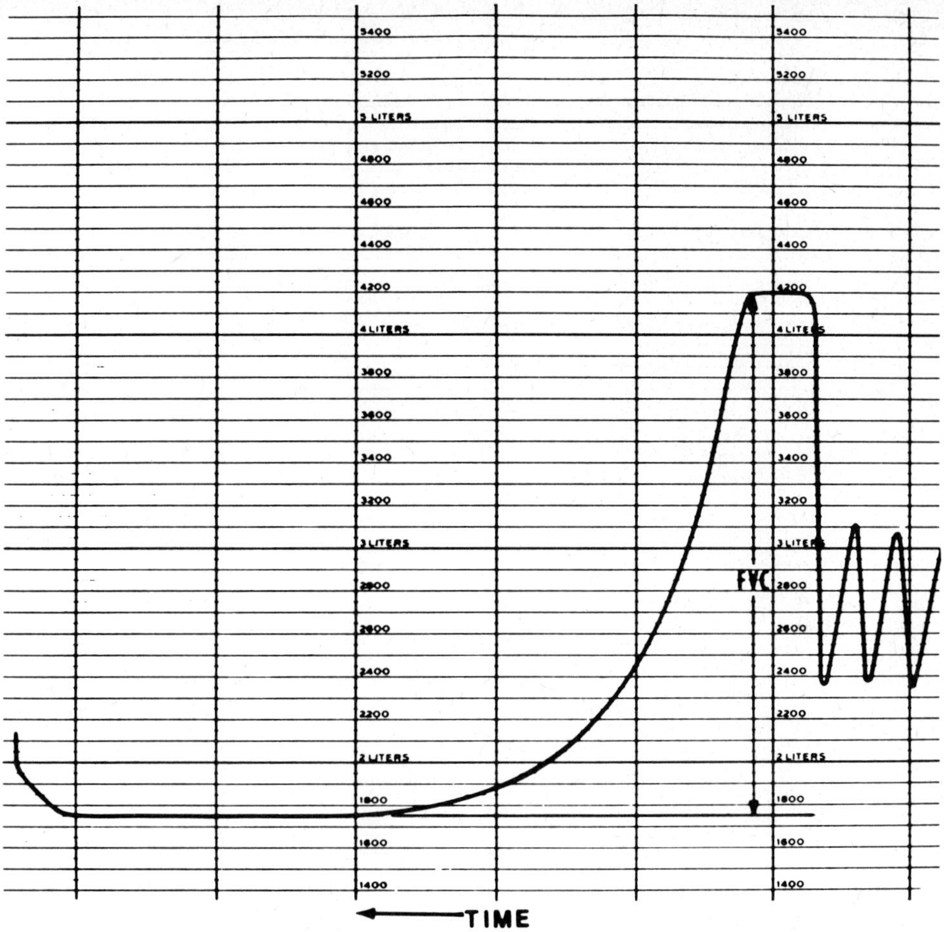

Fig. 25-1. Timed forced vital capacity spirogram. *(Reproduced with permission from Burton GG, Gee GN, Hodgkin JE: Respiratory Care. A Guide to Clinical Practice. Philadelphia, JB Lippincott, 1977)*

point at which exhalation begins may require the use of backward extrapolation to determine zero expiratory time in a timed forced vital capacity maneuver. *Note:* Be certain *not* to include the "plateau" created by an inspiratory pause in the determination of zero expiratory time. An inspiratory pause may produce a plateau when a slight delay occurs in switching the kymograph to high speed following maximum inspiration.

B. From the point of zero exhalation time on the spirogram, measure and mark off 1- and 3-second intervals on the horizontal axis. *Note:* At a kymograph speed of 1920 mm/minute, each large vertical line corresponds to 1 second.

C. At the 1- and 3-second marks, use a straightedge to draw a perpendicular line that intersects the vital capacity curve.

D. Determine the volume that corresponds to the volume of the vital capacity exhaled in 1 and 3 seconds.

E. Multiply the result by the temperature conversion factor (and additional correction factors, if applicable).

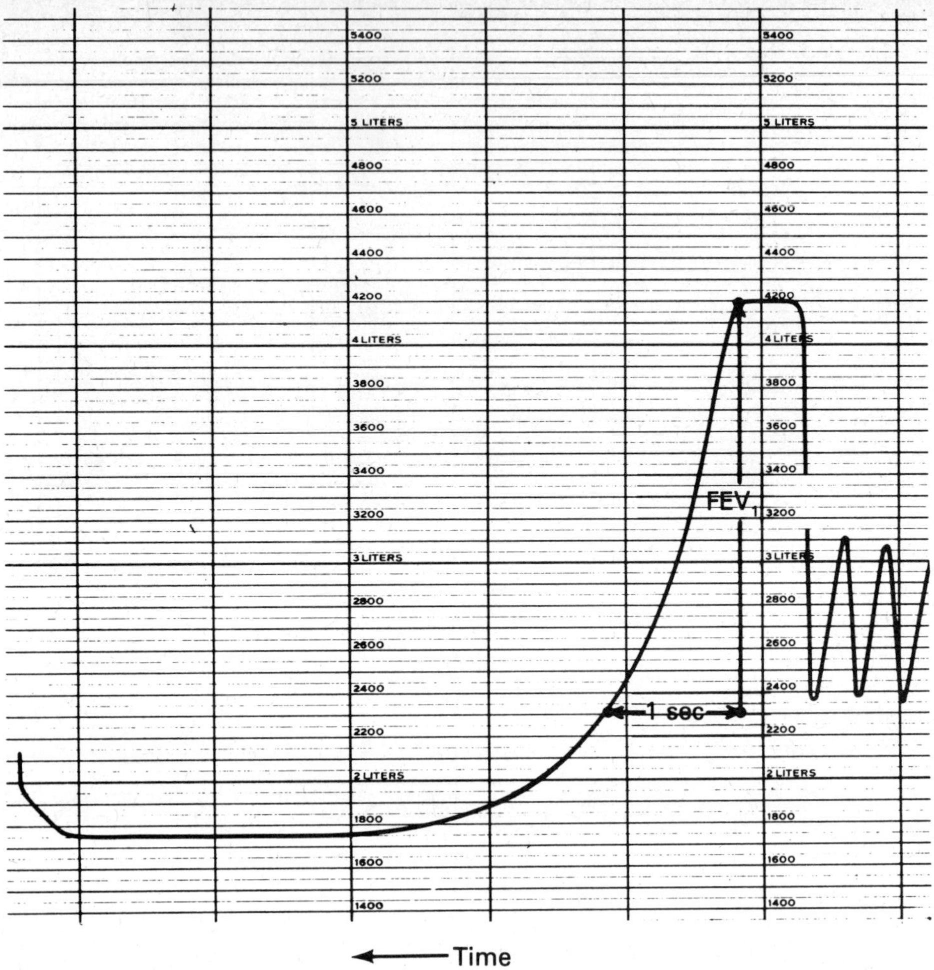

Fig. 25-2. Spirogram of $FEV_{1.0}$. *(Reproduced with permission from Burton GG, Hodgkin JG: Respiratory Care. A Guide to Clinical Practice, 2nd ed. Philadelphia, JB Lippincott, 1984)*

F. Record the results on the laboratory report.

$FEV_{1.0}$ = Calculated $FEV_{1.0}$ × temperature conversion factor × other factor if applicable

$FEV_{3.0}$ = Calculated $FEV_{3.0}$ × temperature conversion factor × other factor if applicable

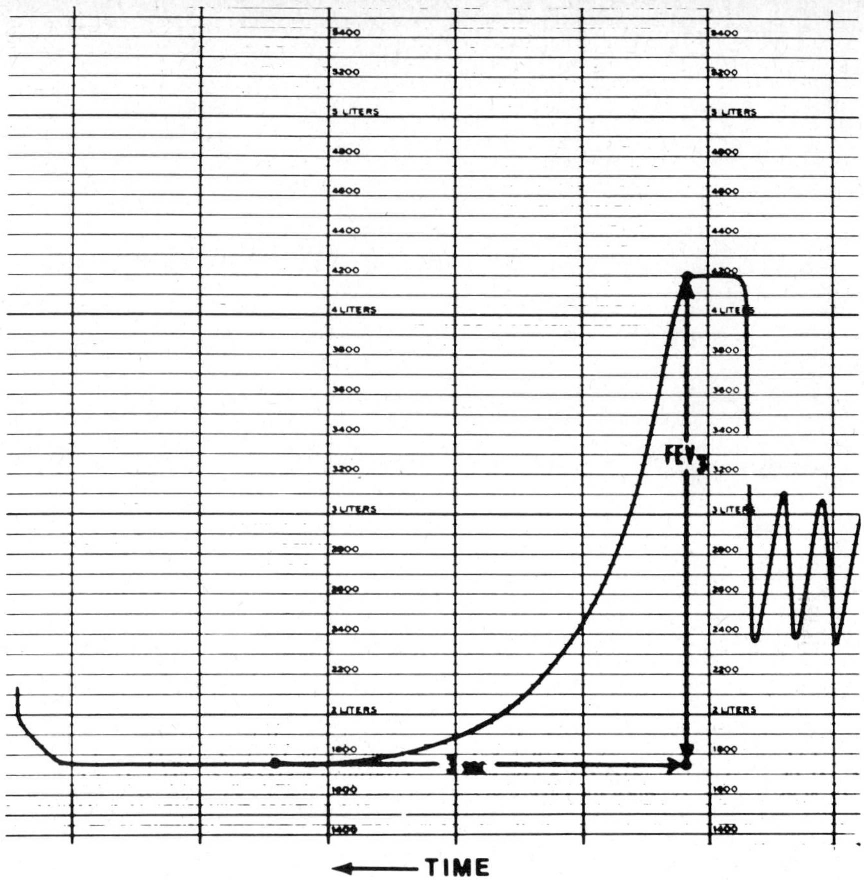

Fig. 25-3. Spirogram of $FEV_{3.0}$. *(Reproduced with permission from Burton GG, Gee GN, Hodgkin JE: Respiratory Care. A Guide to Clinical Practice. Philadelphia, JB Lippincott, 1977)*

Exercise C: Measurement of Forced Expiratory Volume/Forced Vital Capacity (FEV_T/ FVC%)

1. Using the following nomograms for either males or females, determine the predicted vital capacity for your subject. Record the measured and predicted values on the laboratory report.
2. The measured or observed vital capacity derived from the spirogram may be compared to the predicted value by the following formula:

$$\text{Percentage of predicted FVC} = \frac{\text{Measured FVC}}{\text{Predicted FVC}} \times 100$$

3. Record the percent predicted FVC on the laboratory report.

4. Determine the $FEV_T/FVC\%$ by using the following formulas:

$$\frac{FEV_T\%}{FVC} = \frac{FEV_T}{FVC} \times 100$$

$$\frac{FEV_{1.0}\%}{FVC} = \frac{FEV_{1.0}}{FVC\ (measured)} \times 100$$

$$\frac{FEV_{3.0}\%}{FVC} = \frac{FEV_{3.0}}{FVC\ (measured)} \times 100$$

5. The values for $FEV_{1.0}$, $FEV_{3.0}$, and the measured FVC should be temperature corrected before calculations for FEV_T/FVC % are done.
6. Record the results on the laboratory report.

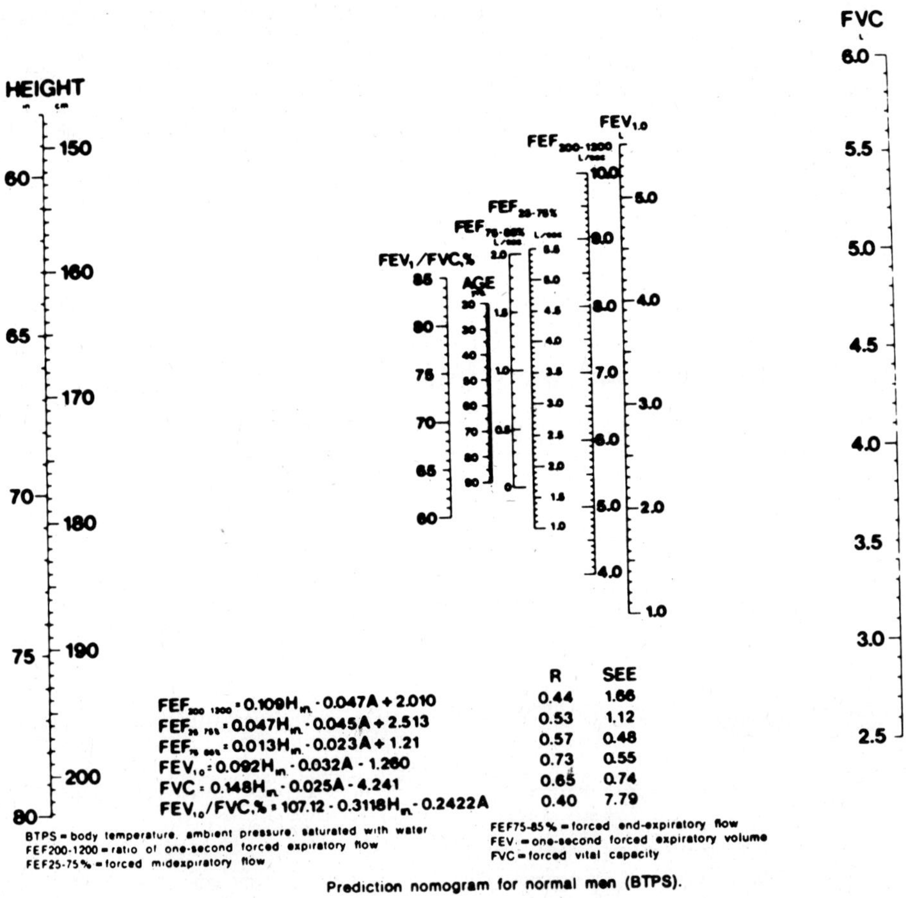

Fig. 25-4. PFT nomogram for normal men. *(Reproduced with permission from Burton GG, Gee GN, Hodgkin JE: Respiratory Care. A Guide to Clinical Practice. Philadelphia, JB Lippincott, 1977)*

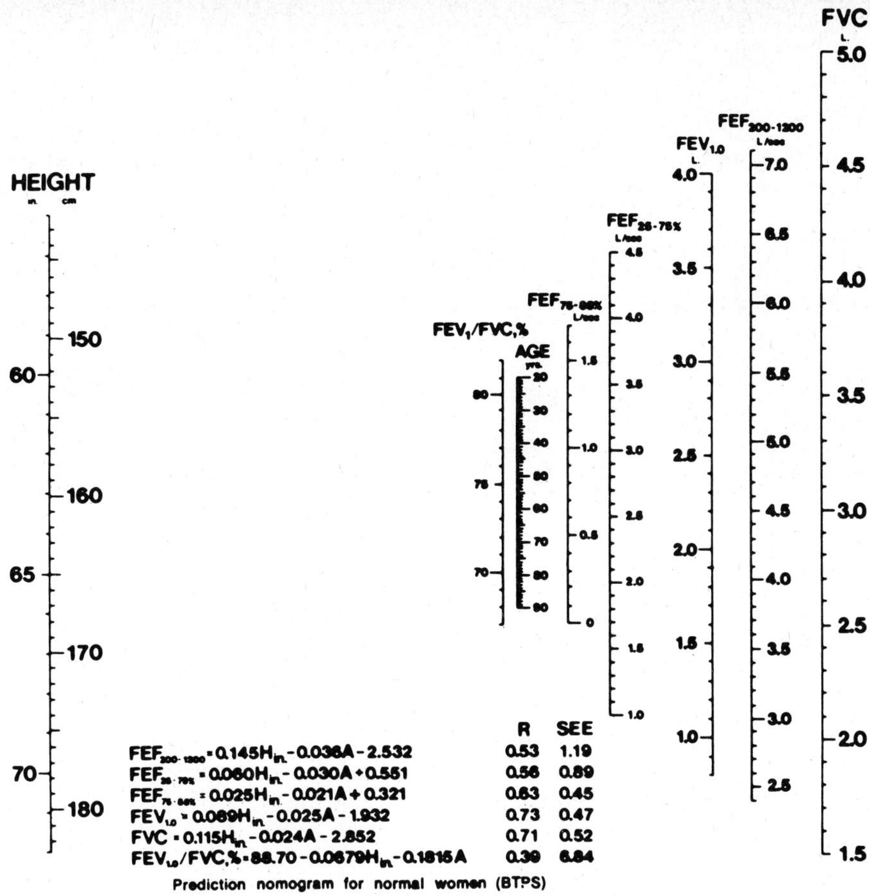

Fig. 25-5. PFT nomogram for normal women. *(Reproduced with permission from Burton GG, Gee GN, Hodgkin JE: Respiratory Care. A Guide to Clinical Practice. Philadelphia, JB Lippincott, 1977)*

Exercise D: Measurement of Forced Expiratory Flow $_{200-1200}$($FEF_{200-1200}$)

1. Obtain a spirogram of a timed forced vital capacity.
2. Determine the point of zero expiratory time (or beginning of expiration).
3. Calculate the $FEF_{200-1200}$ (Fig. 25-6).
4. While referring to the example in Figure 25-6, mark the points on the vital capacity spirogram that correspond to the first 200 ml and 1200 ml exhaled.
5. Using a straightedge, connect the 200 and 1200 points with a straight line such that the drawn line intersects two consecutive vertical time lines. The vertical time lines intersected by the drawn line should correspond to 1 second of time elapsed on the spirogram.

6. Identify the volumes that correspond to the points of intersection of the straight-edge line with the vertical time line.
7. Subtract the low volume from the high volume.
8. Multiply the result by the temperature conversion factor (and other correction factor, if applicable). Record the measured $FEF_{200-1200}$ on the laboratory report.
9. Determine the predicted $FEF_{200-1200}$ from the appropriate nomogram.
10. Calculate the percentage of predicted $FEF_{200-1200}$ using the following formula:

$$FEF_{200-1200} \text{ percent predicted} = \frac{\text{Observed } FEF_{200-1200}}{\text{Predicted } FEF_{200-1200}} \times 100$$

11. Record the percentage of predicted $FEF_{200-1200}$ on the laboratory report.

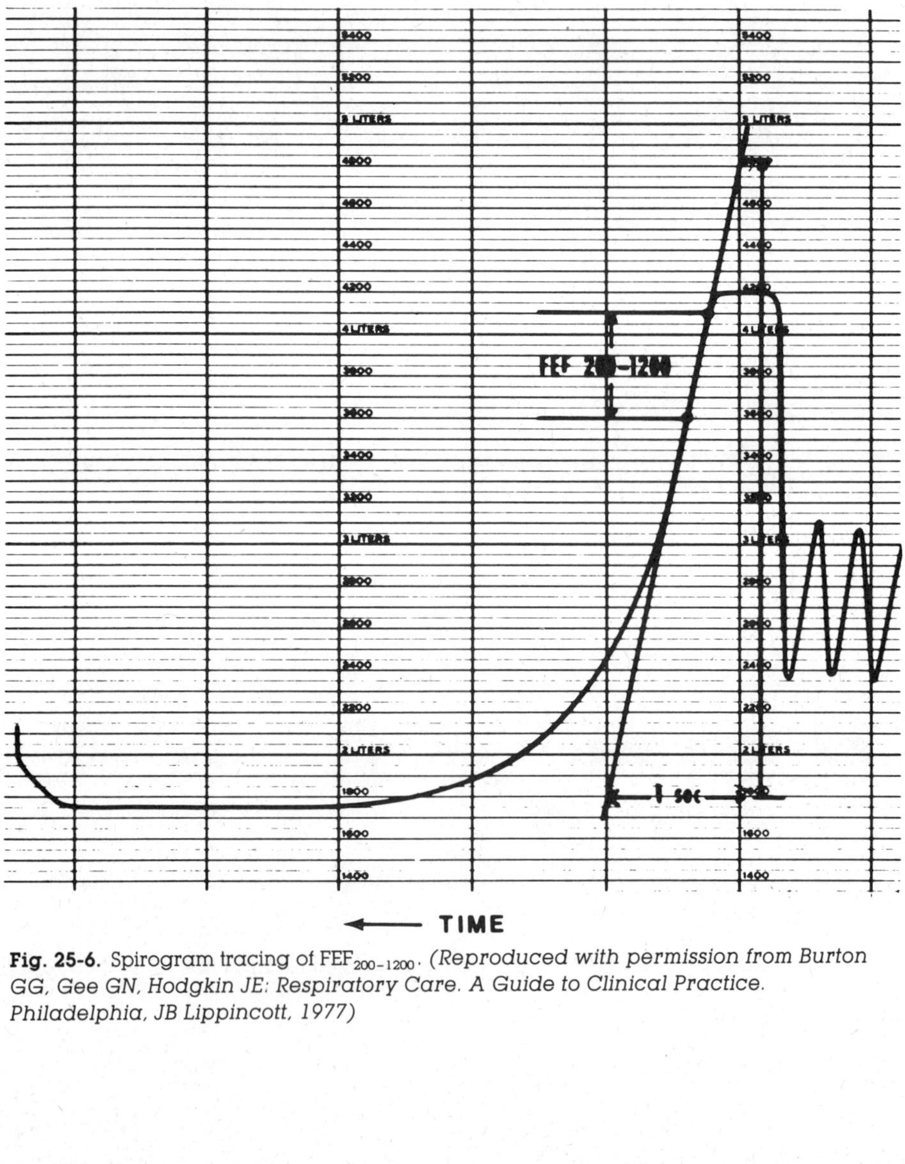

Fig. 25-6. Spirogram tracing of $FEF_{200-1200}$. *(Reproduced with permission from Burton GG, Gee GN, Hodgkin JE: Respiratory Care. A Guide to Clinical Practice. Philadelphia, JB Lippincott, 1977)*

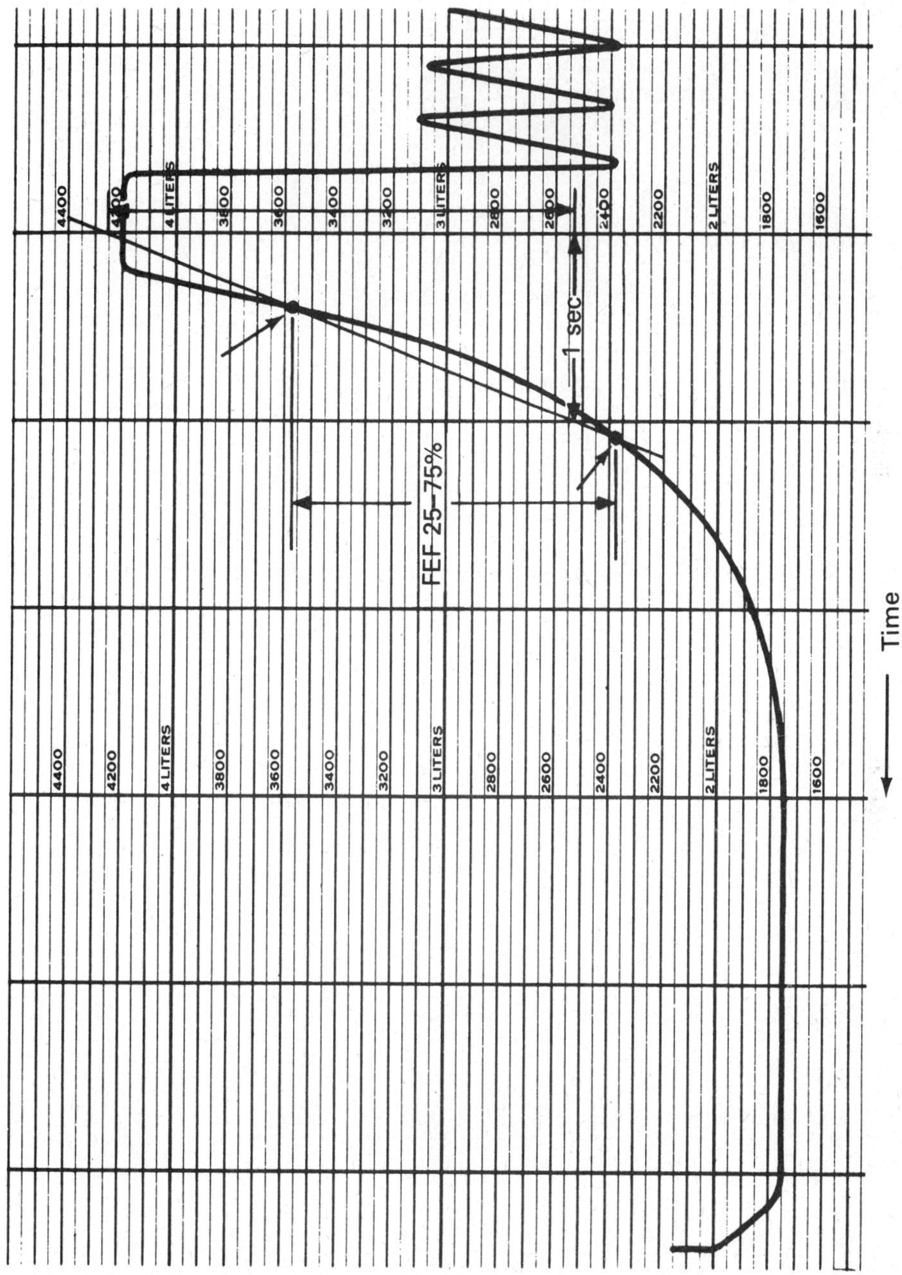

Fig. 25-7. Spirogram tracing of $FEF_{25-75\%}$. *(Reproduced with permission from Burton, GG, Hodgkin JE: Respiratory Care. A Guide to Clinical Practice, 2nd ed. Philadelphia, JB Lippincott, 1984)*

Exercise E: Measurement of Forced Expiratory Flow$_{25\%-75\%}$ ($FEF_{25\%-75\%}$)

1. Obtain a spirogram of a timed forced vital capacity.
2. Determine the point of zero expiratory time (or beginning of expiration).
3. Calculate the $FEF_{25\%-75\%}$ (Fig. 25-7).
4. While referring to the example in Figure 25-7, determine the vital capacity on the spirogram. Multiply the vital capacity by 25% and by 75%, respectively.
5. Mark the points on the spirogram that correspond to the first 25% and 75% of the exhaled vital capacity.
6. Using a straightedge, connect the 25% and 75% points with a straight line such that the drawn line intersects two consecutive vertical time lines. The vertical time lines should correspond to 1 second of time elapsed on the spirogram.
7. Locate the volumes that correspond to the points of intersection between the drawn line and the vertical time line.
8. Subtract the low volume from the high volume.
9. Multiply the result by the temperature conversion factor (and other correction factor, if applicable). Record the corrected $FEF_{25\%-75\%}$ on the laboratory report.
10. Determine the predicted $FEF_{25\%-75\%}$ from the appropriate nomogram.
11. Calculate the percentage of predicted $FEF_{25\%-75\%}$ using the following formula:

$$FEF_{25\%-75\%} \text{ percent predicted} = \frac{\text{Observed } FEF_{25\%-75\%}}{\text{Predicted } FEF_{25\%-75\%}} \times 100$$

12. Record the percentage of predicted $FEF_{25\%-75\%}$ on the laboratory report.

RECOMMENDED READING

Burton GG, Hodgkin JE: Respiratory Care. A Guide to Clinical Practice, 2nd ed. Philadelphia, JB Lippincott, 1984

Kacmarek RM, Dimas S, Mack C: Essentials of Respiratory Therapy, 2nd ed. Chicago, Year Book Medical Publishers, 1985

Ruppel G: Manual of Pulmonary Function Testing, 2nd ed. St Louis, CV Mosby, 1979

Spearman CB, Sheldon RL: Egan's Fundamentals of Respiratory Therapy, 4th ed. St Louis, CV Mosby, 1982

Laboratory Performance Evaluation (#25)

Topic: Pulmonary Function Tests: Flowrates

Student ______________________ Course ______________________

Date ______________________ Section ______________________

Performance Elements	Acceptable	Unacceptable	Not Applicable	Comments
1. Prepares spirometer				
2. Washes hands				
3. Introduces self to subject				
4. Prepares subject for performing a timed forced vital capacity maneuver				
5. Explains procedure to subject				
6. Confirms subject's understanding of procedure				
7. Repeats instructions to subject: A. Inhale maximally B. Exhale forcefully				
8. Operates spirometer correctly				
9. Checks obtained results				
10. Secures spirometer properly				
11. Records obtained results				

Knowledge of Procedure

- ☐ Good; student is knowledgeable about rationale and theory related to procedure
- ☐ Fair; student has adequate understanding of rationale and theory related to procedure
- ☐ Poor; student has inadequate understanding of rationale and theory related to procedure

Performance Deficiencies (check those that apply)

- ☐ Excessive time needed to complete procedure
- ☐ Broke aseptic or sterile technique
- ☐ Gross inaccuracy noted
- ☐ Technique may be harmful to patient
- ☐ Incorrect dosage or gas concentration
- ☐ Incorrect equipment assembly/use
- ☐ Unable to answer questions correctly about rationale and/or theory related to procedure
- ☐ Other ____________________

Evaluation Summary

- ☐ Satisfactory performance
- ☐ Unsatisfactory performance

Recommendations of Evaluator

- ☐ Skills may be applied/observed in clinical setting
- ☐ Specific evaluation deficiencies require correction
- ☐ Complete re-evaluation required
- ☐ Additional laboratory practice required

Signatures:

Evaluator ____________________ Date ____________________

Student ____________________ Date ____________________

Laboratory Report

Student ______________________ Acceptable ______________________

Date ______________________ Unacceptable ______________________

Course ______________________

Topic: Pulmonary Function Tests: Flowrates

Data or Measurements

PFT Test	Measured or Observed (BTPS)	Predicted	% Predicted
FVC			
$FEV_{1.0}$			
$FEV_{3.0}$			
$FEF_{200-1200}$			
$FEF_{25\%-75\%}$			
$FEV_{1.0}/FVC\%$			
$FEV_{3.0}/FVC\%$			

Scenario: As a change of pace, you have been assigned to work in the PFT laboratory. Your first patient is a 5′11″, 49-year-old man weighing 185 pounds who has been smoking 1½ packs of cigarettes per day for the past 30 years, which gives him a ________ pack/year history. He has been referred to the laboratory for evaluation of episodic dyspnea and prebronchodilator and postbronchodilator studies. Please answer the following questions:

1. The subject's observed FVC is 3.7 liters; his predicted FVC is 4.4 liters. Therefore, the observed represents what percentage of the predicted?

2. The same subject's forced expired volume in 1 second ($FEV_{1.0}$) was 2.0 liters. What percentage of the forced vital capacity does the $FEV_{1.0}$ represent?

3. After receiving a bronchodilator, the following results were observed: $FEV_{1.0} = 2.2$ liters; postbronchodilator FVC = 3.7 liters. The $FEV_{1.0}$ represents ________% of the FVC.

4. Did the bronchodilator have a positive response?

5. What percentage increase was observed?

6. What percentage of the vital capacity can normally be exhaled in
   A. 1 second?

   B. 3 seconds?

7. What airflow tests may be used to evaluate gas flow through
   A. large airways?

   B. medium-to-small airways?

8. What is the significance of large decreases in
   A. $FEF_{200-1200}$?

   B. $FEF_{25\%-75\%}$?

chapter 26

Introduction to hemodynamic monitoring for respiratory care

INTRODUCTION

Both noninvasive and invasive methods may be used in hemodynamic monitoring. Relatively simple noninvasive monitoring includes peripheral pulse evaluation, auscultation of heart sounds, and indirect arterial blood pressure measurement.

Invasive hemodynamic monitoring frequently involves the use of a pressure monitoring system. The primary function of a pressure monitoring system is to sample the pressure inside a blood vessel or heart chamber and display it externally. The system comprises three basic components: (1) a transducer to convert pressure into an electrical signal; (2) an amplifier to increase the magnitude of the signal from the transducer; and (3) a recorder or oscilloscope to display the signal. The amplifier and recorder are usually housed within a monitor.

To monitor pressure, the distal end of a catheter is placed in a patient's vessel or heart chamber. The proximal end is connnected to a fluid-filled tubing system. The tubing connects to the transducer, and the transducer connects to the monitor. The system also requires a continuous flush device (*i.e.*, intraflow), and fluid under high pressure is forced through the line to ensure patency.

To ensure accuracy, the transducer/amplifier monitoring system must be zeroed and calibrated prior to patient use. Before the system can be zeroed and calibrated, it must be filled with fluid. This chapter introduces you to both noninvasive and invasive techniques of hemodynamic monitoring for respiratory care.

OBJECTIVES

After completing chapter, you should be able to do the following:

1. *Determine the presence, quality, intensity, and rate of peripheral pulses.*
2. *Identify the heart sounds during chest auscultation.*
3. *Measure arterial blood pressure using sphygmomanometer and stethoscope.*
4. *Demonstrate the correct setup of a pressure monitoring system.*

5. *Demonstrate preparation of a pressure transducer, including the leveling procedure.*
6. *Demonstrate the procedure to zero and calibrate the transducer/amplifier monitoring system.*
7. *Define the three components of a pressure monitoring system and their function.*
8. *Identify the components of a Swan–Ganz catheter.*

EQUIPMENT NEEDED

- ☐ Pressure monitor (*i.e.*, Hewlett–Packard, Mennen 700, Abbott)
- ☐ Blood pressure cuff
- ☐ Mercury manometer
- ☐ Intravenous solution
- ☐ Saline solution plus heparin
- ☐ Pressure transducer
- ☐ Intravenous connecting tubing
- ☐ Intraflow or other flush device
- ☐ Intravenous pole
- ☐ Stethoscope
- ☐ Watch with a second hand
- ☐ Swan–Ganz catheter
- ☐ Tuberculin syringe
- ☐ 10.0 ml syringe

ACTIVITIES

Exercise A: Identification and Palpation of Peripheral Pulses

1. Review the major arteries that may be used for pulse palpation (Fig. 26-1).
2. Identify the following arteries:
   A. Carotid
   B. Brachial
   C. Radial
   D. Femoral
3. Using a laboratory partner, locate and palpate the radial, brachial, and carotid arteries.
4. Palpate the brachial artery for 30 seconds. Note the resting pulse rate and record the results in beats per minute on the laboratory report.
5. While working with a laboratory partner, compare the right and left brachial pulses for rate, rhythm, and quality.

Exercise B: Auscultation of Heart Sounds

1. Using the following illustration, review the areas of the precordium that are conducive to hearing specific heart sounds (Fig. 26-2).
2. Identify the areas that correspond to the location in which sounds may be best transmitted across the chest wall:
   A. Inferior border (mitral area): On left side, located between the 4th and 5th intercostal space proximal to the midclavicular line.
   B. Tricuspsid area: On the right side, located proximal to the xiphoid process.

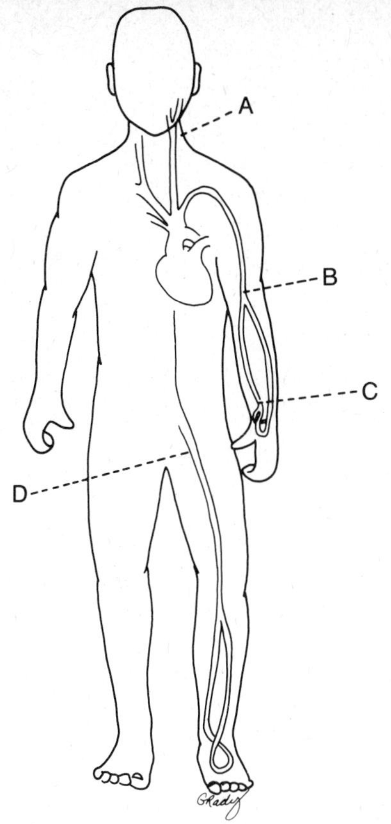

Fig. 26-1. Location of systemic arteries for pulse palpation.

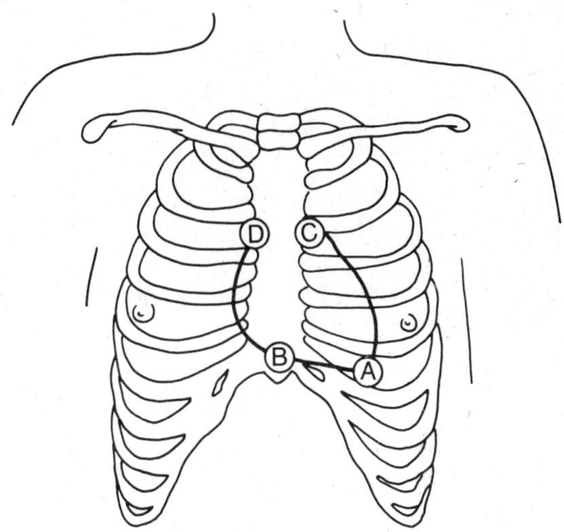

Fig. 26-2. Areas of the precordium conducive to auscultation of heart sounds. *(Modified from Young JA, Crocker D: Principles and Practice of Respiratory Therapy, 2nd ed. Chicago, Year Book Medical Publishers, 1976)*

C. Pulmonary area: On the left side, proximal to the 2nd intercostal space at the sternal border.
D. Aortic area: On the right side, proximal to the 2nd intercostal space at the sternal border.

3. Using a stethoscope, auscultate the precordium of a laboratory partner at rest. Note the intensity, rhythm and rate of the heart sounds. You may request that your partner briefly hold his breath to hear the sounds more clearly.
4. Compare the pulse rate determined by auscultation to that obtained by palpation. You may place the stethoscope over the aortic area to detect the apical heart rate. *Note:* During auscultation of the precordium to detect the pulse rate, two sounds may be heard: The first heart sound, that of systole, usually corresponds to a palpable pulse; the second heart sound, that of diastole, does not correspond to a pulse beat. The second sound is usually shorter and has a higher pitch than the first sound.
5. Record the heart rate obtained by auscultation of the precordium on the laboratory report.

Exercise C: Indirect Measurement of Blood Pressure

1. Request that your laboratory partner assume a supine position. Allow your partner to relax for 3 to 5 minutes.
2. Using a sphygmomanometer, secure the inflatable cuff to the upper arm. Be certain that the location of the cuff tubing corresponds to the location over the brachial

artery. Be certain that the manometer is positioned for ease in monitoring (Fig. 26-3).

3. Palpate the brachial artery.
4. Using the hand bulb, rotate the valve to allow inflation of the cuff. Inflate the cuff to cause occlusion of brachial blood flow (about 200 mm Hg).
5. While auscultating over the antecubital fossa, which corresponds to the area of the brachial pulse, rotate the valve to allow slow deflation of the cuff pressure (about 2–3 mm Hg/heart beat).
6. While slowly deflating the cuff, note the pressure on the manometer at which a pulse sound is first heard. This is the systolic pressure.
7. While continuing to allow cuff deflation, note the pressure at which a definite change or absence of pulse sound occurs. This is the diastolic pressure.
8. Record the systolic and diastolic blood pressure on the laboratory report. Blood pressure as indirectly measured with a sphygmomanometer is traditionally recorded as systolic/diastolic in millimeters of mercury.
   Note: Avoid prolonged occlusion of the brachial artery with the cuff.

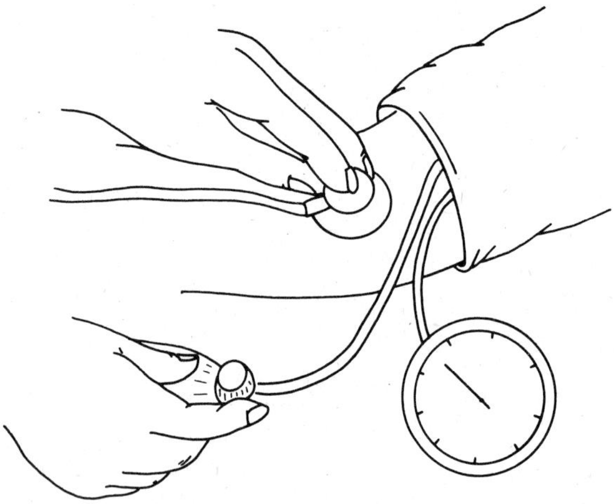

Fig. 26-3. Sphygmomanometer positioned for indirect measurement of blood pressure.

Exercise D: Preparation of a Pressure Transducer

1. A transducer is a device that converts pressure in a catheter to an electrical signal. The typical strain-gauge transducer works on the Wheatstone Bridge principle. The transducer has a dome that has two openings, each with a luer lock fitting. Examine your transducer for the location of these connections.
2. Remove the plastic transducer dome and observe the diaphragm.
3. Fill a 10.0 ml syringe with sterile, 0.9% saline. (In the clinical setting, the solution is heparinized.)
4. Remove the air bubbles from the saline in the syringe.
5. Using the saline from the syringe, form a meniscus in the transducer between the transducer dome and the diaphragm. Be certain that no air bubbles are present.

6. Carefully screw the dome back onto the transducer.
7. Observe the clear dome to ensure there are no air bubbles in the saline solution. Air bubbles will absorb pressure and cause less pressure to be transmitted. Therefore, the pressure reading will be less than the patient's actual pressure when air bubbles exist in the meniscus.
8. If air bubbles are present, repeat steps 2 through 6 above.
9. Mount the transducer on the i.v. pole.
10. When mounted, the transducer must be at the same level as the distal end of the catheter inside an actual patient.
11. Connect the transducer cable into the amplifier.
12. Connect a stopcock to the luer lock fitting on the transducer dome. This stopcock is referred to as stopcock "A."
13. Using the remaining luer connector, attach stopcock "B," an intraflow device and pressurized fluid system, to the other end of the transducer dome (Fig. 26-4).
14. With the stopcock A opened to air, gently pull the red pigtail on the intraflow valve and allow fluid flow in the system. Be certain that stopcock B is turned off toward the catheter to allow fluid flow through the transducer dome and stopcock A.
15. Air bubbles remaining in the transducer dome may be removed by turning the free stopcock (A) straight up and by simultaneously pulling the red pigtail.
16. Turn off stopcock A. Open stopcock B and pull the pigtail to allow fluid flow through the remaining tubing in the system which normally would attach to a catheter.
17. In the clinical setting, after the insertion of a catheter, the fluid-filled tubing eventually would be connected to the catheter following calibration of the system.

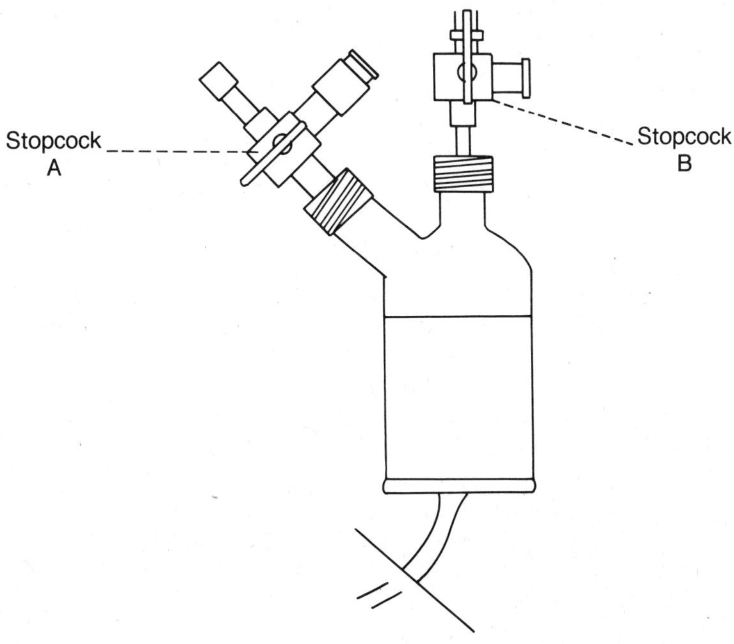

Fig. 26-4. Pressure transducer for measurement of arterial blood pressure.

Exercise E: Calibration of the System

PROCEDURE TO ZERO THE TRANSDUCER/AMPLIFIER

1. Turn the amplifier/monitor on and allow sufficient time to warm up (about 15 minutes). Calibrate the system according to the manufacturer's recommendations.
2. Expose the transducer to atmospheric pressure by opening a port, stopcock A, to room air pressure. The other port, stopcock B, must be closed (turned off toward the pressure transducer).
3. Adjust the amplifier until it reads zero by using the zeroing control knob or by depressing a zeroing button on the casing of the amplifier/monitor.

PROCEDURE TO CALIBRATE THE TRANSDUCER/AMPLIFIER

1. Connect the mercury manometer to the port that was previously open to atmosphere. Pump the manometer to 200 mm Hg (Fig. 26-5).
2. Adjust the monitor to read 200 mm Hg by adjusting the calibration scale factor knob or by depressing a calibration button on the casing of the amplifier.
3. Once you have calibrated the monitor to 200 mm Hg, disconnect the mercury manometer.
4. The monitor should then read zero; if not, repeat the zero and calibration procedure.
5. As an additional check of the calibration procedure, reconnect the mercury manometer. Pump the manometer to 100 mm Hg. The monitor should read 100 mm Hg.
6. Disconnect the mercury manometer and close the stopcock.

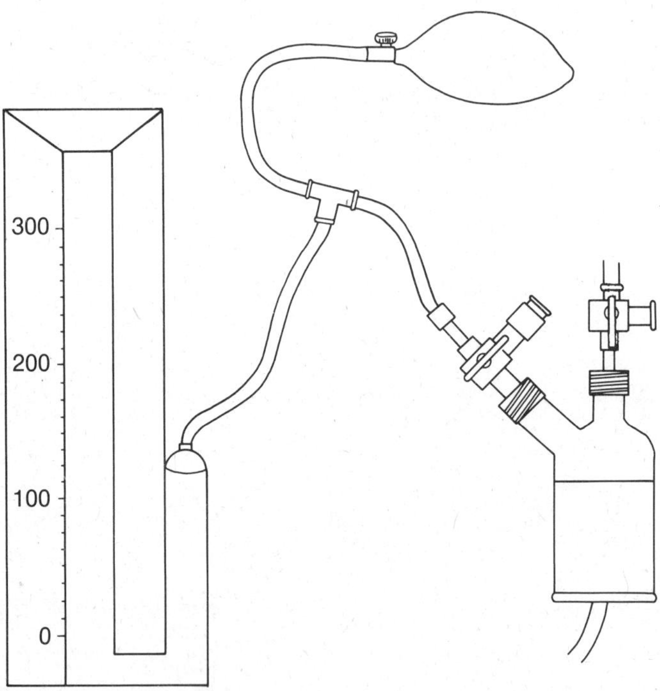

Fig. 26-5. Manometer used for calibration of pressure transducer.

Exercise F: Identification of Swan–Ganz Catheter Components

1. A Swan–Ganz catheter may be connected to a pressure monitoring system in order to measure intracardiac pressure. The catheter may also be used to measure cardiac output and may be used to obtain a sample of mixed venous blood.
2. Examine the components of a Swan–Ganz catheter (Fig. 26-6).
3. Identify the following components of the Swan–Ganz catheter:
   A. Inflation lumen port (red)
   B. Distal lumen port (yellow)
   C. Proximal lumen port (blue)
   D. Thermistor connection for cardiac output computer
   E. Proximal lumen orifice
   F. Thermistor
   G. Balloon
   H. Distal lumen
4. Immerse the tip of the catheter under water.
5. Using a tuberculin syringe, inject 0.8 ml of air into the red inflation lumen port. Check the balloon for leaks. No air bubbles should be observed. Remove the catheter from the water.
6. Using a 10.0 ml syringe, inject 10.0 ml of water into the proximal lumen. Trace the flow of fluid from the proximal lumen orifice to the thermistor.

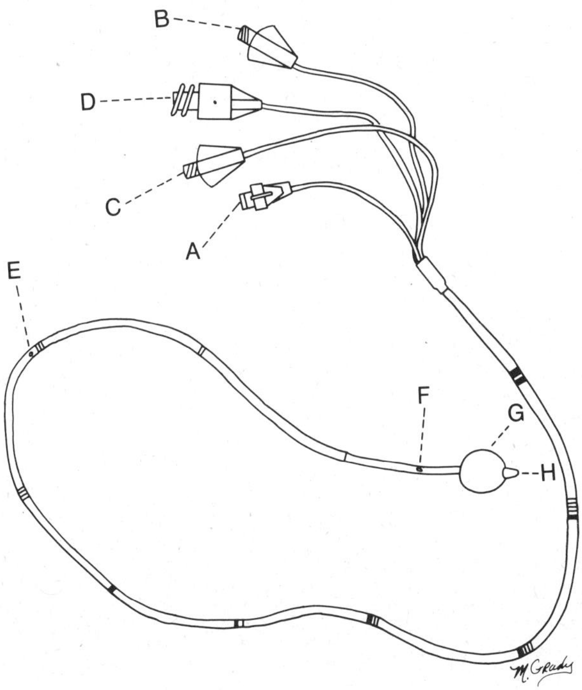

Fig. 26-6. Components of Swan–Ganz catheter.

RECOMMENDED READING

Schroeder JS, Daily EK: Techniques in Bedside Hemodynamic Monitoring. St Louis, CV Mosby, 1976

Spearman CB, Sheldon RL: Egan's Fundamentals of Respiratory Therapy, 4th ed. St. Louis, CV Mosby, 1982

Young JA, Crocker D: Principles and Practice of Respiratory Therapy, 2nd ed. Chicago, Year Book Medical Publishers, 1976

Laboratory Performance Evaluation (#26)

Topic: Introduction to Hemodynamic Monitoring for Respiratory Care

Student ____________________ Course ____________________

Date ____________________ Section ____________________

Performance Elements	Acceptable	Unacceptable	Not Applicable	Comments
1. Obtains necessary equipment				
2. Mounts transducer properly on intravenous pole (proper level)				
3. Connects transducer cable to appropriate amplifier port				
4. Connects stopcocks to appropriate luer lock fittings of the transducer				
5. Opens appropriate stopcock to expose transducer to atmospheric pressure				
6. Adjusts amplifier to "zero"				
7. Attaches a mercury manometer to the transducer				
8. Pressurizes the mercury manometer until a reading of 200 mm Hg has been reached				
9. Calibrates the amplifier until it reads 200 mm Hg				
10. Disconnects the mercury manometer				

Performance Elements	Acceptable	Unacceptable	Not Applicable	Comments
11. Rechecks the "zero" reading				
12. Connects the appropriate "intraflow" device to i.v. tubing, i.v. bag, and indwelling catheter				
13. Checks for adequate flow of i.v. solution from distal port of catheter				

Knowledge of Procedure

- ☐ Good; student is knowledgeable about rationale and theory related to procedure
- ☐ Fair; student has adequate understanding of rationale and theory related to procedure
- ☐ Poor; student has inadequate understanding of rationale and theory related to procedure

Performance Deficiencies (check those that apply)

- ☐ Excessive time needed to complete procedure
- ☐ Broke aseptic or sterile technique
- ☐ Gross inaccuracy noted
- ☐ Technique may be harmful to patient
- ☐ Incorrect dosage or gas concentration
- ☐ Incorrect equipment assembly/use
- ☐ Unable to answer questions correctly about rationale and/or theory related to procedure
- ☐ Other ____________________

Evaluation Summary

- ☐ Satisfactory performance
- ☐ Unsatisfactory performance

Recommendations of Evaluator

- ☐ Skills may be applied/observed in clinical setting
- ☐ Specific evaluation deficiencies require correction
- ☐ Complete re-evaluation required
- ☐ Additional laboratory practice required

Signatures:

Evaluator ______________________ Date ______________________

Student ______________________ Date ______________________

Laboratory Report

Student ____________________ Acceptable ____________________

Date ____________________ Unacceptable ____________________

Course ____________________

Topic: Hemodynamic Monitoring for Respiratory Care

Data or Measurements

Resting pulse rate by palpation __________ (beats/min)

Resting pulse rate by auscultation __________ (beats/min)

Arterial Blood Pressure (systolic/diastolic) __________ mm Hg/__________ mm Hg

Scenario: The medical intensive care unit is your assignment today. You are notified that the emergency room will be sending you a young girl who is a suspected drug overdose victim and who has vomited and aspirated. She is intubated and is being manually ventilated. The unit physician has requested that the following be available when the patient arrives: a volume ventilator and setups for an arterial line and Swan-Ganz catheter. For purposes of efficiency, you write out a list of items needed for the Swan-Ganz catheter and arterial line setups. Please duplicate those lists in the space provided.

1. Swan-Ganz catheter — Arterial line

2. What are the three basic components of a pressure monitoring system?

3. Describe the function of each component named above.

4. What is the function of an intraflow device?

5. How would the presence of air bubbles in a transducer dome affect the patient's pressure reading?

6. At what level should a pressure transducer be when used to measure pulmonary artery pressure?

7. During the indirect measurement of arterial blood pressure with a sphygmomanometer, how are systolic and diastolic pressure determined?

8. What are three uses of a Swan–Ganz catheter?

9. Briefly describe the area of the chest in which sound may best be transmitted for the
   A. mitral area.

   B. aortic area.

chapter 27

Electrocardiography for respiratory care

INTRODUCTION

The recording and the study of the electrical activity of the heart are known as electrocardiography. The heart's electrical activity may be detected by attaching electrodes to the skin. The electrodes, which are connected to an electrocardiograph machine, provide an electrical input to the machine that records the signal on heat-sensitive paper by means of a heated stylus. The signal may also be displayed on an oscilloscope. Electrocardiography may be used for diagnostic and monitoring purposes; as a diagnostic tool, the complete analysis of the electrocardiogram is beyond the scope of this book. In respiratory care, however, it is important to analyze the electrocardiogram for the heart rate and rhythm.

As a monitoring tool, electrocardiography may provide a dynamic display of cardiac electrical activity on an oscilloscope. Since many respiratory care procedures affect cardiac function, the electrocardiogram may be observed to determine the cardiac response to therapeutic intervention. The purpose of this chapter is to introduce you to electrocardiography.

OBJECTIVES

After completing this chapter, you should be able to do the following:

1. *Record a 12-lead electrocardiogram.*
2. *Understand the functions of an electrocardiographic machine.*
3. *Identify the normal heart rate and rhythm.*
4. *Locate the placement of limb and chest leads for a 12-lead electrocardiogram.*
5. *Identify and correct artifact in the electrocardiogram.*

EQUIPMENT NEEDED

- ☐ Electrode pads (or gauze soaked in electrolyte solution)
- ☐ Limb and chest leads
- ☐ Electrocardiograph machine
- ☐ Bed
- ☐ Private room or screen

ACTIVITIES

Preparation of a Subject for an Electrocardiogram: Request that a laboratory partner serve as a subject. A male should not perform a 12-lead electrocardiogram on a female without instructor permission. Adequate privacy should be ensured. The subject should be informed that the procedure is painless, and he should attempt to relax completely before the recording.

Exercise A: Preparation and Attachment of Limb Leads

1. Have the subject remove all jewelry and metal.
2. Request that the subject assume the supine position and relax.
3. Apply either electrolyte gel or pads to the muscular area over both biceps and calves.
4. Apply clean electrodes to the muscular areas over both biceps and calves.
5. The limb leads may be color or alphabetically coded:

Electrode Location	Color Code
Right arm (RA)	White
Right leg (RL)	Green
Left arm (LA)	Black
Left leg (LL)	Red
Chest (C)	Brown

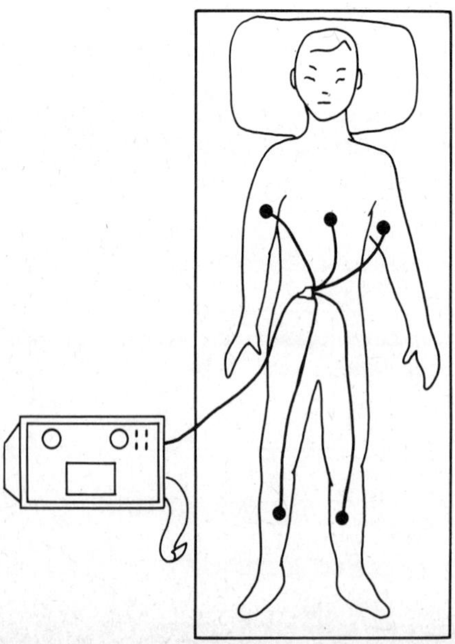

Fig. 27-1. Location of limb leads. *(Modified from Burdick Corp, Milton, WI)*

6. Be certain that the electrode wires do not cross one another (Fig. 27-1).
7. Secure the electrodes to prevent inadvertent disconnection.

Exercise B: Preparation and Attachment of Chest Leads

1. The chest or precordial leads are recorded with either single or multiple electrodes.
2. Place the chest electrode in the following positions (Fig. 27-2).
   V_1: fourth intercostal space at right margin of sternum
   V_2: fourth intercostal space at left margin of sternum
   V_3: midway between positions 2 and 4
   V_4: fifth intercostal space at junction of left midclavicular line
   V_5: at horizontal level of position 4 at left anterior axillary line
   V_6: at horizontal level of position 4 at left midaxillary line
3. If a single chest electrode is used, the electrode must be changed to the proper anatomical site before recording from the precordial leads.
4. Electrolytic gel or an electrolyte pad may be applied to the electrode before placement.
5. Stabilize the chest electrode.

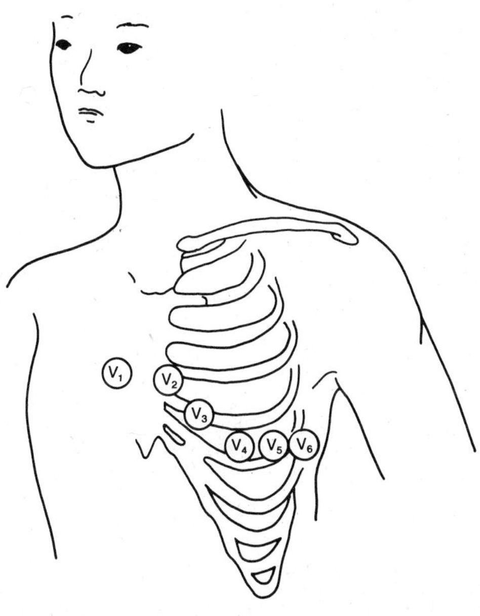

Fig. 27-2. Chest or precordial lead positions. *(Modified from Burdick Corp, Milton, WS)*

Exercise C: Identification of ECG Machine Controls

1. Your instructor will provide you with the appropriate operator's manual or other learning materials. Become thoroughly familiar with the machine controls before recording an electrocardiogram.
2. Examine the electrocardiogram controls (Fig. 27-3).
3. Identify the following controls on the ECG monitor:
   A. On/off switch
   B. Stylus position
   C. Record switch (Amp on/off, run 25, run 50)
   D. Marker
   E. Standard

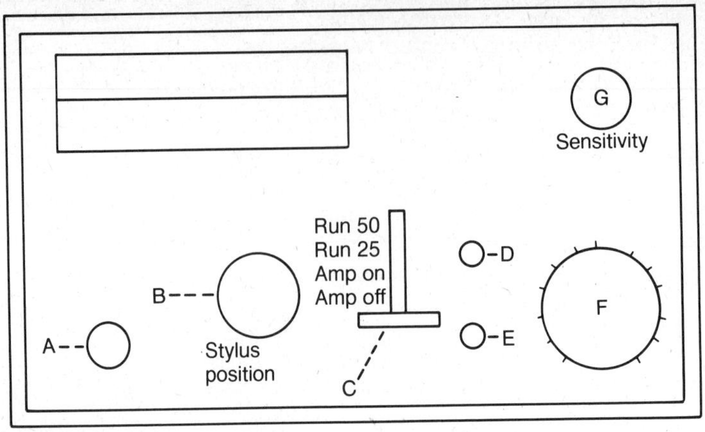

Fig. 27-3. Electrocardiograph controls.

F. Lead selector
G. Sensitivity

Exercise D: Operation of ECG Machine Controls

1. Verify that the machine is properly grounded.
2. Set the lead selector switch to lead 1. The lead selector switch is used to obtain recordings from the desired lead.
3. Turn the record switch to the Amp on position. Rhythmic deflections of the stylus on the heat-sensitive paper should be observed.
4. Turn the record switch to run or record (25 mm/second). The ECG complex may be centered on the paper by using the stylus position control.
5. The sensitivity control may be used for either very high or very low amplitude ECG complexes. If the sensitivity control is used, the standard marker should also be interposed between the "T" wave of one complex and the "P" wave of the following complex.
6. A standardization mark should be included in the recording of each lead.
7. Run about 10 inches of record for leads 1, 2, and 3. For the remaining leads, 5 inches should be sufficient.
8. Turn the record switch to Amp off before changing the position of the chest electrode. Change the electrode to the proper anatomical position, and select the lead to be recorded with the lead selector.
9. Monitor the recording for artifacts or defective recordings. An example of artifact due to body movement during the recording is shown in Figure 27-4.
10. This artifact is prevented by complete patient relaxation and the avoidance of movement during the recording.
11. Another type of artifact results from loose or improperly applied electrodes as in Figure 27-5.

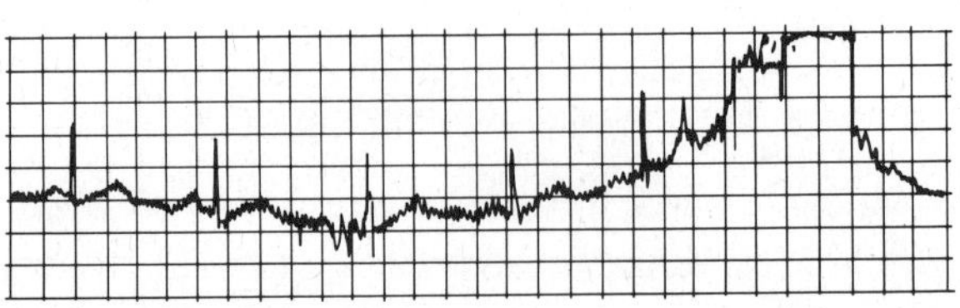

Fig. 24-4. Artifact due to body movement.

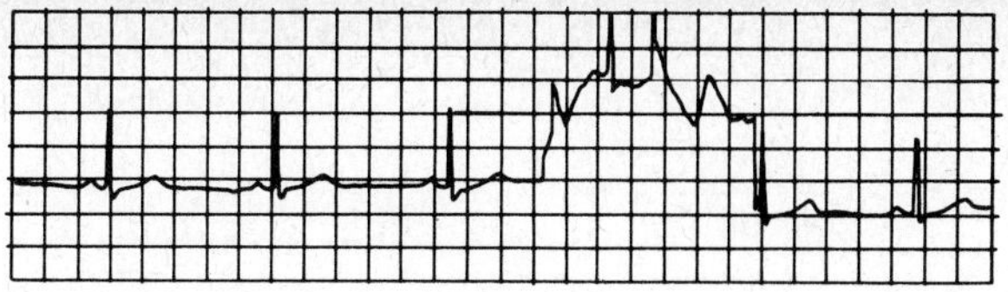

Fig. 27-5. Artifact due to loose electrodes.

12. If this type of artifact is observed, verify that all the electrodes are adequately secured.
13. A drift in the isoelectric baseline may mimic the type of artifact seen with loose electrodes. To prevent baseline drift, allow a few seconds for the electrode voltage to stabililze after selecting a new lead. Before recording in a new lead, leave the record switch in the Amp on position until stabilization occurs.

Exercise E: Analysis of the ECG

1. Identify the P, Q, R, S, and T waves in lead II. Refer to Figure 27-6.
2. Calculate the PR interval, QRS interval, and ST segment. Record the results on the laboratory report.
3. Determine the QRS voltage. Record the results on the laboratory report.
4. Verify that a P wave precedes a QRS complex in all leads.
5. Verify that a T wave follows a QRS complex in all leads.

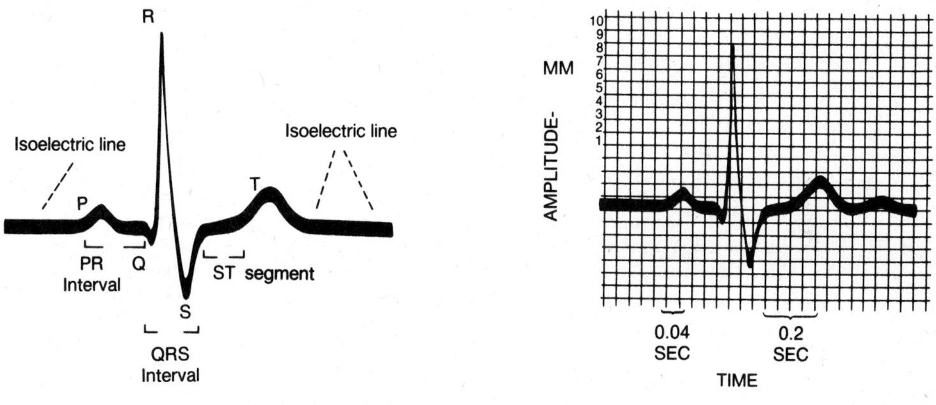

Fig. 27-6. Normal ECG waves, intervals, and segments.

Exercise F: Determination of Cardiac Rate

1. For normal rhythms, locate a QRS complex that has fallen on a dark vertical line in a large square.
2. Determine the R–R interval (R wave to R wave) by counting the number of large squares (0.2 seconds) between the QRS complex on a dark, vertical line and the adjacent QRS complex.
3. Refer to Table 27-1 to determine the heart rate.
4. Determine the heart rate in all leads.
5. Record the results on the laboratory report. *Note:* More precise methods of determining cardiac rate are recommended for arrythmias.

Table 27-1. Heart Rate Table Based on R–R Interval on an Electrocardiogram

Number of Large Squares Between Consecutive R Waves (R–R Interval)	Rate per Minute
1	300
2	150
3	100
4	75 normal sinus rhythm
5	60
6	50

RECOMMENDED READING

Dubin D: Rapid Interpretation of EKGs, 3rd ed. Tampa, Cover Publishing Company, 1984

Kacmarek RM, Dimas S, Mack C: Essentials of Respiratory Therapy, 2nd ed. Chicago, Year Book Medical Publishers, 1985

Schroeder JS, Daily EK: Techniques in Bedside Hemodynamic Monitoring. St Louis, CV Mosby, 1976

Laboratory Performance Evaluation (#27)

Topic: Electrocardiography for Respiratory Care

Student ______________________ Course ______________________

Date ______________________ Section ______________________

Performance Elements	Acceptable	Unacceptable	Not Applicable	Comments
1. Verifies order				
2. Obtains necessary equipment				
3. Identifies simulated patient				
4. Introduces self to simulated patient				
5. Prepares patient properly				
6. Explains procedure to patient				
7. Connects ECG machine power cord to AC outlet				
8. Removes jewelry and metal from patient				
9. Connects limb leads properly				
10. Connects chest leads properly				
11. Runs an ECG Strip of limb leads				
12. Runs an ECG strip of each chest lead				

Knowledge of Procedure

- ☐ Good; student is knowledgeable about rationale and theory related to procedure
- ☐ Fair; student has adequate understanding of rationale and theory related to procedure
- ☐ Poor; student has inadequate understanding of rationale and theory related to procedure

Performance Deficiencies (check those that apply)

- ☐ Excessive time needed to complete procedure
- ☐ Broke aseptic or sterile technique
- ☐ Gross inaccuracy noted
- ☐ Technique may be harmful to patient
- ☐ Incorrect dosage or gas concentration
- ☐ Incorrect equipment assembly/use
- ☐ Unable to answer questions correctly about rationale and/or theory related to procedure
- ☐ Other ______________________________

Evaluation Summary

- ☐ Satisfactory performance
- ☐ Unsatisfactory performance

Recommendations of Evaluator

- ☐ Skills may be applied/observed in clinical setting
- ☐ Specific evaluation deficiencies require correction
- ☐ Complete re-evaluation required
- ☐ Additional laboratory practice required

Signatures:

Evaluator ______________________ Date ______________________

Student ______________________ Date ______________________

Laboratory Report

Student ______________________ Acceptable ______________________

Date ______________________ Unacceptable ______________________

Course ______________________

Topic: Electrocardiography for Respiratory Care

Data or Measurements

PR interval ______________________

R–R interval ______________________

ST segment ______________________

QRS interval ______________________

QRS voltage ______________________

Average rate ______________________

Scenario: In order to refamiliarize you with electrocardiography techniques, you are assigned to the ECG laboratory where regularly scheduled ECGs are performed.

You have just finished with the 10:00 a.m. appointment when you are called to the emergency room stat. "They need a stat 12-lead ECG in Room 1," the nurse said. Arriving in Room 1, you see a mildly obese middle-aged man. He is sitting upright in the stretcher and is obviously distressed. Please respond to the following questions:

1. Describe the method used to prepare the electrode placement sites.

2. Please describe as precisely as possible the location of the electrodes for the precordial leads.

3. Identify, from the above situation, three potential sources of artifact.

   A.

   B.

   C.

4. As the ECG tracing is being produced, you notice two large squares between QRS complexes. An estimate of this patient's heart rate is __________ beats/minute.
5. How many inches of tracing are needed to produce a viable record for interpretation?

6. The __________ wave should *precede* the QRS complex in all leads.
7. The __________ wave should follow the QRS complex in all leads.
8. A drift in the isoelectric baseline may mimic artifact due to what?

9. What are some common causes of artifacts?

10. What are the functions of the
    A. lead selector?

    B. standardization marker?

    C. record switch

11. Define the following terms:
    A. R–R interval

    B. PR interval

    C. ST segment

chapter 28

Introduction to chest radiography for respiratory care

INTRODUCTION

The chest radiograph may provide valuable information in the diagnosis and evaluation of chest conditions. In conjuction with information obtained from the history and physical examination, blood gas analysis, pulmonary function tests, and appropriate laboratory tests, the chest radiograph may be used as one of several diagnostic tools. In respiratory care, a radiograph of the chest may also be used to evaluate the effectiveness of therapeutic techniques and to locate the position of artificial airways and intravascular catheters.

A chest radiograph is produced when radiographic film is exposed to ionizing, electromagnetic radiation or roentgen rays. Radiographic film appears white before exposure to roentgen rays. After exposure to radiation, the film appears black. The characteristic black and white radiographic appearance of a chest film occurs because of differences in roentgen ray absorption and penetration. In general, tissue density determines the degree of penetration or absorption of roentgen rays. When roentgen rays are directed through the chest, dense tissue such as bone absorbs radiation and creates a white appearance on the chest film. In contrast, the air-filled lung parenchyma allows radiation to penetrate the tissue to create a black appearance on the chest film. In the normal chest radiograph, the white appearance of radiopaque ribs contrasts sharply with the black appearance of the radiolucent, air-filled lung fields.

In this chapter, you are introduced to a systematic evaluation of the chest film. Although a few common pathologic patterns are mentioned, the radiographic appearance of structures within the chest film of a normal healthy adult is emphasized.

OBJECTIVES

After completing this chapter, you should be able to do the following:

1. *Understand the common projections used to produce chest films.*
2. *Evaluate a chest film for bilateral symmetry, right versus left side, and phase of respiration.*

3. *Identify the structures found within the chest film of a healthy adult.*
4. *Locate the carina to determine the relative position of an artificial airway.*
5. *Define the terminology commonly used to describe chest films.*

ACTIVITIES

Exercise A: Orientation to the Chest Film

Several projections may be used to produce a chest film. A projection refers to the positioning of the subject with respect to the beam of roentgen rays and the radiographic film. Four projections commonly used are the anteroposterior (A-P), postero anterior (P-A), lateral, and lateral decubitus projections (Fig. 28-1).

In the A-P projection, roentgen rays pass through the subject from front to back, and the film cassette is placed posterior to the subject's back. In the P-A projection, the roentgen rays penetrate the chest from back to front, and the film cassette is located

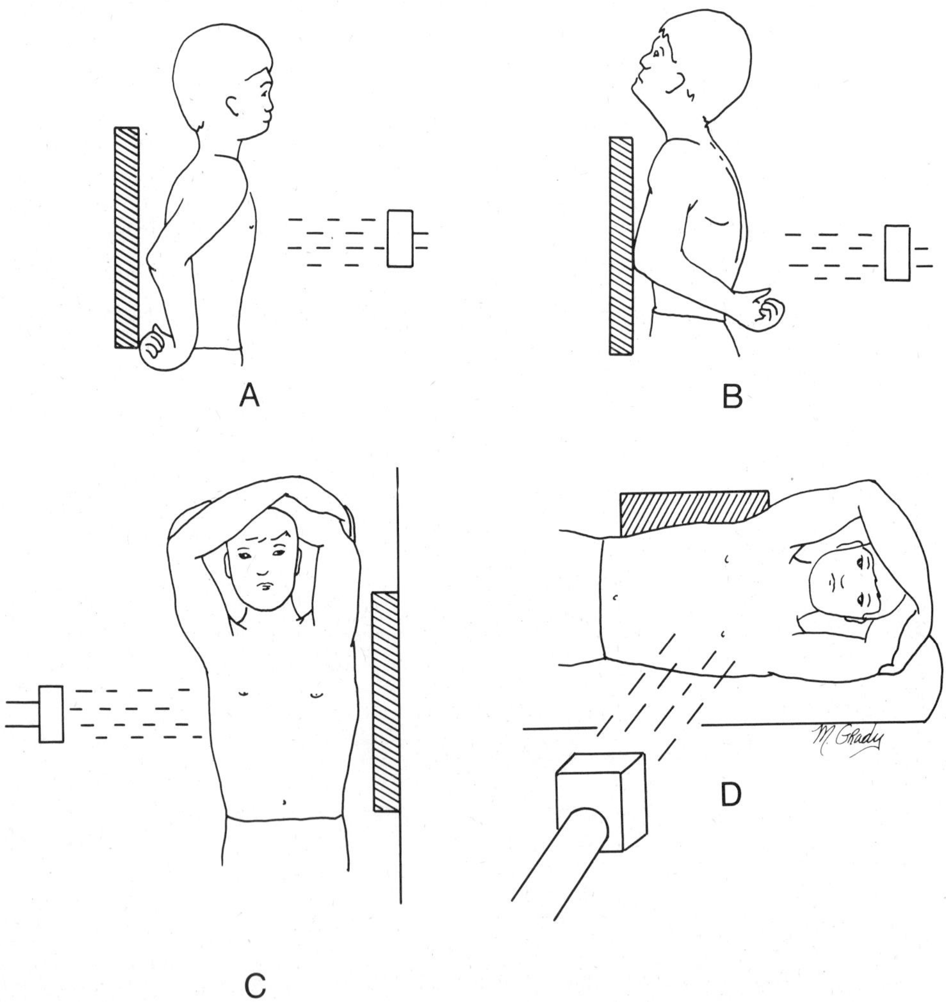

Fig. 28-1. Location of subject, film, and roentgen rays in (A) A-P projection, (B) P-A projection, (C) lateral projection, and (D) lateral decubitus projection.

anterior to the chest. The beam of roentgen rays enters one side of the chest and exits the opposite side in the lateral position. In the lateral decubitus position, the subject lies on the affected side to allow "layering" of fluid. The roentgen beam penetrates the chest in a horizontal tangent to "layered" fluid in the lateral decubitus position.

1. Your instructor will provide you with actual chest films, slides, or other learning materials. In the materials provided, determine the projection and visualize the path of of roentgen rays as they penetrate and exit the chest (Fig. 28-2).
2. When viewing the film, the right and left sides of the film refer to the subject's right and left sides. The location of the gastric bubble usually indicates the left side. In addition, most chest films are marked as to the right and left sides. In the materials provided by your instructor, locate the right and left sides of the film.
3. In an A-P projection of the chest, the position of the subject and degree of rotation may be evaluated by comparing the right and left sternoclavicular junctions to the midline. When bilateral symmetry is present, each sternoclavicular junction is equidistant to the midline. When significant rotation is present, the distance from the right and left sternoclavicular junction to the midline is unequal. Observe the materials provided for bilaterial symmetry in an A-P or P-A projection.

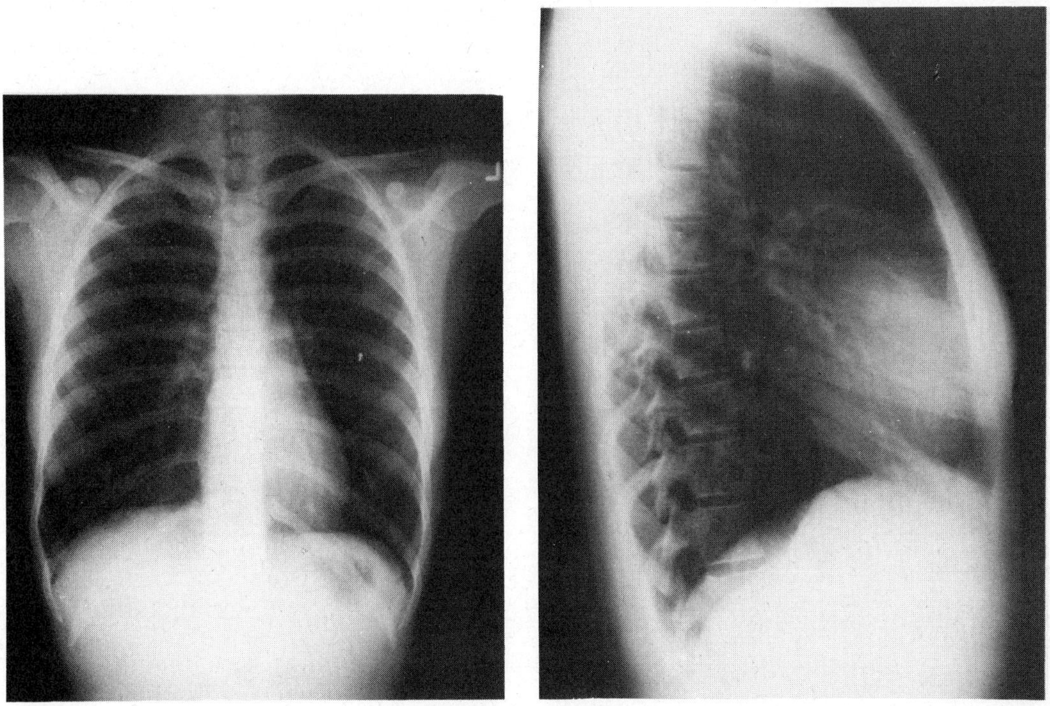

A B

Fig. 28-2. Normal chest films in the (A) A-P and (B) lateral projections.

Exercise B: Identification of Bony Structures in the Thorax

1. Using the diagram provided, examine the bony structures of the thorax that may be present on a chest radiograph (Fig. 28-3).
2. Identify the following bony structures:
   A. Clavicles (right and left)

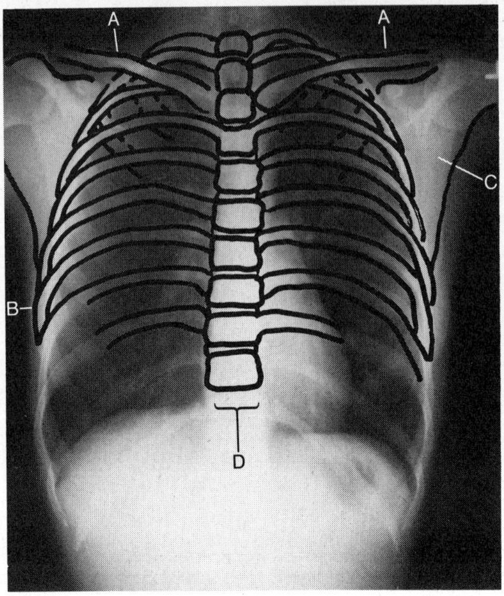

Fig. 28-3. Bony structures in the thorax.

   B. Ribs
   C. Scapulae
   D. Vertebrae
   E. Sternum (not shown)
3. In the chest films, slides, or learning materials provided by your instructor, locate the bony structures of the thorax.
4. Observe the length of the clavicles.
5. Locate the first rib. The intercostal spaces are numbered by the rib on top. The first intercostal space is beneath the first rib and above the second rib.
6. Identify and count the remaining ribs. Look for fractures, lesions, deformities, or abnormal notching of the ribs.
7. Locate the first thoracic vertebral body. Identify and count the remaining vertebrae.
8. Locate the area near the fourth and fifth thoracic vertebrae. In the normal adult, this area corresponds to the carina and is an important landmark for determining artificial airway position.

Exercise C: Identification of the Heart and Vasculature

1. Using the diagram provided, examine the appearance of the heart, hila, and vasculature (Fig. 28-4).
2. Identify the following structures:
   A. Superior vena cava
   B. Inferior vena cava
   C. Right atrium
   D. Right hilum
   E. Aortic arch
   F. Left hilum
   G. Left ventricle
3. In the chest films or slides provided by your instructor, locate the aforementioned structures.
4. Observe the shape, width, and borders of the heart. At the level of the diaphragms,

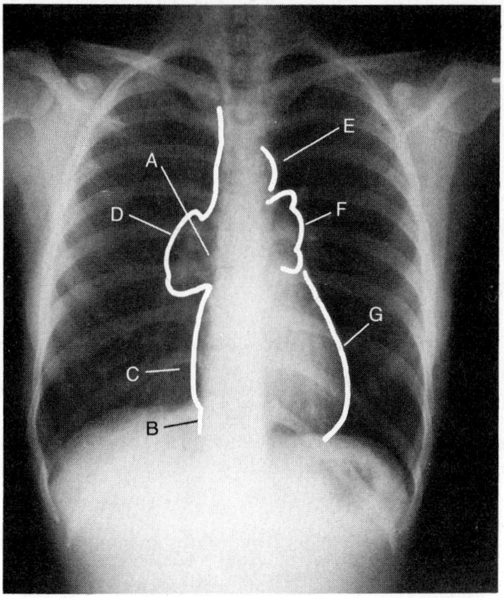

Fig. 28-4. The heart, vasculature, and C-T ratio.

compare the transverse width of the heart to that of the inner thoracic diameter (the cardio-thoracic or C-T ratio). In the healthy adult, the C-T ratio is less than 50%, or less than a 1 : 2 ratio in the P-A projection.

5. Locate the right and left hilar regions. In the healthy adult, the left hilum is usually about 2 cm higher than the right hilum. Compare hila regions.

Exercise D: Identification of the Trachea, Bronchi, and Carina

1. Using the diagram provided, examine the appearance of the trachea, bronchi, and carina (Fig. 28-5).

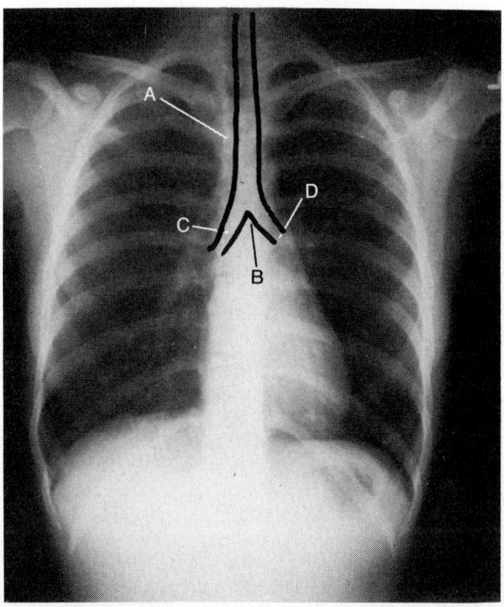

Fig. 28-5. Tracheobronchial tree and carina.

2. Identify the following structures:
   A. Trachea
   B. Carina
   C. Right main-stem bronchus
   D. Left main-stem bronchus
3. In chest films or slides provided by your instructor, locate the aforementioned structures.
4. Determine the position of the carina. Compare the position of the carina to the area between the fourth and fifth thoracic vertebrae in an adult chest film, and to the area between the third and fourth thoracic vertebrae in a neonate's chest film.
5. Locate the area between the second and third anterior ribs in an adult chest film. Compare this area to the location of the carina.
6. If the chest films provided by your instructor show the radiopaque line located at the distal end of a tracheostomy or endotracheal tube, determine the tube tip position relative to the carina.

Exercise E: Identification of the Diaphragmatic Domes, Pleura, and Costophrenic Angles

1. Using the diagram provided, examine the appearance of the diaphragmatic domes and costophrenic angles (Fig. 28-6).
2. Identify the position of the following structures:
   A. Right hemidiaphragm
   B. Left hemidiaphragm
   C. Right costophrenic angle
   D. Left costophrenic angle
3. In the chest films or slides provided by your instructor, locate the aforementioned structures.
4. Both the right and left costophrenic angles should appear as sharp, distinct, clearly demarcated structures. The abnormal presence of a pleural effusion may cause blunting or haziness of the costophrenic angles.

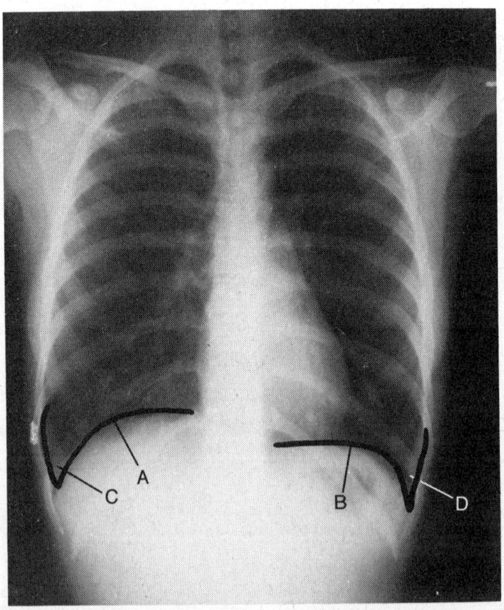

Fig. 28-6. Diaphragm domes and costophrenic angles.

5. Compare the positions of each hemidiaphragm. The right hemidiaphragm is normally about 2 cm higher than the left hemidiaphragm. Flattening of the hemidiaphragms may be associated with lung hyperinflation.
6. Determine the phase of respiration during which the chest film was taken by comparing the position of the hemidiaphragms to the anterior ribs. During a deep inspiration, which is usually requested when a chest film is made, the right hemidiaphragm normally lies near the sixth anterior rib or tenth posterior rib.
7. The pleura are not usually visible. In the presence of a pneumothorax or air in the pleural space, the visceral pleura may appear as a thin line circling the lung.

Exercise F: Identification of the Lung Fields

1. Using the diagram provided, examine the appearance of the lung fields and soft tissues (Fig. 28-7).
2. Identify the following structures:
   A. Right horizontal fissure (if applicable)
   B. Right oblique fissure (if applicable)
   C. Left oblique fissure (if applicable)
   D. Women's breast shadows (if applicable)
3. Using the chest films or slides provided by your instructor, locate the fissures or breast shadows if they are apparent on the radiograph.
4. Several pathologic conditions may affect the radiographic appearance of the lung fields. The following terminology is used to describe these conditions.

Lung Field Pathology	Radiographic Appearance
Infiltrate	Increase radiodensity in lung field; may be diffuse or localized "fluffy" alveolar patterns. Interstitial patterns may appear as "net"- or "web"-like reticular densities.
Pulmonary nodule	Coin lesion, well-circumscribed and demarcated, increased radiodensity.

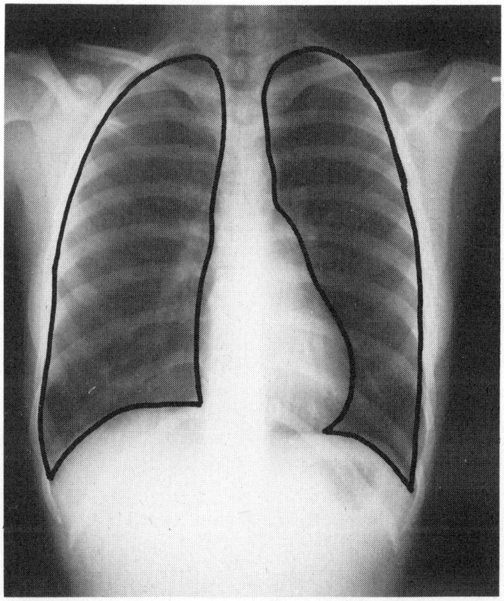

Fig. 28-7. Lung fields.

Lung Field Pathology	Radiographic Appearance
Cavity	Radiolucent hole in lung parachyma.
Cyst	Thin-walled, radiolucent cavity that may be filled with fluid.
Bleb	Radiolucent subpleural collection of air.
Bullae	Radiolucent air space larger than 1 cm in diameter.
Atelectasis	Increased radiodensity, displaced interlobular fissures, elevation of diaphragm on affected side. Deviation of trachea and mediastinum toward affected side. Hyperaeration of unaffected side.
Hyperinflation	Radiolucent lung fields, flattened diaphragms, widening of intercostal spaces, increased retrosternal air space; bullous changes possible.
Pneumothorax	Shift of trachea away from affected side; displaced interlobular fissures; increased radiolucency in pleural space; lung collapse on affected side with appearance of visceral pleura; depressed diaphragm on affected side.

5. Request the assistance of your instructor in locating examples of lung field abnormalities.

RECOMMENDED READING

Burton GG, Hodgkin JE: Respiratory Care. A Guide to Clinical Practice, 2nd ed. Philadelphia, JB Lippincott, 1984

Hinshaw C, Murray JF: Diseases of the Chest, 4th ed. Philadelphia, WB Saunders, 1980

Shapiro BA, Harrison RA, Kacmarek RM, Cane RD: Clinical Applications of Respiratory Care, 3rd ed. Chicago, Year Book Medical Publishers, 1985

Spearman CB, Sheldon RL: Egan's Fundamentals of Respiratory Therapy, 4th ed. St. Louis, CV Mosby, 1982

Laboratory Performance Evaluation (#28)

Topic: Chest Radiography for Respiratory Care

Student ______________________ Course ______________________

Date ______________________ Section ______________________

Performance Elements	Acceptable	Unacceptable	Not Applicable	Comments
1. Positions chest film correctly on light box for viewing				
2. Determines "right" and "left" on chest film				
3. Determines phase of breathing present during chest film production				
4. Evaluates symmetry of chest appropriately				
5. Identifies bony structures				
6. Identifies heart and vasculature markings				
7. Identifies tracheobronchial tree and carina				
8. Identifies domes of diaphragm and costophrenic angles				
9. Evaluates overall lung fields				
10. Records observations				

Knowledge of Procedure

☐ Good; student is knowledgeable about rationale and theory related to procedure

☐ Fair; student has adequate understanding of rationale and theory related to procedure

☐ Poor; student has inadequate understanding of rationale and theory related to procedure

Performance Deficiencies (check those that apply)

☐ Excessive time needed to complete procedure

☐ Broke aseptic or sterile technique

☐ Gross inaccuracy noted

☐ Technique may be harmful to patient

☐ Incorrect dosage or gas concentration

☐ Incorrect equipment assembly/use

☐ Unable to answer questions correctly about rationale and/or theory related to procedure

☐ Other ____________________

Evaluation Summary

☐ Satisfactory performance

☐ Unsatisfactory performance

Recommendations of Evaluator

☐ Skills may be applied/observed in clinical setting

☐ Specific evaluation deficiencies require correction

☐ Complete re-evaluation required

☐ Additional laboratory practice required

Signatures:

Evaluator ____________________ Date ____________________

Student ____________________ Date ____________________

Laboratory Report

Student ______________________ Acceptable ______________________

Date ______________________ Unacceptable ______________________

Course ______________________

Topic: Chest Radiography for Respiratory Care

Scenario: Immediately after morning report, you accompany the physician in charge of the critical care unit to the x-ray department, where the chest films of the patients residing on the unit are reviewed.

One of the first patients reviewed is a young lady who was admitted to the unit 48 hours ago with a diagnosis of drug overdose and aspiration. Another patient suffers from severe emphysema and currently has a right lower lobe pneumonia, whereas a third patient has pulmonary edema. All of these patients are endotracheally intubated.

1. Please describe the x-ray appearance of the "properly" placed endotracheal tube.

2. How would the x-ray appear if the endotracheal tube was in the right main-stem bronchus?

3. List four projections commonly used in chest radiography.

4. How may the right and left side and respiration phase be determined from a chest radiograph?

5. Define the following and briefly describe the radiographic appearance of
   A. cardio-thoracic ratio

   B. infiltrate

   C. nodule

   D. costophrenic angle

6. From a chest radiograph, where is the carina located in a healthy, normal adult and neonate?

7. What radiographic patterns may be associated with
   A. right upper lobe atelectasis?

   B. right-sided pneumothorax?

C. bilateral hyperinflation?

D. interstitial infiltrate due to pulmonary edema?

chapter 29

Infection control

INTRODUCTION

One of the greatest risks inherent in the delivery of patient care is microbial contamination with subsequent infection. In respiratory care, a variety of activities are directed toward controlling the spread of potentially harmful micro-organisms and preventing infection. The purpose of this chapter is to introduce the student to the technique of infection control in respiratory care.

OBJECTIVES

After completing this chapter, you should be able to do the following:

1. *Describe the decontamination and processing techniques for contaminated respiratory therapy equipment.*
2. *Understand the significance of proper handwashing technique.*
3. *Identify methods used to evaluate the effectiveness of equipment processing techniques.*
4. *Identify the attire for strict and respiratory isolation*
5. *Describe a procedure for processing contaminated equipment obtained from a simulated highly contagious patient in a strict isolation setting.*
6. *Decontaminate and process equipment provided by the laboratory instructor.*

EQUIPMENT NEEDED

☐ Contaminated laboratory equipment
☐ Culture swab and agar plate
☐ Detergent
☐ Sterilizing/disinfectant agent
☐ Brush
☐ Sterile gloves and field

☐ Equipment basins
☐ Sterile distilled water

ACTIVITIES

Exercise A: Identification of Equipment Decontamination and Processing Area

1. The area for cleaning and processing laboratory equipment and supplies will be designated by your laboratory instructor.
2. Locate and identify the following features of an equipment processing area (Fig. 29-1).
   A. Dirty (contaminated) equipment entrance
   B. Clean (decontaminated) equipment exit
   C. Large contaminated equipment deposit area
   D. Small contaminated equipment deposit area
   E. Contaminated equipment disassembly table or shelf
   F. Double basin sink/wash area
   G. Disinfection/sterilization area
   H. Chemical, steam autoclave, ethylene oxide, pasteurization equipment
   I. Dryer or drying area

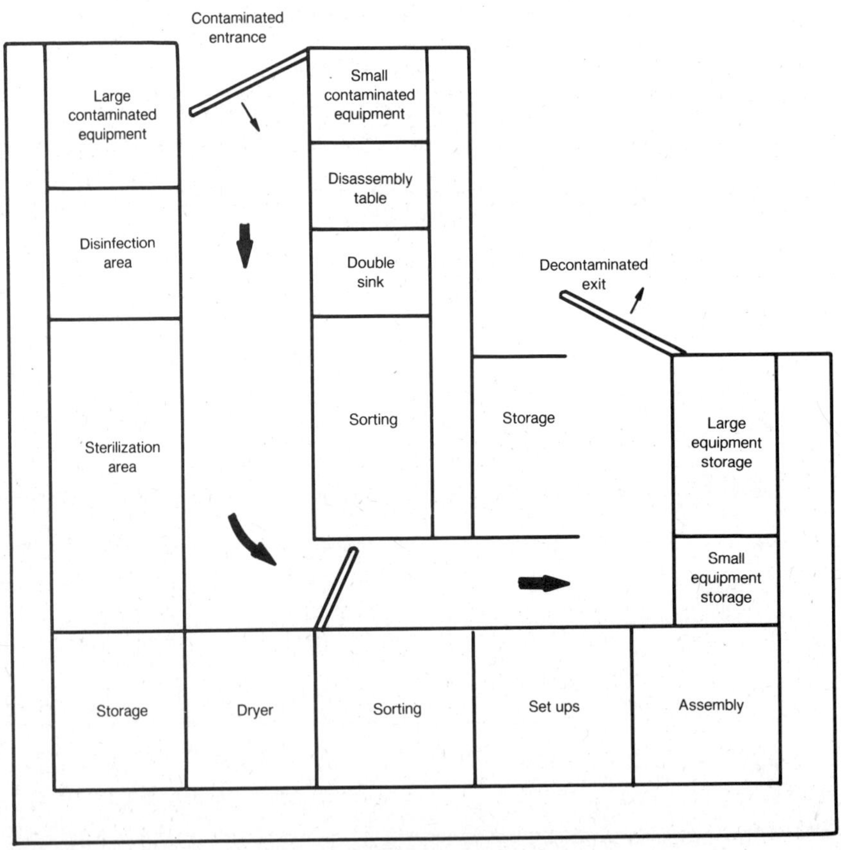

Fig. 29-1. Design of equipment decontamination and processing area. *(Modified from Young JA, Crocker D: Principles and Practice of Respiratory Therapy, 2nd ed. Chicago, Year Book Medical Publishers, 1976)*

J. Equipment assembly area
K. Disinfected/sterilized equipment storage area or shelves

3. On the laboratory report, diagram and label the equipment processing area for laboratory equipment. Be sure to indicate the intended "flow" of equipment from contaminated to clean equipment areas.

Exercise B: Equipment Cleaning and Processing (Decontamination)

1. Your instructor will provide you with contaminated laboratory equipment or supplies that require disinfection or sterilization.
2. Put on rubber gloves.
3. Completely disassemble the equipment.
4. Using one basin (or half of a double-basin sink), fill the sink with hot water and add an appropriate amount of detergent to the running water.
5. Place the disassembled equipment in the wash basin.
6. Allow the equipment to soak thoroughly in the detergent solution for a few minutes.
7. Using a brush, scrub the contaminated equipment. All visible organic material must be removed from the equipment (Fig. 29-2).
8. Using a second basin (or the remaining half of a double basin sink), use hot water for rinsing the equipment.
9. After thoroughly cleaning the equipment, prepare a chemical solution for disinfection or sterilization (or follow the directions of your laboratory instructor for pasteurization, steam autoclaving, or ethylene oxide sterilization).
10. Record on your laboratory report the amounts and ingredients used in preparing the chemical sterilization solution.
11. Place the cleaned equipment and chemical solution into a covered container. Allow the equipment to soak in the solution according to the manufacturer's

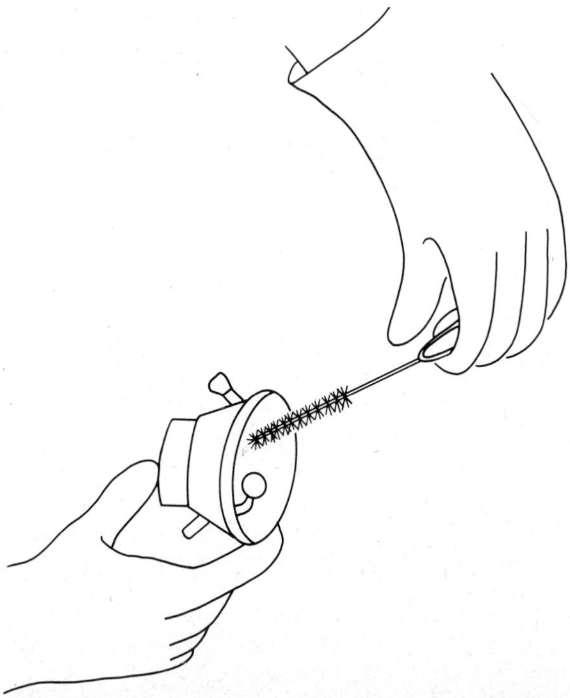

Fig. 29-2. Equipment cleaning.

specifications for disinfection or for sterilization to occur. Record the date and time of the solution preparation. Clearly label the covered container with the date of preparation of the solution and the contents of the solution.

12. After allowing an appropriate amount of time for disinfection or sterilization, remove the cover from the chemical container.
13. Wash your hands and put on sterile gloves.
14. Prepare a sterile field for the equipment.
15. Remove the equipment from the chemical solution and thoroughly rinse several times with sterile water.
16. Place the sterilized equipment on the sterile field to air dry, or use sterile dryers.
17. After the equipment has dried, reassemble the equipment with sterile technique.
18. Package the equipment in sterile plastic bags.
19. Store the packaged equipment in the appropriate area.
20. Clean and disinfect the equipment cleaning area. Verify that all supplies are appropriately stored.

Exercise C: Equipment Culture

1. After disinfection or sterilization of the equipment, the effectiveness of the technique can be monitored by mocrobial culture.
2. Obtain a sterile swab and culture tube. Moisten the swab with sterile water. Swab the disinfected or sterilized equipment. Label the swab and culture tube (Fig. 29-3).

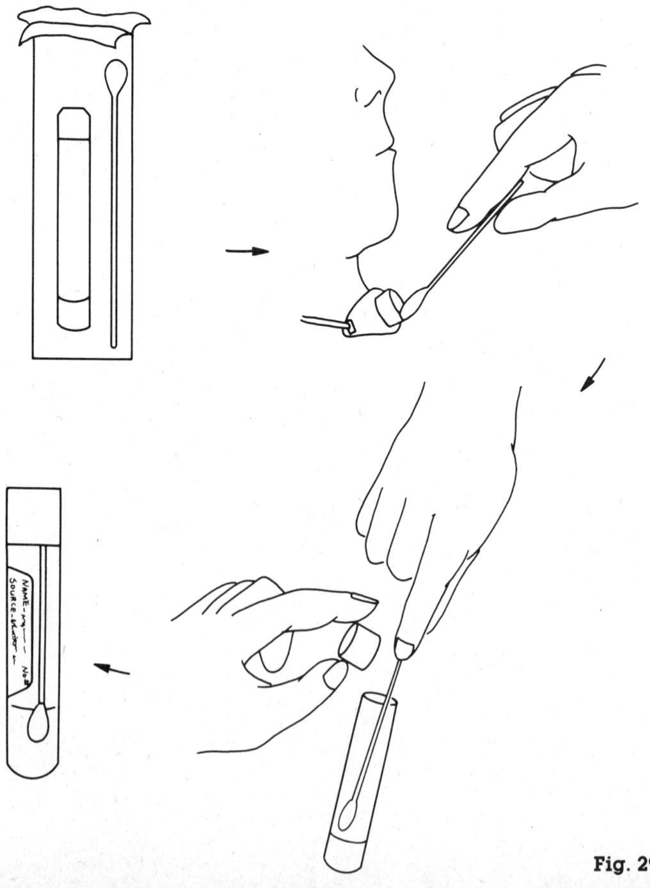

Fig. 29-3. Swab culture technique.

3. After microbiologic identification, record the results and report to your laboratory instructor.
4. Activated aerosol and humidified gas delivery systems may be cultured by exposing an agar plate and bacteriologic growth medium to the aerosol.
5. Assemble the aerosol or humidified gas apparatus.
6. Allow several minutes of operation before sampling.
7. Direct the flow of aerosol or humidified gas to the agar plate. A funnel may be used to minimize accidental contamination with airborne microbes. If a funnel is not used, direct the flow of aerosol or humidified gas to the agar plate by displacing the agar plate cover at an angle (Fig. 29-4).
8. Label the culture with the equipment samples, the date, and your initials.
9. Equipment may also be monitored for microbial contamination by a nutrient broth rinse technique.
10. Obtain the equipment to be cultured. Using the prepared nutrient broth, rinse the equipment with the broth. A small amount of broth may be used inside the tubing and collected in a culture tube (Fig. 29-5).

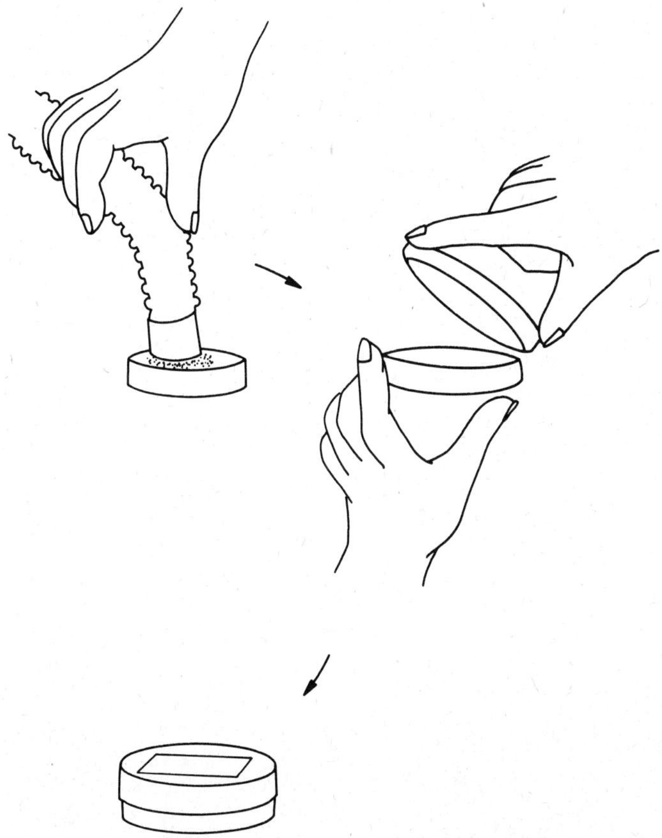

Fig. 29-4. Culture of gas or aerosol. *(Modified from Blodgett D: Manual of Respiratory Care Procedures. Philadelphia, JB Lippincott, 1980)*

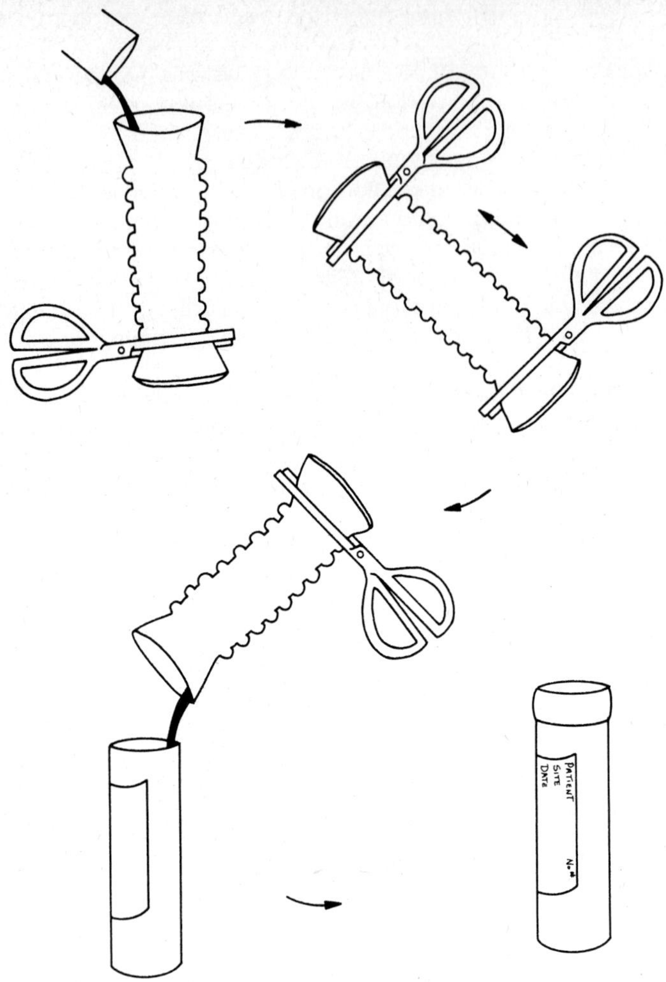

Fig. 29-5. Broth rinse culture technique. *(Modified from Blodgett D: Manual of Respiratory Care Procedures. Philadelphia, JB Lippincott, 1980)*

Exercise D: Handwashing

1. Using either foot-pedal controls or faucets, adjust the water to the desired flow and temperature.
2. Remove all jewelry, and remove your watch.
3. While directing your hands below the level of your elbows, wet the hands and wrists thoroughly.
4. Obtain a generous portion of iodophor soap and begin the scrubbing process.
5. Scrub *all* surfaces of the hands and fingers for a minimum of 15 seconds.
6. Nails may be cleaned by working them against the palms or by using plastic nail cleaners.
7. Rinse your hands thoroughly by positioning them to allow water to flow down off the fingertips. Verify that all soap solution has been removed.
8. Dry your hands with paper towels, working from the fingertips to the wrists.
9. If faucets are used to control water flow, use a paper towel to turn off the faucet (Fig. 29-6). Be careful not to contaminate cleaned hands by touching the faucets or sink.

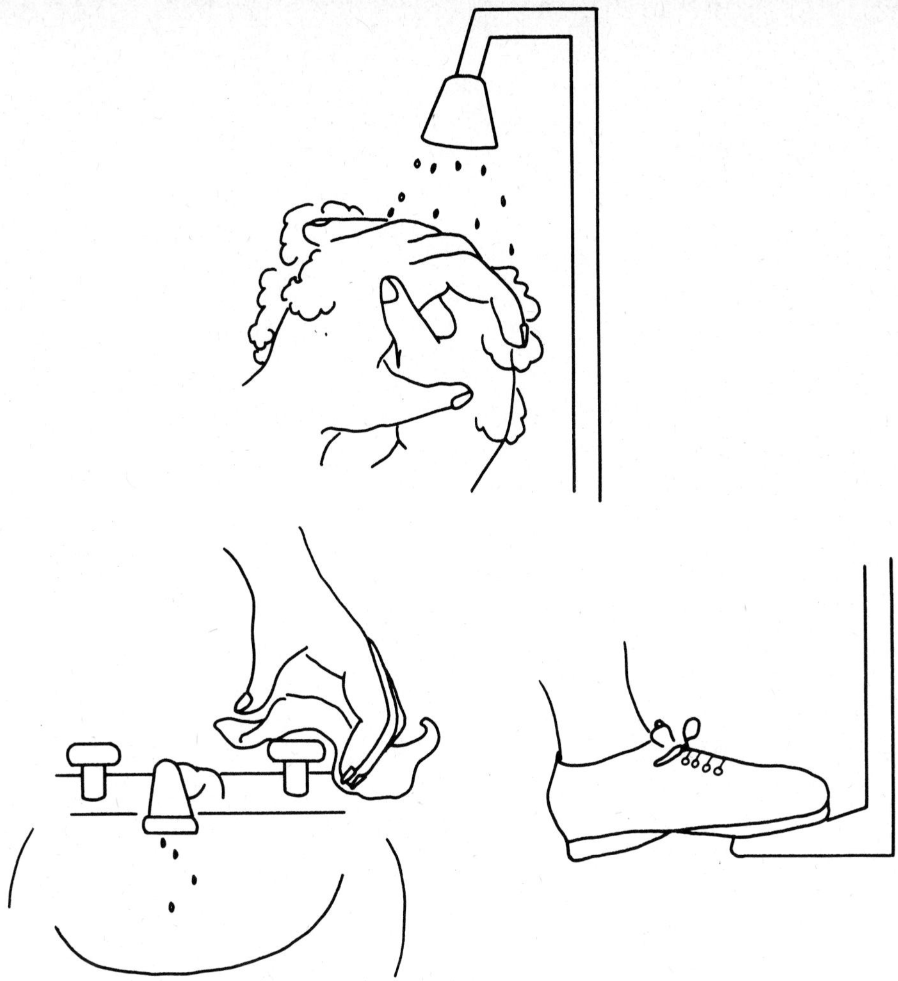

Fig. 29-6. Avoidance of recontamination after handwashing.

The following guidelines on handwashing are recommended:

A. The hands should be kept clean at all times and should be washed before and after contact with each patient.

B. Fingernails should be kept short and clean.

C. When frequent handwashing is necessary, antiseptic lotion can be used to prevent chapping.

D. Gloves or tongs should be used for handling contaminated articles.

E. Jewelry should not be worn in isolation areas.

Exercise E: Isolation Attire

1. Identify and procure the attire recommended by the Centers for Disease Control (CDC) for each type of isolation technique (Table 29-1).
2. Assume that strict isolation technique is required to process contaminated equipment of a simulated patient with a confirmed diagnosis of pneumonic plague.
3. Put on shoe and hair coverings. Be certain that *all* of your hair is covered.
4. Wash your hands using the aforementioned technique.
5. Put on a gown. Fasten the gown with ties or buttons.

Table 29-1. Isolation Technique and Attire

Type of Isolation Technique	Isolation Attire	Handwashing	Private Room
Strict isolation	Gowns, masks, gloves	Hands must be washed when entering and leaving room	Necessary; door must be kept closed
Respiratory isolation	Masks must be worn by persons entering room unless that person is not susceptible to the disease. Gowns and gloves not necessary	Hands must be washed when entering and leaving room	Necessary; door must be kept closed
Protective isolation	Gowns and masks. Gloves required for direct patient contact	Hands must be washed when entering and leaving room	Necessary; door must be kept closed
Wound and skin precautions	Gowns needed for direct contact with patient. Masks necessary only for dressing changes. Gloves necessary for contact with infected area	Hands must be washed when entering and leaving room	Desirable
Enteric precautions	Gowns needed for direct patient contact. Masks not necessary. Gloves necessary for direct contact with articles contaminated by fecal matter	Hands must be washed when entering and leaving room	Necessary only for children

6. Apply a mask by securing the ties to the back of the head (not over the head). Be certain that the mask snugly covers the nose and mouth by adjusting the malleable metal nose piece. Do not use a wet mask. Should a mask become wet because of sweating or water, replace the mask.
7. Put on gloves (Fig. 29-7).
8. Proceed to the isolation room or area designated by your laboratory instructor.
9. Deposit contaminated disposable supplies in a designated waste disposal bag.
10. Place contaminated equipment inside a large, clear plastic bag. Seal the bag, then place the sealed bag inside a second plastic bag and clearly label it *Isolation* (Fig. 29-8).
11. Sterilize the double-bagged, contaminated equipment immediately, without opening the bags. Avoid contact with other equipment until sterilization has been completed. *Note:* Assistance from a second person outside the room is helpful in double-bagging equipment.
12. Review the infection control guidelines for the care of AIDS patients in Table 29-2.

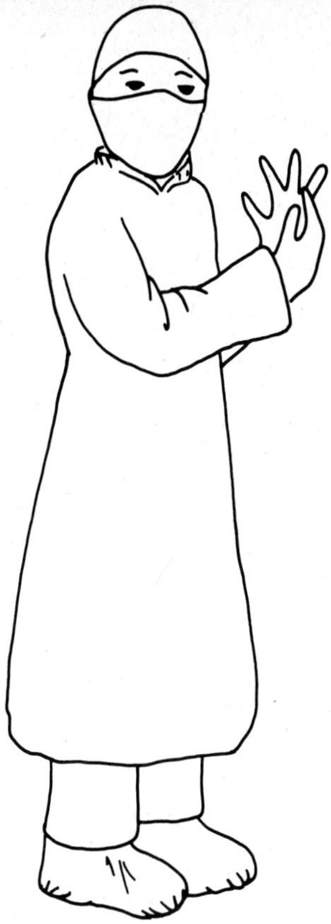

Fig. 29-7. Strict isolation attire consisting of mask, gown, gloves, hair, and shoe covers.

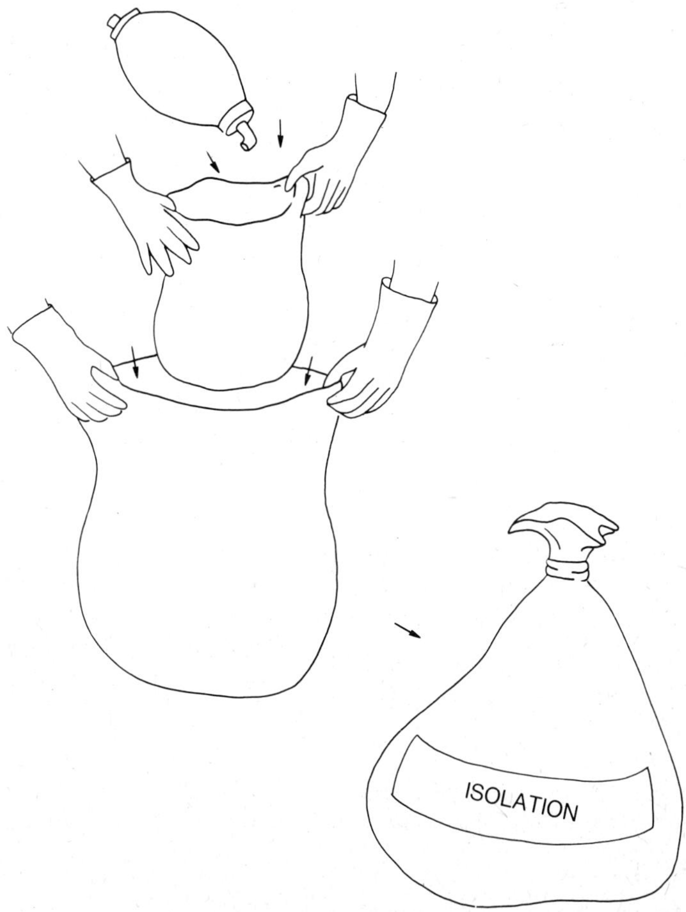

Fig. 29-8. Processing equipment from a strict isolation setting.

Table 29-2. Infection Control Guidelines for the Care of AIDS Patients

1. Wash hands before and after contact with blood or body fluid, and wear gloves.
2. All specimens should be marked with a warning label of the biohazard type that does not mention a specific disease and should be placed in a waterproof bag or container for transport.
3. Wear gowns for direct contact with blood or body fluids.
4. Clean contaminated environmental surfaces promptly with 0.5% to 1% sodium hypochlorite (*e.g.*, 1 : 10 dilution of 5.25% stock).
5. Wearing of masks by patients with a cough is indicated when they must leave their rooms. Wearing of masks is indicated for visitors or care providers of a coughing patient, or for one being suctioned (*e.g.*, if splattering or spraying of any body fluid is a risk, goggles are also indicated, such as for all personnel involved in bronchoscopy, gastrointestinal endoscopy, or endotracheal tube placement or care).
6. Needles and syringes should be disposed of in rigid, puncture-resistant containers. Do *not* recap needles or bend them.
7. Linens and disposable items visibly soiled with blood or body fluids should be considered "infectious waste" and identified as such. Contaminated linen should be double bagged.
8. A private room is not necessary if the patient is cooperative and is neither a risk to, nor placed at risk by, his roommate.
9. In the case of CPR, manual resuscitation bags and masks or disposable devices for respiratroy resuscitation instead of mouth-to-mouth resuscitation should be available, and all care providers should be trained in their use.

(Courtesy of Charles Ellenboggen, M.D.)

Exercise F: Processing Equipment from Isolation Setting

1. Your laboratory instructor will designate a room or area as an isolation area. You will be provided with the simulated patient's diagnosis and the type of isolation technique.
2. You are to process contaminated equipment from the designated isolation area.

RECOMMENDED READING

Burton GG, Hodgkin JE: Respiratory Care. A Guide to Clinical Practice, 2nd ed. Philadelphia, JB Lippincott, 1984

Kacmarek RM, Dimas S, Mack C: Essentials of Respiratory Therapy, 2nd ed. Chicago, Year Book Medical Publishers, 1985

US Department of Health, Education, and Welfare, Public Health Service, Center for Disease Control. Isolation Techniques for Use in Hospitals, 2nd ed. Washington DC, US Government Printing Office, 1975

Young JA, Crocker D: Principles and Practice of Respiratory Therapy, 2nd ed. Chicago, Year Book Medical Publishers, 1976

Laboratory Performance Evaluation (#29)

Topic: Infection Control

Student ______________________ Course ______________________

Date ______________________ Section ______________________

Performance Elements	Acceptable	Unacceptable	Not Applicable	Comments
1. Washes hands				
2. Wears appropriate isolation attire: A. Gown B. Mask C. Gloves D. Shoes/hair cover				
3. Places contaminated isolation equipment in appropriate container				
4. Labels container bag				
5. Avoids contamination of any other equipment				
6. Equipment processing: A. Obtains equipment B. Disassembles equipment C. Washes equipment D. Rinses equipment E. Dries equipment F. Disinfects/sterilizes equipment G. Cultures equipment H. Reassembles equipment I. Packages assembled equipment J. Stores equipment in appropriate area				
7. Cleans and disinfects processing area				

Knowledge of Procedure

- ☐ Good; student is knowledgeable about rationale and theory related to procedure
- ☐ Fair; student has adequate understanding of rationale and theory related to procedure
- ☐ Poor; student has inadequate understanding of rationale and theory related to procedure

Performance Deficiencies (check those that apply)

- ☐ Excessive time needed to complete procedure
- ☐ Broke aseptic or sterile technique
- ☐ Gross inaccuracy noted
- ☐ Technique may be harmful to patient
- ☐ Incorrect dosage or gas concentration
- ☐ Incorrect equipment assembly/use
- ☐ Unable to answer questions correctly about rationale and/or theory related to procedure
- ☐ Other ________________

Evaluation Summary

- ☐ Satisfactory performance
- ☐ Unsatisfactory performance

Recommendations of Evaluator

- ☐ Skills may be applied/observed in clinical setting
- ☐ Specific evaluation deficiencies require correction
- ☐ Complete re-evaluation required
- ☐ Additional laboratory practice required

Signatures:

Evaluator ________________ Date ________________

Student ________________ Date ________________

Laboratory Report

Student ______________________ Acceptable ______________________

Date ______________________ Unacceptable ______________________

Course ______________________

Topic: Infection Control

Data or Measurements

1. Disinfection/sterilization agent: ______________________

2. Composition of chemical solution

   *p*H solution life ______________________

   ____

   ____

   ____

3. Date prepared: ______________________

4. Time required for disinfection: ______________________

5. Time required for sterilization: ______________________

Scenario: Mr. Reynolds, a 28-year-old man, arrived in the emergency room in a weakened, emaciated state. His breathing was stertorial. Chest x-ray film revealed what appeared to be a full-blown pneumonia, requiring that he be immediately intubated endotracheally. As laboratory results and the chart from his past admissions became available, it was learned that Mr. Reynolds is the victim of autoimmune deficiency syndrome (AIDS). He is now on the medical intensive care unit in an isolation room. Mr. Reynolds has been placed on a volume ventilator. Because of his precarious status and instability, he requires frequent endotracheal suctioning and frequent arterial blood sampling. Please answer the following questions:

1. What type of isolation would this situation require?

2. Please describe the preparations made before entering his room.

3. Please describe in detail the isolation techniques taken when suctioning this patient.

4. What isolation procedures would you use when obtaining arterial blood samples, given this situation?

5. It is 96 hours later, and Mr. Reynolds has died. Please discuss the methods used to retrieve and decontaminate the equipment and supplies in his room.

6. What is the most important technique for controlling the spread of potentially harmful microbes?

7. Define the following:
   A. Contamination

   B. Infection

   C. Disinfection

   D. Sterilization

E. Decontamination

8. What type of isolation attire is recommended by the National Centers for Disease Control for
   A. strict isolation?

   B. respiratory isolation?

   C. reverse isolation or protective isolation, neutropenic?

   D. wound/skin isolation?

   E. enteric isolation?

chapter 30

Airway patency and artificial airways

INTRODUCTION

A device that may be used to maintain a clear path for gas flow between the upper and lower airways is termed an artificial airway. Several types of artificial airways exist: oropharyngeal, nasopharyngeal, and esophageal obturator airways. In addition, endotracheal and tracheostomy tubes may be classified as artificial airways that are directly inserted into the trachea. Since the establishment and maintenance of a patent airway are fundamental responsibilities in respiratory care, it is essential for you to become thoroughly familiar with these devices. The purpose of this chapter is to introduce you to artificial airways.

OBJECTIVES

After completing this chapter, you should be able to do the following:

1. *Identify the following artificial airways:*
   A. *Oropharyngeal airway*
   B. *Nasopharyngeal airway*
   C. *Endotracheal tube*
   D. *Tracheostomy tube*
   E. *Esophageal obturator airway*
2. *Identify the components of endotracheal and tracheostomy tubes.*
3. *Test the cuff on endotracheal and tracheostomy tubes.*
4. *Perform the following manual techniques:*
   A. *Neck hyperextension*
   B. *Chin lift*
   C. *Jaw thrust*
   D. *Triple airway maneuver*
5. *Insert and stabilize a nasopharyngeal or an oropharyngeal airway.*

EQUIPMENT NEEDED

- ☐ Endotracheal tube
- ☐ Tracheostomy tube
- ☐ Oral airway (oropharyngeal)
- ☐ Nasopharyngeal airway
- ☐ Adult mannequin
- ☐ Tape
- ☐ 10 ml syringe
- ☐ Lubricant
- ☐ Esophageal obturator airway

ACTIVITIES

Exercise A: Manual Techniques for the Establishment of Airway Patency

1. Review the manual techniques for establishing a patent airway without using adjunctive equipment (see Chap. 1).
2. Using an adult mannequin, practice the head tilt–neck lift, head tilt–chin lift, and jaw thrust maneuvers.
3. The triple airway maneuver consists of
   A. head tilt–neck lift;
   B. jaw thrust or mandibular displacement;
   C. separation of lips and teeth.
4. Practice the triple airway maneuver using an adult mannequin.

Exercise B: Oropharyngeal Airway Insertion

1. Select the appropriate-sized oropharyngeal airway for an adult mannequin. *Note:* An excessively large oropharyngeal airway may compress the epiglottis and create rather than relieve airway obstruction.

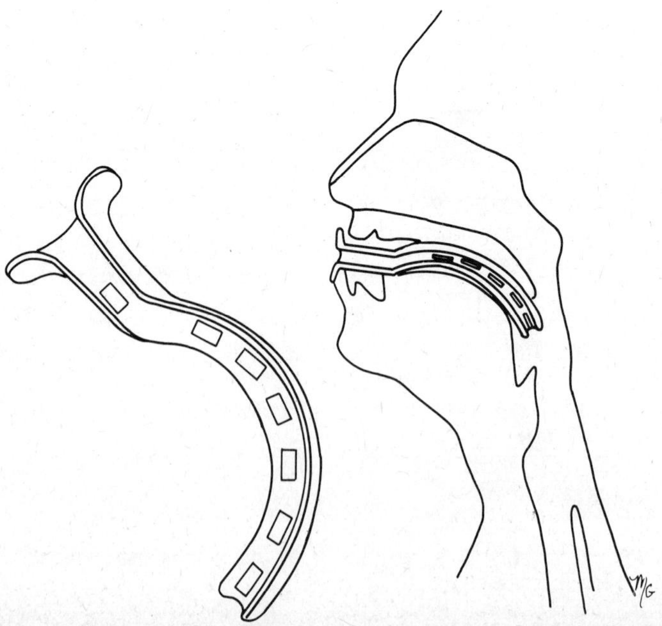

Fig. 30-1. Oropharyngeal airway and proper positioning in the hypopharynx.

2. Open the airway manually using the head tilt–neck lift technique. The mouth may be opened by crossing the finger and thumb while separating the upper and lower teeth. *Caution:* Your fingers should never be inserted between the teeth of a conscious or semiconscious patient.
3. While retracting the lips from the teeth, insert the oropharyngeal airway. The airway may be inserted either directly to the posterior position at the base of the tongue or upside down (at a 180° angle) and rotated into position.
4. Verify adequate positioning of the airway (Fig. 30-1).
5. Secure the airway by applying tape to the external flange. Be certain that the tape does not occlude the airway. *Note:* In the clinical setting, artificial airways are usually secured by tape to the maxillary area rather than to the mandible because movement of the jaw may result in inadvertent displacement of the airway.

Exercise C: Nasopharyngeal Airway Insertion

1. Select the appropriate-sized nasopharyngeal airway for use with an adult mannequin. Verify that both the length and diameter are adequate.
2. Lubricate the airway with water-soluble lubricant.
3. Simulate the determination of nasal patency by alternately occluding each nostril and listening for air flow. Lubricate the nasopharyngeal airway with sterile, water-soluble lubricant.
4. Insert the tip of the nasopharyngeal airway into the external nares. The bevel of the airway should face upward during insertion.
5. Throughout the insertion, rotate the airway gently to conform to the shape of the pharynx.
6. After insertion, the tip of the airway should be located in the posterior hypopharynx at the base of the tongue (not at the uvula) (Fig. 30-2).
7. Stabilize the airway by applying tape to the flange. A safety pin may be inserted through the flange for additional stability.

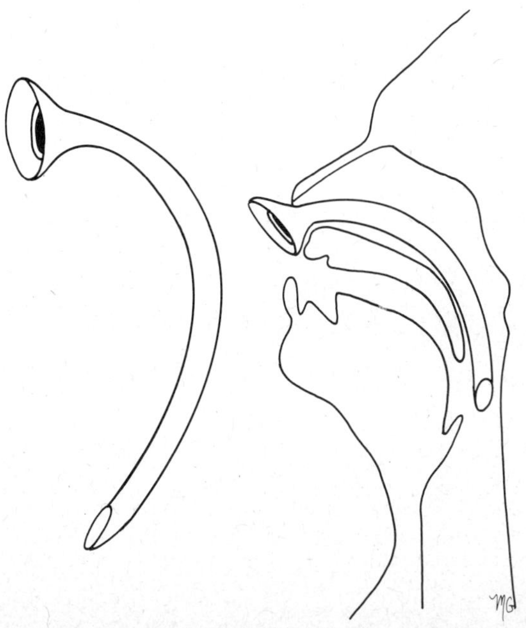

Fig. 30-2. Nasopharyngeal airway and proper positioning in the hypopharynx.

Exercise D: Esophageal Obturator Airway Insertion

1. Obtain an esophageal obturator airway.
2. Verify that a mannequin is placed in the supine position with the neck and head midline. Do not manually open the airway in order to allow intubation of the esophagus.
3. Insert the tip of the esophageal airway into the esophagus until the mask creates a tight seal on the face.
4. Using a 10 ml syringe, inflate the pilot balloon.
5. Ventilate through the esophageal obturator airway by mouth-to-tube breathing or by using a manual bag.
6. Verify the position of the airway by looking at the chest and by listening for exhaled air flow (Fig. 30-3).
7. If the stomach inflates during inspiration, the trachea probabley has been accidentally intubated. If the trachea was intubated, deflate the cuff and insert the tube into the esophagus.
8. *Note:* In clinical practice, if you encounter a patient with an esophageal obturator airway in place (usually during resuscitation in the emergency room), intubate the trachea *before* removing the esophageal obturator airway.

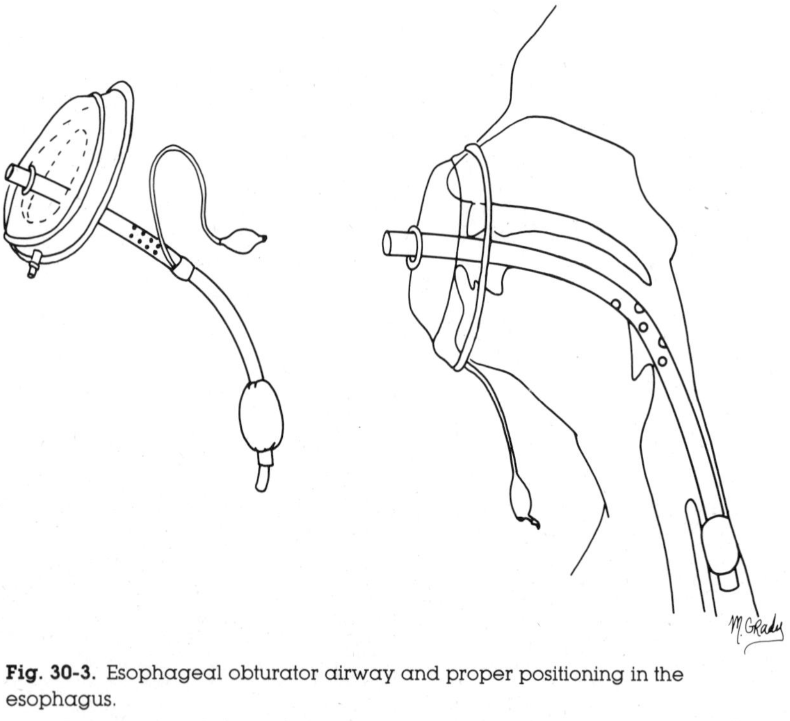

Fig. 30-3. Esophageal obturator airway and proper positioning in the esophagus.

Exercise E: Identification of Endotracheal Tube Components

1. Obtain an endotracheal tube. Examine the components and tube markings of an endotracheal tube (Fig. 30-4).
2. Identify the following parts:
   A. Cuff
   B. Murphy eye
   C. 15 mm adapter

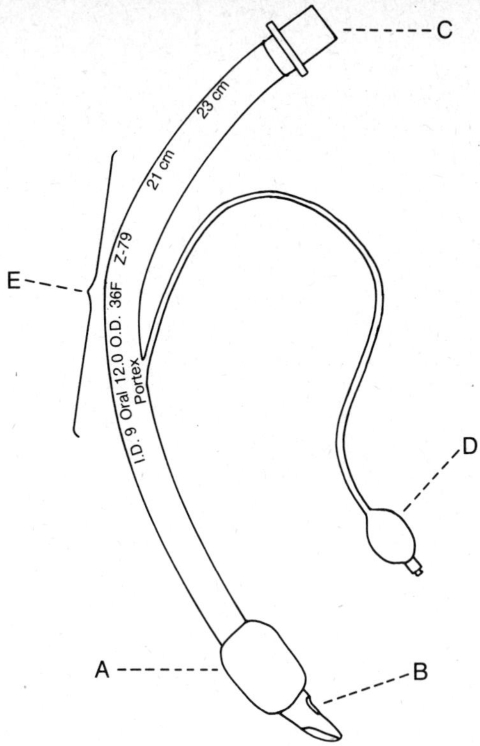

Fig. 30-4. Endotracheal tube.

D. Pilot balloon

E. Tube markings:

1) Brand name
2) Internal and external diameter
3) Radiopaque line
4) Depth markings
5) Oral or nasal
6) Z-79: Mark of Standards Committee for Anesthesia Equipment
7) Mark indicating that tube material is nontoxic

3. Attach a 10 ml syringe to the pilot balloon. Inject an adequate volume of air into the cuff to check for gas leaks. Record the volume injected into the cuff on the laboratory report. *Note:* A one-way valve may be located in the pilot balloon adapter that the syringe must activate in order to allow inflation and deflation of the cuff.
4. Obtain a size 3.0 mm ID neonateal endotracheal tube. Compare and contrast the neonatal tube with an 8.0 mm ID adult tube.
5. On the laboratory report, diagram and label an enlarged endotracheal tube.

Exercise F: Identification of Tracheostomy Tube Components

1. Obtain a tracheostomy tube. Examine the components of a tracheostomy tube (Fig. 30-5).
2. In addition to the similar structures found on an endotracheal tube, identify the following:

A. outer cannula

B. pilot balloon

C. inner cannula

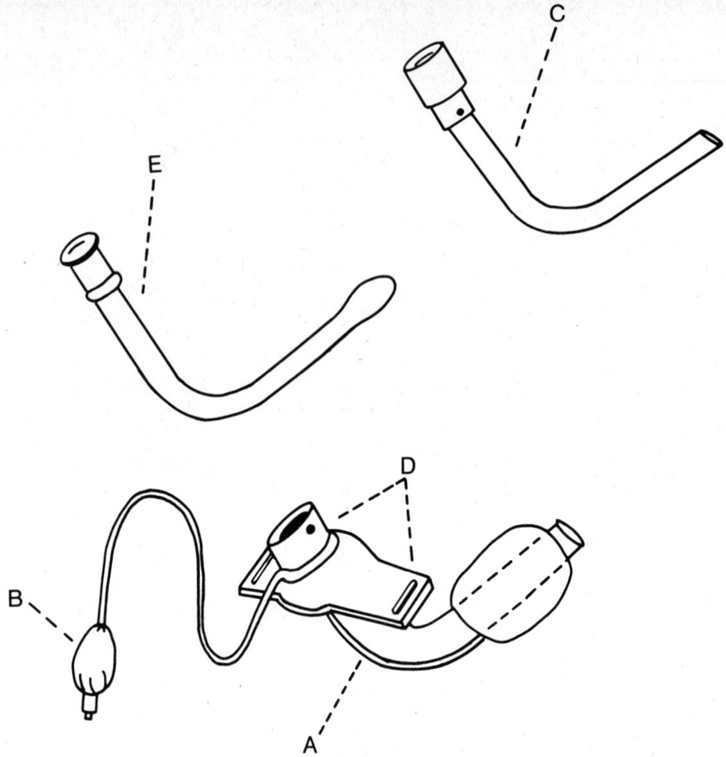

Fig. 30-5. Tracheostomy tube.

D. flange
E. obturator

3. Insert the obturator into the outer cannula. Remove the obturator.
4. Insert the inner cannula inside the outer cannula. Lock the inner cannula to the outer cannula (if applicable).
5. Using a syringe, check the cuff for gas leaks by inserting an adequate volume of air. Observe the pilot balloon during maximum cuff inflation and during complete deflation.
6. Diagram and label an enlarged tracheostomy tube on the laboratory report.

RECOMMENDED READING

Applebaum EL, Bruce DL: Tracheal Intubation. Philadelphia, WB Saunders, 1976

Burton GG, Hodgkin JE: Respiratory Care. A Guide to Clinical Practice, 2nd ed. Philadelphia, JB Lippincott, 1984

McPherson SP, Spearman CB: Respiratory Therapy Equipment, 3rd ed. St. Louis, CV Mosby, 1985

Shapiro BA, Harrison RA, Kacmarek RM, Cane RD: Clinical Application of Respiratory Care, 3rd ed. Chicago, Year Book Medical Publishers, 1985

Laboratory Performance Evaluation (#30)

Topic: Airway Patency and Artificial Airways

Student ______________________ Course ______________________

Date ______________________ Section ______________________

Performance Elements	Acceptable	Unacceptable	Not Applicable	Comments
1. Obtains patent airway: **A.** Neck hyperextension **B.** Chin lift **C.** Jaw thrust **D.** Triple airway maneuver				
2. Inserts and stabilizes pharyngeal airways: **A.** Nasopharyngeal airway **B.** Oropharyngeal airway				
3. Inserts esophageal obturator airway				
4. Identifies endotracheal tube components and size				
5. Identifies tracheostomy tube components and size: **A.** Inserts obturator **B.** Inserts and locks inner cannula **C.** Tests cuff on endotracheal and tracheostomy tubes				

Knowledge of Procedure

- ☐ Good; student is knowledgeable about rationale and theory related to procedure
- ☐ Fair; student has adequate understanding of rationale and theory related to procedure
- ☐ Poor; student has inadequate understanding of rationale and theory related to procedure

Performance Deficiencies (check those that apply)

- ☐ Excessive time needed to complete procedure
- ☐ Broke aseptic or sterile technique
- ☐ Gross inaccuracy noted
- ☐ Technique may be harmful to patient
- ☐ Incorrect dosage or gas concentration
- ☐ Incorrect equipment assembly/use
- ☐ Unable to answer questions correctly about rationale and/or theory related to procedure
- ☐ Other ______________________________

Evaluation Summary

- ☐ Satisfactory performance
- ☐ Unsatisfactory performance

Recommendations of Evaluator

- ☐ Skills may be applied/observed in clinical setting
- ☐ Specific evaluation deficiencies require correction
- ☐ Complete re-evaluation required
- ☐ Additional laboratory practice required

Signatures:

Evaluator ______________________ Date ______________________

Student ______________________ Date ______________________

Laboratory Report

Student ______________________ Acceptable ______________________

Date ______________________ Unacceptable ______________________

Course ______________________

Topic: Airway Patency and Artificial Airways

Data or Measurements

Endotracheal tube cuff volume ______________________

Tracheostomy tube cuff volume ______________________

Scenario: The nurse on the neurosurgical unit has asked for your consultation on a postoperative craniotomy patient. Arriving at the patient's room, you notice a frankly obese middle-aged man whose loud snoring is interrupted when he stops breathing, at which time he exhibits visible retractions. Please answer the following questions:

1. What manual technique would be useful in overcoming his immediate airway obstruction?

2. In the above situation, which would probably work better, an oral airway or a nasopharyngeal airway?

3. A patient who has undergone oromaxillary surgery and who has wired jaws would benefit from which type of airway?

4. Why may a nasopharyngeal airway benefit a patient who requires frequent nasotracheal suctioning?

5. Why is the size of an oropharyngeal airway important?

6. Describe the proper position for the tip of a nasopharyngeal airway.

7. Describe briefly the function of the following endotracheal tube structures and markings:
   A. Radiopaque line

   B. Depth markings

   C. 15 mm adapter

   D. Cuff

   E. Pilot balloon

8. Explain briefly the Z-79 label on artificial airways.

9. Why is an artificial airway stabilized to the maxillary area of the face?

chapter 31

Oral endotracheal intubation

INTRODUCTION

Endotracheal intubation—the insertion of an endotracheal tube into the trachea—is a common method of obtaining a patent airway. Endotracheal intubation may be accomplished either through the nose or through the mouth. Oral endotracheal intubation frequently is the route of choice in an emergency situation such as a respiratory or cardiac arrest. During oral intubation, the glottic landmarks are visualized with a laryngoscope. In neonates, oral endotracheal intubation frequently is preferred over the nasal route because of the risk of hemorrhage from adenoid tissue located in the nasopharynx. The purpose of this chapter is to introduce you to the procedure of oral endotracheal intubation in the adult and infant.

OBJECTIVES

After completing this chapter, you should be able to do the following:

1. *Perform oral endotracheal intubation on adult and infant mannequins.*
2. *Identify the anatomical landmarks in the airway for oral intubation.*
3. *Evaluate proper placement of the endotracheal tube.*
4. *Describe head and neck positioning before orotracheal intubation.*
5. *Identify the equipment necessary for intubation.*
6. *Identify the components of a laryngoscope.*
7. *Compare and contrast the use of straight and curved laryngoscope blades.*

EQUIPMENT NEEDED

- ☐ Oxygen source and flowmeter
- ☐ Manual ventilation bag
- ☐ Suction source and catheters
- ☐ Intubation mannequins (adult and infant) or animal model
- ☐ Oral airways

- ☐ Endotracheal tubes
- ☐ Magill forceps
- ☐ Stylet (rarely needed)
- ☐ Syringe
- ☐ Laryngoscope and blades
- ☐ Tape
- ☐ Hemostat

ACTIVITIES

Exercise A: Equipment Assembly and Function Check

1. Assemble the needed equipment and check the functions of the following:
   - A. Bag–valve–mask unit and oxygen flow
   - B. Endotracheal tube cuff
   - C. Laryngoscope blade bulb
   - D. Suction catheter
2. *Note:* Since oral intubation usually is an emergency procedure, equipment function should *not* be checked at the time it is needed. In the clinical setting, intubation equipment usually is checked at pre-determined intervals.

Exercise B: Adult Oral Intubation

1. Stand at the head of the mannequin.
2. Elevate the head above the level of the shoulders by placing a small pillow under the head. Extend the head by moving the chin up and back. This position is known as the "sniffing position" and allows for direct exposure of the glottis (Fig. 31-1).
3. Position the head and neck midline. The nose, chin, and thyroid cartilage should be aligned.
4. If necessary, clear the oropharynx with a suction catheter and remove dentures.
5. Hold the laryngoscope handle in the left hand.
6. Retract the lower lip with the right thumb. The structures in the oropharynx will appear as in the diagram (Fig. 31-2).
7. Insert the laryngoscope blade on the right side of the mouth.

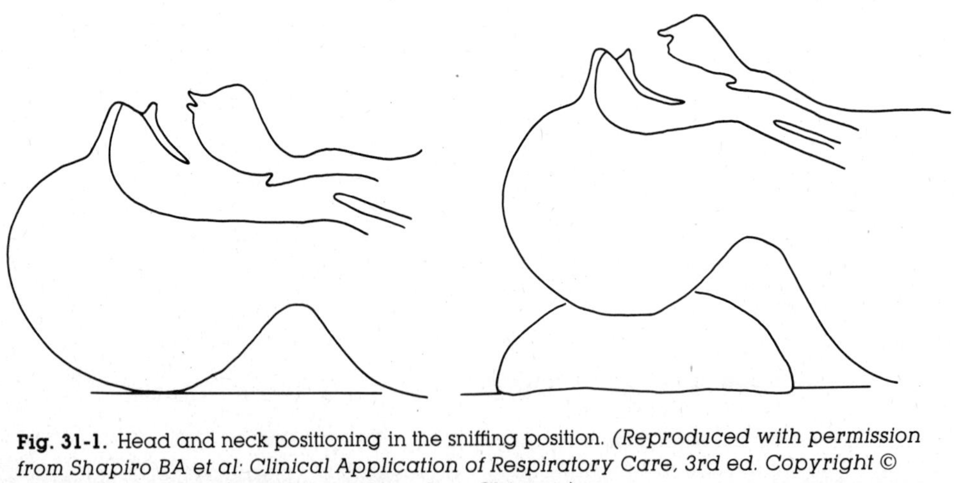

Fig. 31-1. Head and neck positioning in the sniffing position. *(Reproduced with permission from Shapiro BA et al: Clinical Application of Respiratory Care, 3rd ed. Copyright © 1985 by Year Book Medical Publishers, Inc., Chicago)*

8. After insertion of the laryngoscope blade into the oropharynx, be certain to maintain an adequate distance from the mouth. The laryngoscopist must visualize glottic landmarks with both eyes open to allow the advantage of depth perception.
9. After visualization of the epiglottis, bring the blade and tongue midline (Fig. 31-3).
10. While keeping the left wrist straight, and by lifting *only* the shoulder and arm, lift the base of the tongue and epiglottis anteriorly to expose the glottis.
11. Expose the glottis without using the teeth as a fulcrum.
12. A straight laryngoscope blade will directly displace the epiglottis. A curved blade will indirectly expose the glottis by insertion into the vallecula. The techniques are shown in the following diagram (Fig. 31-4).
13. Identify the glottic landmarks:
    A. Epiglottis
    B. Arytenoid cartilages
    C. Vocal cords
14. Hold the endotracheal tube about ¾ of the tube length from the cuff. If the endotracheal tube is held in the right hand during insertion of the laryngoscope blade, you may avoid groping for the tube and inadvertent displacement of the glottic landmarks.
15. Insert the endotracheal tube into the right side of the mouth
16. Simultaneously advance the tube toward the vocal cords while "twirling" the tube between two fingers in order to direct the tip of the tube anteriorly toward the glottis. The natural curvature of the endotracheal tube combined with a rotating or twirling motion is often sufficient to avoid the use of a stylet.
17. Advance the endotracheal tube forward and through the vocal cords during direct visualization. *Caution:* If you do not visualize the glottis, do *not* advance the tube. Extensive trauma (and permanent damage) to the larynx and soft tissues may occur from blind "probing" attempts during intubation.

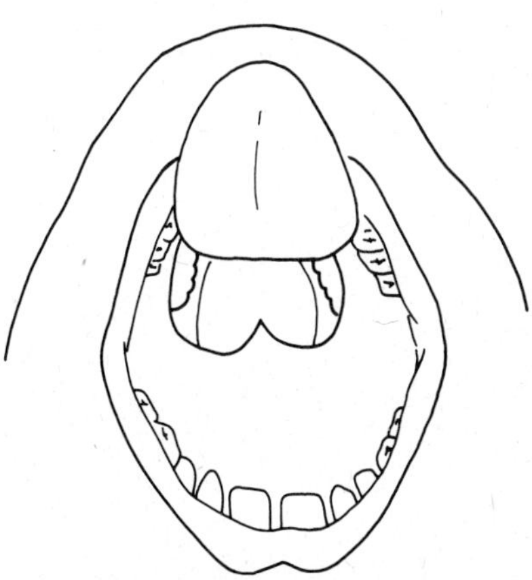

Fig. 31-2. Appearance of the oropharynx when viewed by the intubator. *(Modified from Spearman CB, Sheldon RL: Egan's Fundamentals of Respiratory Therapy, 4th ed. St Louis, CV Mosby, 1982)*

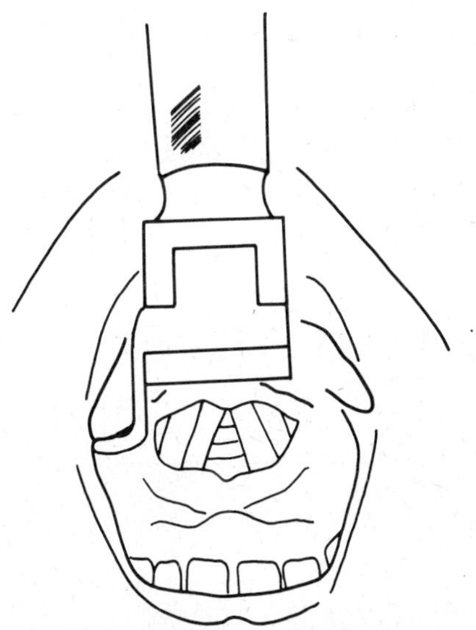

Fig. 31-3. Anatomical landmarks for oral intubation. *(Reproduced with permission from Shapiro BA et al: Clinical Application of Respiratory Care, 3rd ed. Copyright © 1985 by Year Book Medical Publishers, Inc, Chicago)*

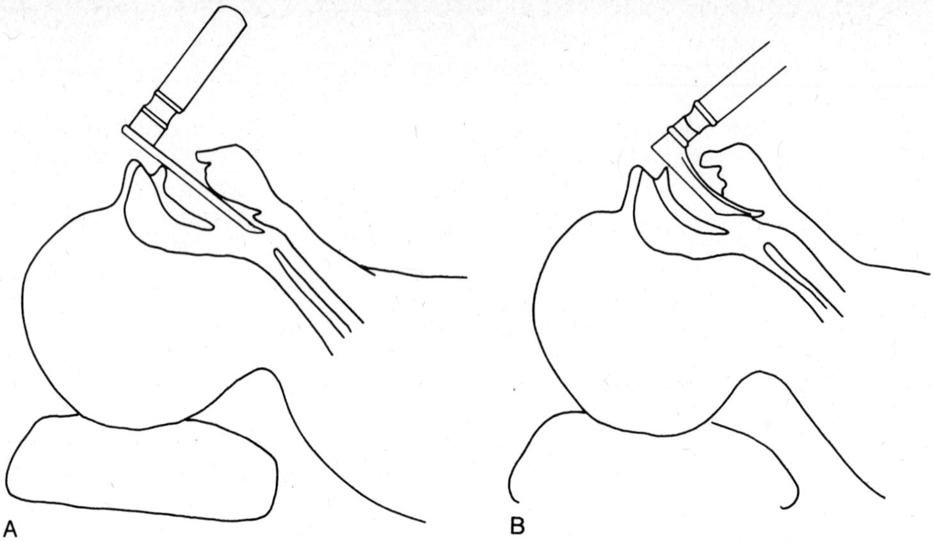

Fig. 31-4. Use of the (A) straight and (B) curved larnygoscope blade. *(Reproduced with permission from Shapiro BA et al: Clinical Application of Respiratory Care, 3rd ed. Copyright © 1985 by Year Book Medical Publishers, Inc, Chicago)*

18. After the tube passes through the glottis, advance the tube an additional 2 inches under direct visualization, or until the cuff disappears from view.
19. Gently remove the laryngoscope blade while securing the tube.
20. Immediately inflate the tube cuff and ventilate.

Exercise C: Infant Oral Intubation

1. Prepare the equipment needed for endotracheal intubation. Verify that neonatal-sized laryngoscope blades, endotracheal tubes, and suction catheters are present and functional.
2. Endotracheal intubation of the neonate is similar to that of the adult, with the following differences:
   A. Elective and emergency intubation of the neonate usually is done using the oral route. Infants rarely are intubated through the nose because of the large amount of adenoid tissue.
   B. Before attempting laryngoscopy of an infant, the neck may be extended by placing a towel or diaper roll under the neonate's shoulders (Fig. 31-5).

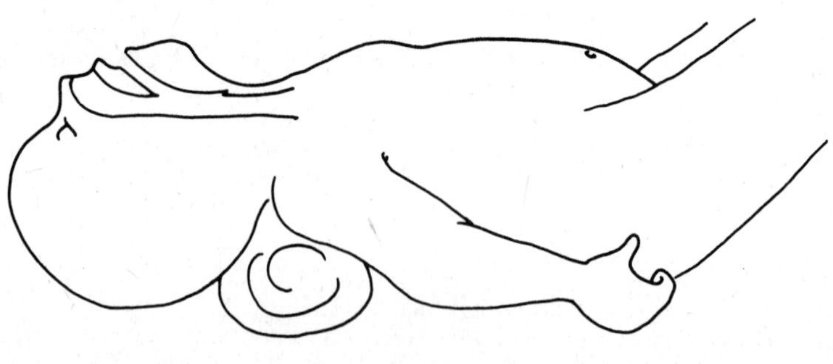

Fig. 31-5. Positioning of an infant before oral intubation. *(Modified from Lough MD, Williams TJ, Rawson J: Newborn Respiratory Care. Chicago, Year Book Medical Publishers, Inc., 1979)*

3. Verify that the infant's nose, mouth, and thyroid cartilage are midline. The neck should be neither flexed nor hyperextended.
4. Hold the laryngoscope handle with your thumb and one or two fingers only. The laryngoscope is held in the left hand.
5. Hold the endotracheal tube in your right hand.
6. While retracting the infant's lower lip, gently advance the laryngoscope blade into the right corner of the mouth.
7. Upon visualization of the epiglottis, swing the blade midline and gently lift anteriorly, thereby retracting the tongue. This maneuver creates room on the right side of the mouth for the endotracheal tube.
8. The laryngoscope blade is inserted into the vallecula in neonates. Because the epiglottis is relatively "fragile," it should not be directly displaced regardless of the blade type. The technique of neonatal laryngoscopy is shown in the following diagram (Fig. 31-6).
9. Advance the endotracheal tube through the glottis while the vocal cords are open.
10. After the tip of the tube passes through the vocal cords, advance the tube an additional 1 cm to 2 cm.
11. After intubation, the tube may be stabilized by inserting a finger into the mouth and pressing the tube against the palate. The tube is then stabilized with tape to the neonate's face.

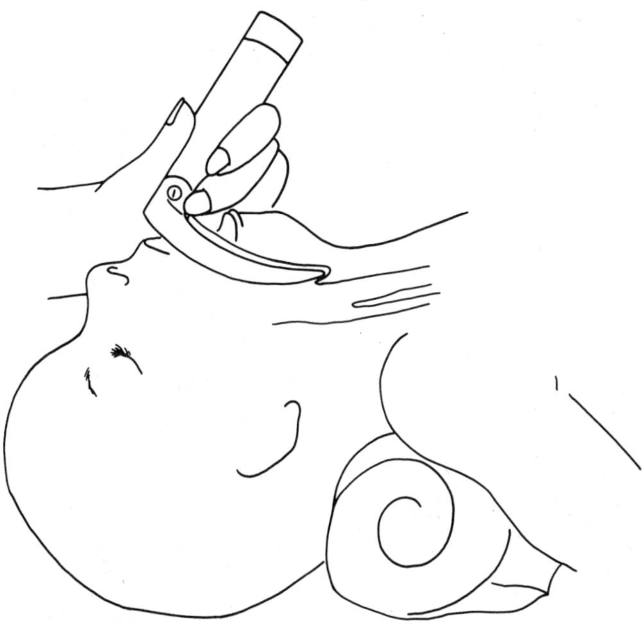

Fig. 31-6. Position of laryngoscope blade in vallecula during infant oral intubation.

Exercise D: Evaluation of Tube Position

1. After intubation, inflate the tube cuff.
2. Evaluate endotracheal tube position by the following:
   - A. Auscultation (equal bilateral breath sounds)
   - B. Observation (symmetrical chest movement)
   - C. Palpation of tube cuff
   - D. Chest x-ray film (tip should be located proximal to the second anterior rib or between the third and fourth thoracic vertebral bodies (in adults)
   - E. Direct visualization of tube through cords

Exercise F: Stabilization of Endotracheal Tube

1. After determining proper endotracheal tube placement, note the depth marking.
2. Stabilize the endotracheal tube by preparing the maxillary area with tincture of benzoin.
3. Tape the endotracheal tube to the maxillary area.
4. Separately insert and stabilize an oral airway in the oropharynx. *Note:* In the event that an intubation attempt is unsuccessful after 30 seconds, clear the airway and provide several breaths by means of the bag–valve–mask unit. Repeat the intubation attempt.

RECOMMENDED READING

Applebaum EL, Bruce DL: Tracheal Intubation. Philadelphia, WB Saunders, 1976

Burton GG, Hodgkin JG: Respiratory Care. A Guide to Clinical Practice, 2nd ed. Philadelphia, JB Lippincott, 1984

Shapiro BA, Harrison RA, Kacmarek RM, Cane RD: Clinical Application of Respiratory Care, 3rd ed. Chicago, Year Book Medical Publishers, 1985

Laboratory Performance Evaluation (#31)

Topic: Oral Endotracheal Intubation

Student ______________________ Course ______________________

Date ______________________ Section ______________________

Performance Elements	Acceptable	Unacceptable	Not Applicable	Comments
1. Assembles needed materials				
2. Checks function of equipment (bag, cuff, light)				
3. Positions head, neck, and shoulders (sniffing position)				
4. Inserts oral airway				
5. Preoxygenates and ventilates with bag and mask				
6. Holds laryngoscope in left hand, inserts blade on right side				
7. Brings blade to midline after visualizing epiglottis				
8. Exposes glottis without "fulcrum" pressing on incisor teeth				
9. Inserts tube through vocal cords by means of direct visualization				
10. Inflates cuff				
11. Stabilizes tube to maxillary area				
12. Stabilizes oral airway separately				

Performance Elements	Acceptable	Unacceptable	Not Applicable	Comments
13. Checks tube placement: **A.** Equal, bilateral breath sounds **B.** Symmetrical chest expansion on inspirationtr				
14. Intubation attempt lasts a maximum of 30 seconds				
15. If attempt is unsuccessful, ventilation and oxygen are accomplished by bag-valve-mask before next attempt				

Knowledge of Procedure

☐ Good; student is knowledgeable about rationale and theory related to procedure

☐ Fair; student has adequate understanding of rationale and theory related to procedure

☐ Poor; student has inadequate understanding of rationale and theory related to procedure

Performance Deficiencies (check those that apply)

☐ Excessive time needed to complete procedure

☐ Broke aseptic or sterile technique

☐ Gross inaccuracy noted

☐ Technique may be harmful to patient

☐ Incorrect dosage or gas concentration

☐ Incorrect equipment assembly/use

☐ Unable to answer questions correctly about rationale and/or theory related to procedure

☐ Other ______________________________

Evaluation Summary

☐ Satisfactory performance

☐ Unsatisfactory performance

Recommendations of Evaluator

- ☐ Skills may be applied/observed in clinical setting
- ☐ Specific evaluation deficiencies require correction
- ☐ Complete re-evaluation required
- ☐ Additional laboratory practice required

Signatures:

Evaluator ______________________ Date ______________________

Student ______________________ Date ______________________

Laboratory Report

Student ______________________ Acceptable ______________________

Date ______________________ Unacceptable ______________________

Course ______________________

Topic: Oral Endotracheal Intubation

Scenario: You are for the first time carrying the "bag" that contains all of the equipment necessary for performing an emergency intubation. This means that *you* will be responding to emergencies and intubating when indicated. Upon receiving the bag, your first task is to inventory the contents and check all of the equipment for proper function.

You had just completed your equipment check when you are paged stat to the emergency room. "You better get a tube for that one," someone said, pointing toward the crash room. The patient in the crash room is a young man, an obvious accident victim, who has suffered multiple facial lacerations. He is bleeding from his nose. Just as you open the bag and secure your equipment, he becomes apneic.

Please answer the following questions:

1. List the equipment that must be checked before performing an oral intubation.

2. What are the consequences of *not* checking your equipment before using it?

3. In the emergency room, your first intubation attempt is unsuccessful. Describe what you would do.

4. Compare and contrast oral intubation of the adult with that of a neonate.

5. Describe briefly how tube position may be determined.

6. Why should a functional suction catheter be available during the intubation procedure?

7. Which airway reflexes may be stimulated during oral intubation?

8. Please list the anatomical "landmarks" for performing this intubation.

9. After having successfully intubated the patient, a chest x-ray film is obtained. Describe in radiographic terms the proper location of the endotracheal tube.

chapter 32

Nasal endotracheal intubation

INTRODUCTION

In contrast to the emergency oral route, nasal endotracheal intubation is frequently performed as an elective procedure. A nasal endotracheal tube may be placed in the following situations:

1. A conscious or alert patient
2. A patient who can breathe spontaneously for a brief period and requires intubation
3. Convulsions, trismus, or rigidity of the mandible
4. Oral trauma or oral surgery

The technique of nasal intubation involves the insertion of an endotracheal tube through the nose and into the trachea either with direct visualization of the glottic landmarks or using a "blind" technique. Blind nasotracheal intubation refers to the insertion of an endotracheal tube while listening to air flow through the tube. The purpose of this chapter is to introduce you to nasal endotracheal intubation.

OBJECTIVES

After completing this chapter, you should be able to do the following:

1. *Perform nasal endotracheal intubation on an adult mannequin using both blind and direct visualization techniques.*
2. *Identify the procedure for premedication before elective intubation*
3. *Compare and contrast blind and direct visualization elective intubation procedures.*
4. *Evaluate proper endotracheal tube position.*

EQUIPMENT NEEDED

- ☐ Oxygen source and flowmeter
- ☐ Manual ventilation bag

☐ Suction source and catheters
☐ Adult intubation mannequin
☐ Oral airway
☐ Magill forceps
☐ Nasal decongestant, topical anesthetic gel
☐ Stylet
☐ Syringe
☐ Laryngoscope blade
☐ Tape

ACTIVITIES

Exercise A: Equipment Selection, Assembly, and Function Check

1. Assemble the needed equipment and check the functions of the following:
   A. Bag-valve-mask unit and oxygen flow
   B. Endotracheal tube cuff
   C. Laryngoscope blade light bulb
   D. Suction catheter patency and pressure

Exercise B: Site Preparation

1. Administer a decongestant by spraying an aerosol into both sides of the nasopharynx.
2. Administer a topical anesthetic into the nasopharynx and oropharynx by means of an atomizer (Fig. 32-1). Spray the anesthetic to the lingual tonsillar area near the base of the tongue. Request that the patient swallow a small volume of anesthetic solution.
3. Administer 100% oxygen by rebreathing mask.
4. Verify that the continuous ECG monitor and intravenous line are functional.
5. Establish a baseline heart rate and rhythm.
6. A tranquilizer may be administered. *Note:* Before performing this exercise, your instructor may modify an intubation mannequin to simulate spontaneous breathing (See Chap. 19 for recommended modification procedure).

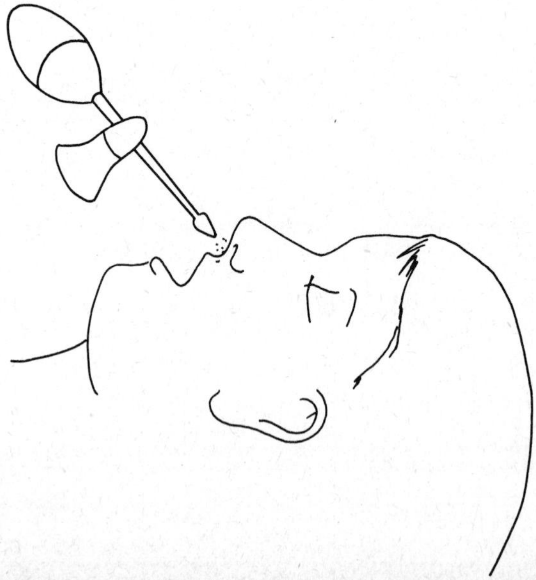

Fig. 32-1. Administration of topical anesthetic by atomizer.

Exercise C: Blind Nasal Endotracheal Intubation

1. Explain the procedure to a conscious patient using simple terms.
2. Position the head and neck in the "sniffing" position.
3. Position the rebreathing mask so that it covers the mouth and exposes the external nares.
4. Maintain supplemental oxygen throughout the procedure (Fig. 32-2).
5. Apply anesthetic gel to the endotracheal tube.
6. Insert the tip of the endotracheal tube into the external nares with the bevel up.
7. Insert the tube. Advance the tube away from the basal turbinates.
8. Gently add a slight, constant pressure to advance the tube through the internal nares. Do *not* use excessive force. If a great deal of resistance is met, slightly withdraw the tube and extend the head farther. Advance the tube again.
9. Rotate the tube according to the volume of exhaled breath sounds through the tube.
10. Continue to advance the tube until breath sounds are loudest.
11. Observe the chest while advancing the tube (Fig. 32-3). Note that the chest is observed for movement while simultaneously listening for air flow through the tube.
12. Request that the patient stick his tongue out (if applicable). Advance the tube through the vocal cords on inspiration.
13. Note that the vocal cords are farthest apart during inspiration and the glottis is at its widest diameter. *If stimulation of the larynx induces a cough, the tube may be advanced between the vocal cords during the deep inspiration immediately following the cough (Fig. 32-4).
14. Advance the tube an additional 2.0 cm after insertion through the vocal cords.
15. Inflate the cuff.
16. Immediately provide ventilation and supplemental oxygen by means of a manual ventilation bag.
17. Reassure the patient and stabilize the tube to the maxillary area.
18. Verify that the endotracheal tube position is above the carina by observing chest movement and by auscultation.

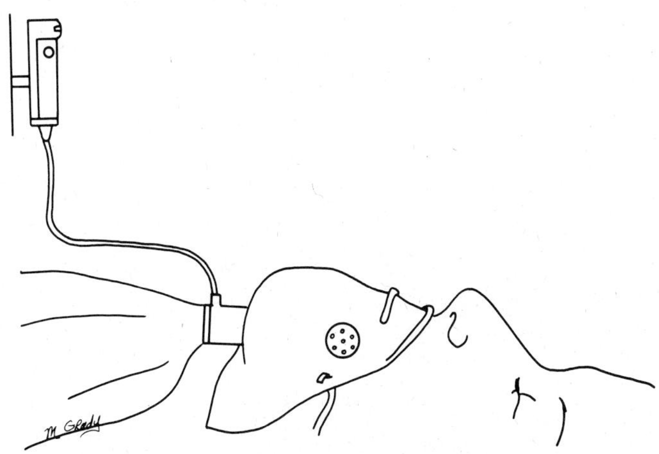

Fig. 32-2. Administration of oxygen during nasotracheal intubation.

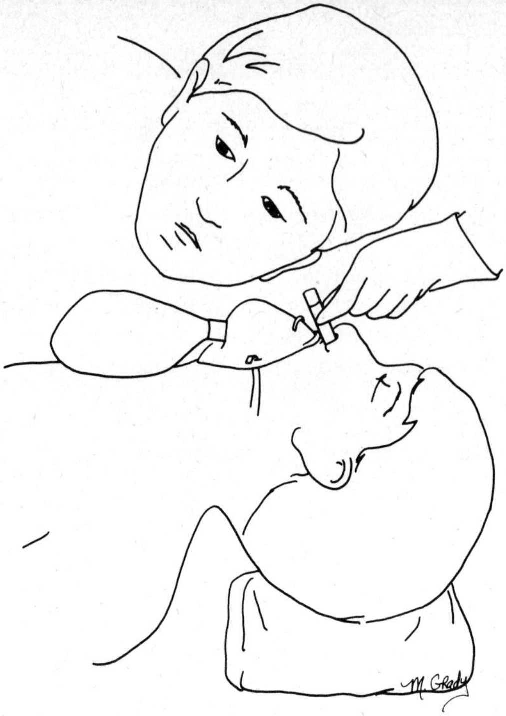

Fig. 32-3. Observation of the chest during blind nasotracheal intubation.

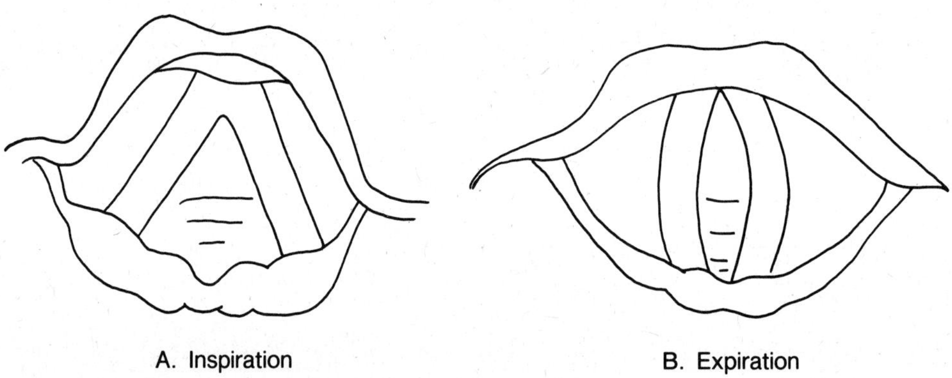

Fig. 32-4. Position of vocal cords during (A) inspiration and (B) expiration. *(Modified from Spearman CB, Sheldon RL: Egan's Fundamentals of Respiratory Therapy, 4th ed. St Louis, CV Mosby, 1982)*

Exercise D: Nasal Intubation Under Direct Visualization

1. The procedure is similar to blind intubation and is usually performed when blind intubation is unsuccessful.
2. Follow steps 1 through 8 in the blind elective endotracheal intubation procedure (see above).
3. After the tube has passed the uvula, expose the oropharynx with a laryngoscope.
4. Under direct visualization by laryngoscopy, grasp the tip of the endotracheal tube with Magill forceps. *Note:* Avoid grasping the cuff with the forceps.
5. Steer the tip of the tube into the glottis. Have an assistant advance the tube into the oropharynx while you hold the laryngoscope with your left hand and Magill forceps with your right hand (Fig. 32-5).
6. Advance the tube cuff beyond the vocal cords.
7. Inflate the cuff and immediately provide manual ventilation.
8. Verify endotracheal tube position.

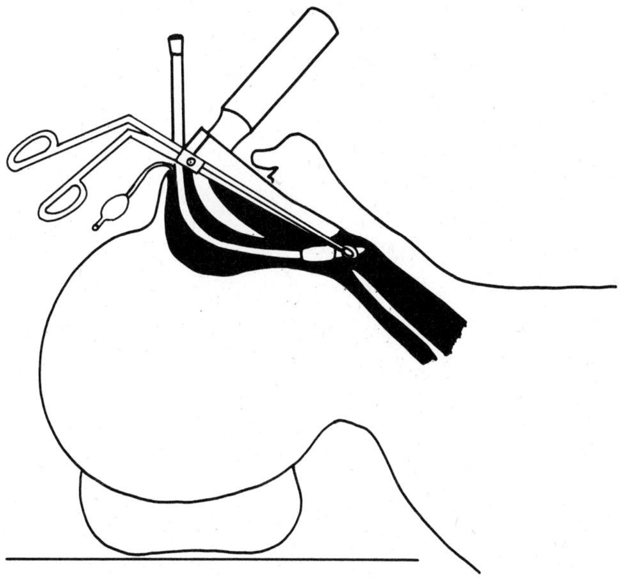

Fig. 32-5. Nasotracheal intubation during direct visualization of glottis. *(Reproduced with permission from Shapiro BA et al: Clinical Application of Respiratory Care, 3rd ed. Copyright © 1985 by Year Book Medical Publishers, Inc, Chicago)*

Exercise E: Evaluation of Tube Position and Stabilization

1. After intubation, evaluate the tube position by auscultation and observation of the chest for symmetrical chest movement.
2. Stabilize the endotracheal tube by taping it to the maxillary area of the face.

RECOMMENDED READING

Applebaum EL, Bruce DL: Tracheal Intubation. Philadelphia, WB Saunders, 1976

Burton GG, Hodgkin JE: Respiratory Care. A Guide to Clinical Practice, 2nd ed. Philadelphia, JB Lippincott, 1984

Shapiro BA, Harrison RA, Kacmarek RM, Cane RD: Clinical Application of Respiratory Care, 3rd ed. Chicago, Year Book Medical Publishers, 1985

Laboratory Performance Evaluation (#32)

Topic: Nasal Endotracheal Intubation

Student ______________________ Course ______________________

Date ______________________ Section ______________________

Performance Elements	Acceptable	Unacceptable	Not Applicable	Comments
1. Assembles material for oral intubation in addition to the following: A. Topical anesthetic (gel or spray) B. Stylet C. Magill forceps				
2. Assures proper function of equipment				
3. Monitors cardiopulmonary system for baseline values				
4. Identifies self and simulated patient				
5. Explains procedure				
6. Positions head, neck, and shoulders (sniffing position)				
7. Preoxygenates with 100% oxygen				
8. Maintains supplemental oxygen throughout procedure				
9. Anesthetizes nasopharynx and oropharynx				
10. Inserts endotracheal tube into nostril (bevel up)				
11. Attempts to proceed along turbinates				

Performance Elements	Acceptable	Unacceptable	Not Applicable	Comments
12. Uses mild but constant pressure advancing into internal nares				
13. Rotates tube				
14. Advances tube until breath sounds exiting tube are loudest (manipulates tube past cartilage)				
15. Advances tube between vocal cords during inspiration				
16. Inflates cuff				
17. Reassures patient, stabilizes tube to maxilla				
18. Checks for tube placement by observation and auscultation				

Knowledge of Procedure

☐ Good; student is knowledgeable about rationale and theory related to procedure

☐ Fair; student has adequate understanding of rationale and theory related to procedure

☐ Poor; student has inadequate understanding of rationale and theory related to procedure

Performance Deficiencies (check those that apply)

☐ Excessive time needed to complete procedure

☐ Broke aseptic or sterile technique

☐ Gross inaccuracy noted

☐ Technique may be harmful to patient

☐ Incorrect dosage or gas concentration

☐ Incorrect equipment assembly/use

☐ Unable to answer questions correctly about rationale and/or theory related to procedure

☐ Other ______________________________

Evaluation Summary
☐ Satisfactory performance ☐ Unsatisfactory performance

Recommendations of Evaluator
☐ Skills may be applied/observed in clinical setting ☐ Specific evaluation deficiencies require correction ☐ Complete re-evaluation required ☐ Additional laboratory practice required

Signatures:

Evaluator ____________________ Date ____________________

Student ____________________ Date ____________________

Laboratory Report

Student ______________________ Acceptable ______________________

Date ______________________ Unacceptable ______________________

Course ______________________

Topic: Nasal Endotracheal Intubation

Scenario: Not long after your first successful oral endotracheal intubation, you are summoned to the cardiac care unit to intubate a patient who is in fulminating pulmonary edema. Although confused, the patient is quite alert and cognizant. Please answer the following questions:

1. What are the indications for elective nasal intubation?

2. Briefly compare and contrast the indications for elective nasal intubation with emergency oral intubation.

3. What is the function of Magill forceps in elective intubation?

4. What would you do if the patient experiences asystole after you have advanced a nasal tube through the external nares?

5. What ECG changes would indicate the need for immediately discontinuing the nasal intubation attempt and re-establishing ventilation with a bag–valve–mask system?

6. Which airway reflexes may be stimulated during nasal intubation?

7. After inserting the tip of the endotracheal about 3 cm to 4 cm into the right nostril, you are met with a considerable amount of resistance. What would you do?

8. When performing a blind nasal endotracheal intubation, how do you determine when you have entered the trachea?

9. What method is used to ascertain whether an adequate amount of topical anesthetic has been administered before performing the intubation?

chapter 33

Manual ventilation

INTRODUCTION

Respiratory bags or bag–valve–mask units are devices that can be manually compressed to produce ventilation. Many clinical circumstances may necessitate the use of a manual bag, including resuscitation, intrahospital and interhospital patient transport, artificial airway intubation and extubation, tracheobronchial aspiration, and mechanical ventilator malfunction. Since a manual bag may be used in emergency situations, it is necessary to understand the mechanical function of each device before use in the clinical setting.

Although many brands of manual bags exist, the following characteristics may be found in the "perfect" bag:

1. Nonrebreathing valve that does not jam with high oxygen flowrates and allows for spontaneous breathing without bag compression.
2. Standard 15/22 mm adapter for connection to endotracheal tubes or mask.
3. Adapters that allow for measurement of proximal airway pressure and PEEP delivery.
4. Transparent material to allow monitoring of gas flow during ventilation.
5. Oxygen filling and reservoir system to provide nearly 100% oxygen during different ventilatory patterns.
6. Component parts that are easy to disassemble, clean, and reassemble.
7. Pressure relief valve.
8. Adult, pediatric, and neonatal sizes.

In addition, manual bags may be either flow- or self-refilling. The purpose of this chapter is to introduce you to manual ventilation using respiratory bags.

OBJECTIVES

After completing this chapter, you should be able to do the following:

1. *Provide ventilation to adult and infant mannequins wth a self- and flow-inflating manual ventilation bag.*

2. *Understand the factors that affect the oxygen concentration delivered by a manual bag.*
3. *Identify and understand the functions of the primary conponents in manual bags.*
4. *Identify manual bags through which spontaneous breathing is possible.*

EQUIPMENT NEEDED

- ☐ Several brands of manual ventilation bags
- ☐ Wright spirometer
- ☐ Gas source and flowmeter
- ☐ Oxygen analyzer
- ☐ Adult and infant mannequins
- ☐ Adult or infant lung simulator
- ☐ Oropharyngeal airway

ACTIVITIES

Exercise A: Identification and Assembly of a Manual Ventilation Bag

1. Select a self-refilling manual ventilation bag (Fig. 33-1).
2. Identify the following components:
   A. Nonrebreathing valve
   B. Oxygen inlet
   C. Pressure relief valve
   D. 15 mm/22 mm universal connector
   E. Reservoir system
3. Compress the bag and observe the valve in position during inspiration and expiration.

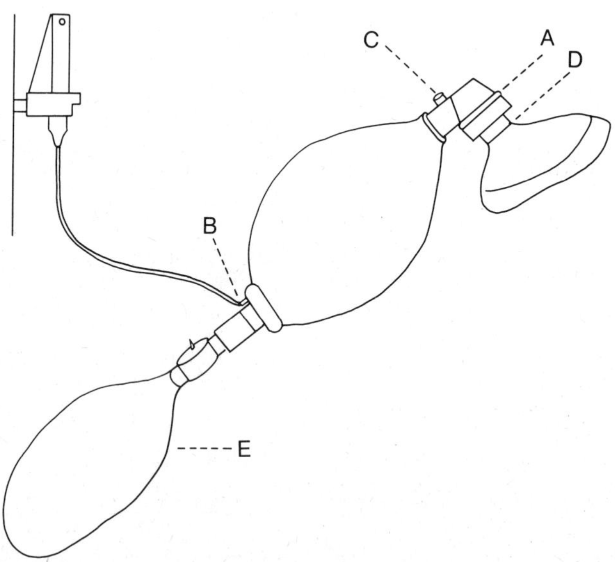

Fig. 33-1. Self-refilling manual ventilation bag.

4. On the laboratory report, diagram and label the valve position during inspiration and expiration from the manual bags provided by your instructor. Trace the gas flow through each valve.
5. Obtain a flow-inflating manual bag (Fig. 33-2).
6. Identify the following components:
   A. 15/22 mm connector
   B. Bag
   C. Oxygen tubing connection
   D. Pressure relief valve
7. Completely disassemble and reassemble the manual bags provided by your instructor. After reassembly, verify the proper function of the unit by occluding the patient connection and compressing the bag.

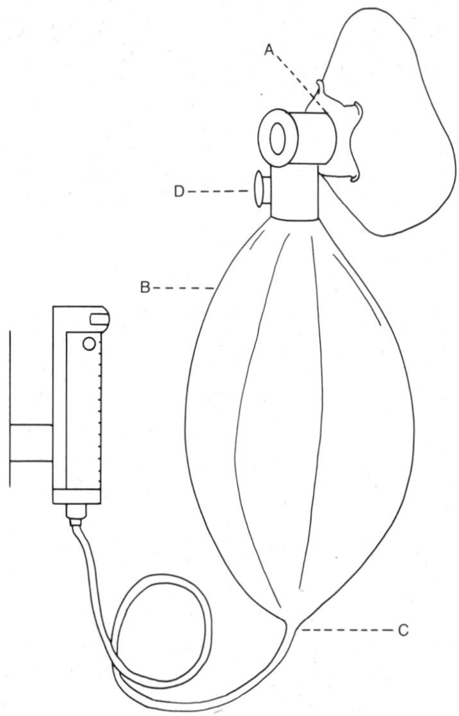

Fig. 33-2. Flow-inflating manual ventilation bag.

Exercise B: Measurement of Delivered Tidal Volume

1. Connect each adult manual bag to a spirometer or a lung simulator (settings R_1 and C_1).
2. Maximally compress the bag with one hand. *Note:* Avoid rapid compression, which may damage the spirometer.
3. Record the delivered tidal volume on the laboratory report.
4. Maximally compress the bag with two hands.
5. Record the delivered tidal volume.

Exercise C: Manual Bag and Mask Ventilation

1. Assume that the simulated patient (recording CPR mannequin) is apneic. Completely assemble the bag and connect to oxygen at flowrate of 12 liters/minute.
2. Open the airway by neck hyperextension.

3. Encircle the mask with the index and thumb of the left hand. With the remaining fingers, perform the chin lift maneuver for opening the airway. *Note:* When maintaining airway patency with the chin lift maneuver, be certain to lift the bony portion of the chin and *not* the soft tissue beneath the chin.
4. Compress the bag with the right hand (Fig. 33-3).
5. Perform manual ventilation at a rate of 12 breaths/minute for 2 minutes.

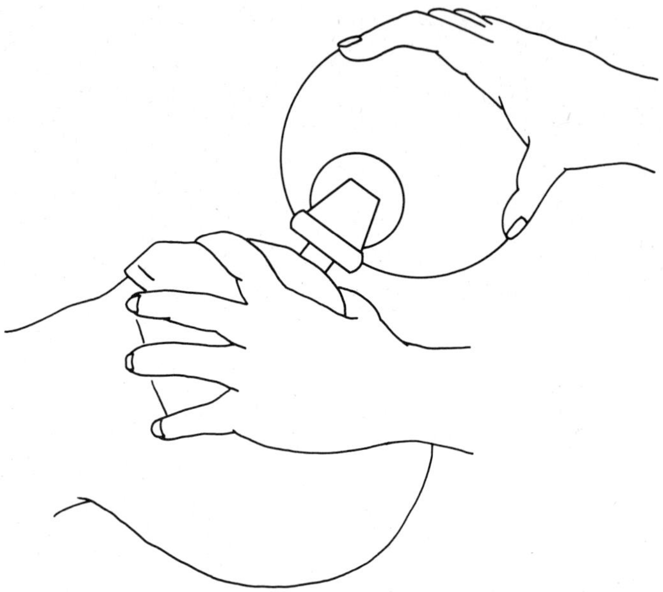

Fig. 33-3. Positioning of the airway and mask application during manual ventilation.

Exercise D: Manual Ventilation of an Intubated Mannequin with a Self-Inflating Bag

1. Completely assemble the manual bag and check for proper function.
2. Connect the bag to oxygen tubing and adjust the flow to that which does not cause the valve to jam.
3. Connect the 15 mm adapter to the endotracheal tube.
4. Perform manual ventilation for 2 minutes (Fig. 33-4).

Exercise E: Manual Ventilation of a Mannequin with a Flow-Inflating Bag

1. Completely assemble a flow-inflating neonatal manual bag. Verify proper function of the bag and pressure relief valve.
2. Connect the 15 mm adapter to an intubated neonatal mannequin.
3. Ventilate the mannequin at a rate of about 30 breaths/minute. Adjust the oxygen flowrate to provide adequate bag refilling while maintaining a rate of 30 breaths/minute.
4. If applicable, connect a manometer to the universal connector. Determine the average peak airway pressure delivered while ventilating with the flow-inflating bag (Fig. 33-5).
5. Record the oxygen flowrate required and the average peak airway pressure on the laboratory report.

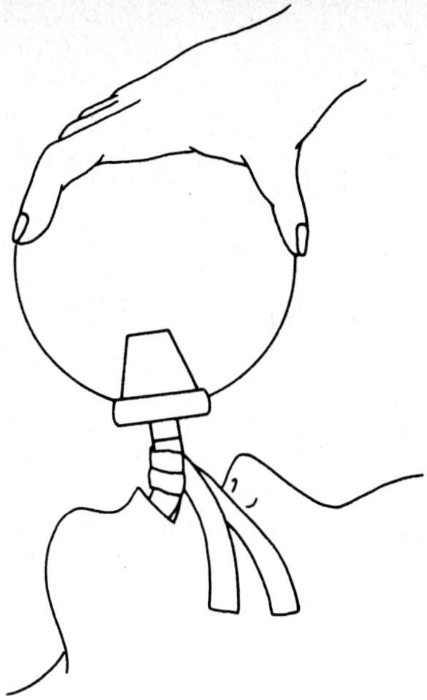

Fig. 33-4. Manual ventilator bag connected to an endotracheal tube.

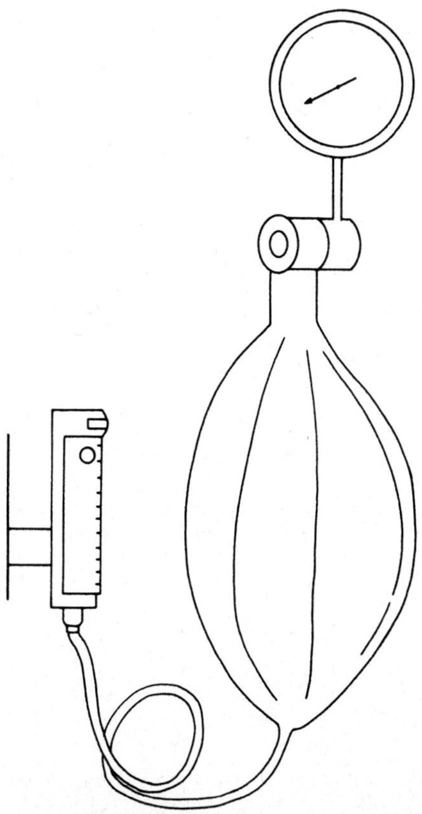

Fig. 33-5. Method for measuring proximal airway pressure during manual ventilation.

RECOMMENDED READING

Applebaum EL, Bruce DL: Tracheal Intubation. Philadelphia, WB Saunders, 1976

Burton GG, Hodgkin JE: Respiratory Care. A Guide to Clinical Practice, 2nd ed. Philadelphia, JB Lippincott, 1984

McPherson SP, Spearman CB: Respiratory Therapy Equipment, 3rd ed. St Louis, CV Mosby, 1985

Shapiro BA, Harrison RA, Kacmarek RM, Cane RD: Clinical Application of Respiratory Care, 3rd ed. Chicago, Year Book Medical Publishers, 1985

Laboratory Performance Evaluation (#33)

Topic: Manual Ventilation

Student ______________________ Course ______________________

Date ______________________ Section ______________________

Performance Elements	Acceptable	Unacceptable	Not Applicable	Comments
1. Assembles manual bag: A. Assembles valve B. Connects bag C. Attaches reservoir D. Connects oxygen tubing E. Regulates gas flowrates F. Tests bag function G. Attaches face mask				
2. Demonstrates effective ventilation on mannequin using the following: A. Face mask B. Endotracheal tube and connector C. Tracheostomy tube and connector				

Knowledge of Procedure

- ☐ Good; student is knowledgeable about rationale and theory related to procedure
- ☐ Fair; student has adequate understanding of rationale and theory related to procedure
- ☐ Poor; student has inadequate understanding of rationale and theory related to procedure

Performance Deficiencies (check those that apply)

- ☐ Excessive time needed to complete procedure
- ☐ Broke aseptic or sterile technique
- ☐ Gross inaccuracy noted
- ☐ Technique may be harmful to patient
- ☐ Incorrect dosage or gas concentration
- ☐ Incorrect equipment assembly/use
- ☐ Unable to answer questions correctly about rationale and/or theory related to procedure
- ☐ Other ______________________

Evaluation Summary

- ☐ Satisfactory performance
- ☐ Unsatisfactory performance

Recommendations of Evaluator

- ☐ Skills may be applied/observed in clinical setting
- ☐ Specific evaluation deficiencies require correction
- ☐ Complete re-evaluation required
- ☐ Additional laboratory practice required

Signatures:

Evaluator ______________________ Date ______________________

Student ______________________ Date ______________________

Laboratory Report

Student ____________________ Acceptable ____________________

Date ____________________ Unacceptable ____________________

Course ____________________

Topic: Manual Ventilation

Measurements or Data

1. Diagrams and labeling of manual bag valves during inspiration and expiration.

	Inspiration	Expiration
A.		
B.		
C.		
D.		
E.		

2. Measurement of tidal volume

	Adult Bag			Neonatal Bag	
Brand	One-Hand	Two-Hand	Brand	One-Hand	Two-Hand
1.			1.		
2.			2.		
3.			3.		
4.			4.		
5.			5.		
Average	________ and ________		Average	________ and ________	

3. Ventilation with a flow-inflating bag:

Oxygen flowrate ____________________

Peak airway pressure ____________________

Scenario: The emergency room has asked that you be on standby for a cardiac arrest patient being transported via rescue squad. The patient's anticipated arrival is about 7 to 10 minutes. The patient, a large obese man whose age appears to be in the mid-to-late-50s, is apparently in full cardiac arrest. You assume responsibility for manually ventilating the patient while the EMTs move the patient from the vehicle onto the emergency room receiving dock. Please respond to the following questions:

1. In a manual ventilation bag, what is the function of the
   A. 15 mm connection?

   B. nonrebreathing valve?

   C. 22 mm connection?

   D. reservoir system?

2. Why is it essential to have a tight seal between the patient's face and the mask when manually ventilating?

3. Why is it useful to have an oral airway in place when manually ventilating a patient?

4. What determines the fraction of inspired oxygen available when using a bag and mask to ventilate manually?

5. In this situation, how many breaths per minute would you provide?

6. Compare and contrast a self-refilling bag with a flow-refilling bag.

The patient you received in the emergency room was successfully resuscitated and is now residing on the coronary care unit. You are about to leave when you are notified to go to the emergency room stat, this time for the unannounced arrival of a premature infant who is to be admitted directly to the intensive care nursery. Immediately upon arrival in the emergency room, you assume responsibility for manually ventilating the baby with a mask and bag.

7. How many breaths per minute will you provide to the baby?

8. What complication(s) may be produced when an intubated neonate is ventilated with a flow-inflating bag?

9. In both situations, how is the immediate adequacy of ventilation determined?

chapter 34

Artificial airway maintenance

INTRODUCTION

A variety of techniques may be involved in the maintenance of an artificial airway. Since an artificial airway may bypass the normal conditioning functions of the upper respiratory tract, adequate humidification of inspired gas may be produced by heated humidifiers or aerosol generating equipment. Because a cough may be impossible with either an endotracheal or a tracheostomy tube in place, adequate bronchial hygiene is dependent upon tracheobronchial aspiration or suctioning. In order for medications to be administered to a spontaneously breathing patient with an artificial airway, IPPB or nebulizer equipment modifications may be necessary. Since an artificial airway effects a seal of the trachea by means of a cuff, routine maintenance requires the measurement and regulation of intracuff pressure and volume. Finally, excessive tube movement may be minimized by proper stabilization methods. The purpose of this chapter is to introduce you to techniques that may be employed in the maintenance of artificial airways.

OBJECTIVES

After completing this chapter, you should be able to do the following:

1. *Provide adequate humidification for an artificial airway.*
2. *Perform tracheal lavage and suctioning through an artificial airway.*
3. *Measure cuff volume and pressure of a tracheostomy or endotracheal tube.*
4. *Administer medications through an artificial airway by means of a medication or an IPPB nebulizer.*
5. *Add or remove mechanical deadspace to an artificial airway.*
6. *Stabilize an artificial airway using adapters.*

EQUIPMENT NEEDED

- ☐ Suction catheter kit (gloves, catheter, sterile field)
- ☐ Oxygen source, flowmeter, connecting tubing
- ☐ Manual ventilation bag and mask
- ☐ Lubricant
- ☐ Vacuum source and suction bottle
- ☐ 5 or 10 ml syringe with saline
- ☐ Manometer
- ☐ Three-way stopcock
- ☐ Calibrated syringe
- ☐ Endotracheal tube connectors or stabilizing adapters
- ☐ Glass test tube or simulated trachea
- ☐ Cascade humidifier
- ☐ Heated jet nebulizer
- ☐ Intubated adult mannequin
- ☐ Adult endotracheal and tracheostomy tubes

ACTIVITIES

Exercise A: Artificial Airway Humidification

1. Your instructor will provide you with an intubated adult mannequin. You may assume that the mannequin is breathing spontaneously.
2. Assemble a heated cascade humidifier with an FI_{O_2} of 0.35 and a total gas flowrate of 40 liters/minute. Verify the FI_{O_2} by analysis. Adjust the proximal airway temperature to 36°C. Deliver the gas to the mannequin by means of a T-tube.
3. Assemble a jet nebulizer to deliver an FI_{O_2} of 0.65 with a total gas flowrate of 40 liters/minute. Either a T-tube or tracheostomy mask may be used for an endotracheal or tracheostomy tube, respectively. Analyze the FI_{O_2}.

Exercise B: Suctioning Through Endotracheal and Tracheostomy Tubes

1. Assemble the equipment needed for suctioning.
2. Prepare oxygenation apparatus. Determine baseline heart rate and rhythm.
3. Wash hands with antimicrobial preparation.
4. Open catheter package. Deposit on sterile surface.
5. Hyperoxygenate patient with six or seven breaths of 100% oxygen or allow spontaneous breathing of oxygen.
6. Glove one hand with a sterile glove. Aseptically grasp the catheter with the sterile glove. *Note:* When initially practicing tracheobronchial aspiration, wear only one glove in order to clearly establish aseptic technique. In the clinical setting, however, gloves should be worn on both hands when suctioning to avoid secretion contact and to minimize the risk of herpetic Whitlow infection of the hands and nails.
7. Test catheter patency. Test negative suction pressure by occluding the connecting tubing and checking the manometer.
8. Aseptically introduce catheter into airway *without* negative pressure. Advance the catheter until slight resistance is met.
9. Withdraw catheter 1 or 2 cm.

10. Apply negative pressure while rotating and withdrawing catheter.(Do not rotate catheter unless catheter is within the endotracheal tube) (Fig. 34-1).
11. Limit suction time to 15 seconds.
12. Hyperoxygenate and hyperinflate the lungs after suction.
13. Assess patient status:
    A. Auscultation (change in breath sounds)
    B. ECG (change in heart rate and rhythm) or pulse
    C. Color (presence of cyanosis)
14. Repeat as indicated. *Note:* If the patient has tenacious secretions, 5 to 10 ml of sterile normal saline may be injected into the tube before suctioning, followed by bag breathing and hyperinflation before and after suctioning (Fig. 34-2).
15. Review the suction pressures typically used for adults, children, and infants in Table 34-1.
16. Completely occlude the suction tubing when initially adjusting the amount of negative pressure needed.

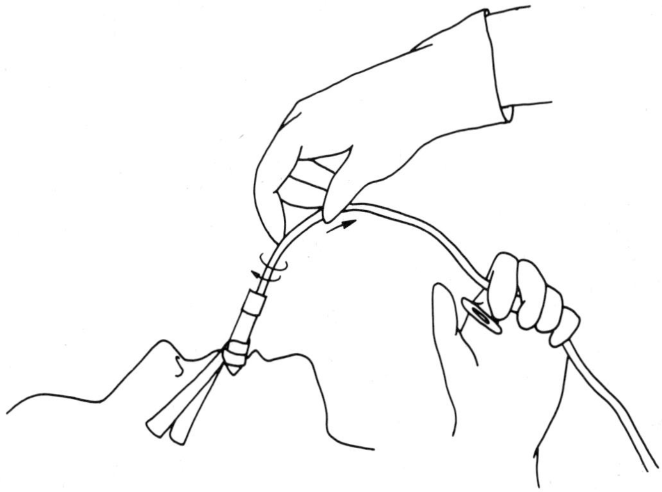

Fig. 34-1. Suctioning through an endotracheal tube.

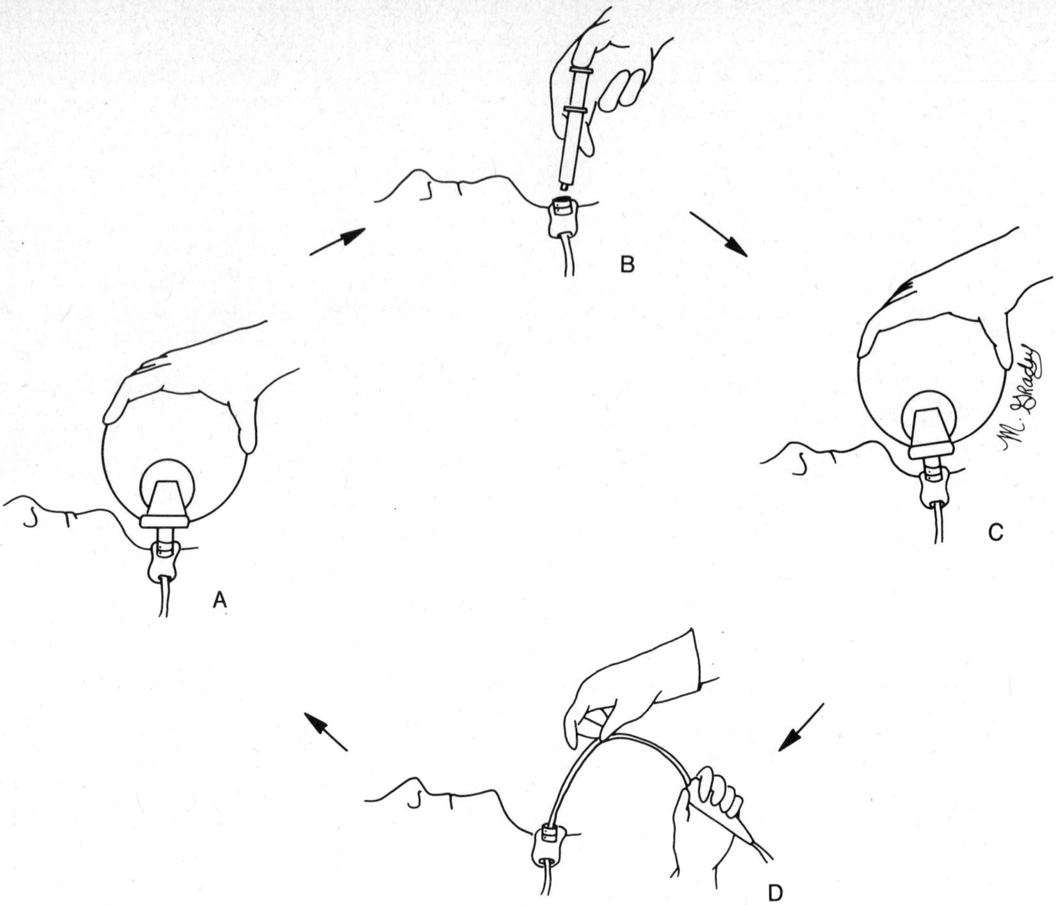

Fig. 34-2. Sequence of steps in tracheal lavage and suction. Note that lung hyperinflation and oxygenation is performed before suctioning, after saline instillation, and after suction.

Table 1-1. Suction Pressures Recommended for Adults, Children, and Infants

Age Group	Negative Pressure (mm Hg)
Adult	120–150
Child	80–120
Infant	50–100

Exercise C: Medication Administration Through Artificial Airways

1. Practice the administration of 5.0 ml of saline by assembling a nebulizer incorporated into a mechanical ventilator breathing circuit.
2. Activate the nebulizer. Connect the circuit to an intubated mannequin.
3. Assemble an IPPB breathing circuit. Inject the saline into the nebulizer. Cycle the ventilator on and verify adequate aerosol output. Connect the IPPB circuit to an intubated mannequin by means of a flex tube and 15 mm adapter.

4. Practice the administration of 5.0 ml of saline via a medication nebulizer and a T-tube. Connect the medication nebulizer to the T-tube with a piece of flex tubing (Fig. 34-3).
5. Be certain that the gas flow from both the jet nebulizer and medication nebulizer is adequate.

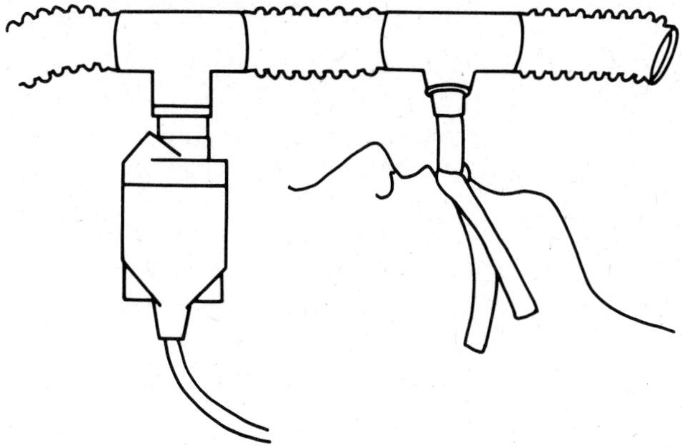

Fig. 34-3. Medication administration using a small-volume nebulizer for an artificial airway.

Exercise D: Intracuff Pressure and Volume Measurement

1. Insert the stopcock into the pilot line (in the closed position).
2. Attach tubing from the manometer to the stopcock.
3. Attach the syringe to the third opening on the stopcock (Fig. 34-4).
4. Suction the pharynx to remove any accumulated secretions above the cuff.

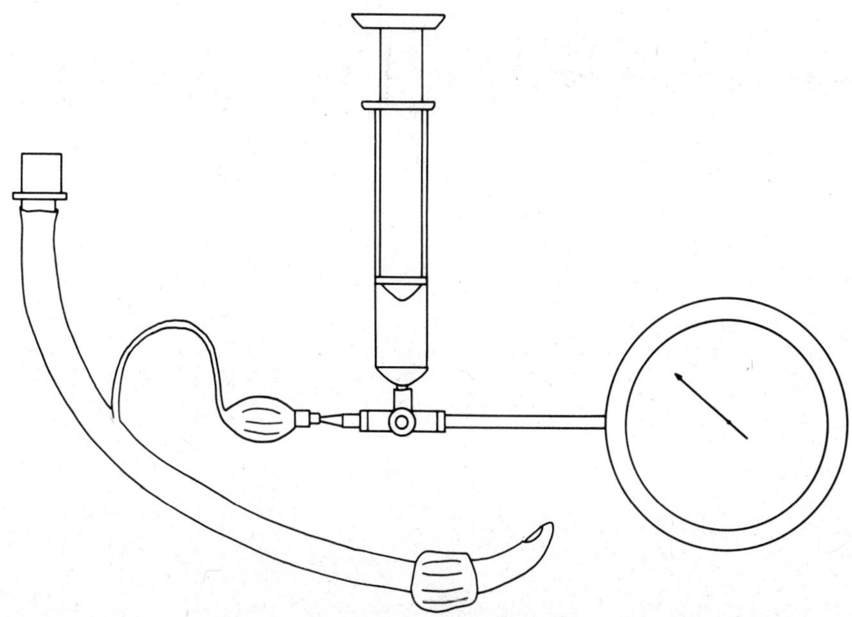

Fig. 34-4. Apparatus for measurement of cuff volume and pressure.

5. Rotate the stopcock to allow passage of air from the cuff into the syringe.
6. Aspirate the entire volume of air from the cuff and measure the volume.
7. Reinsert the air back into the cuff.
8. Rotate the stopcock to allow the pressure in the cuff to be read on the manometer.
9. Note the pressure reading.
10. The initial pressure reading may be falsely *low* and is a preliminary step only.
11. Again rotate the stopcock to allow passage of air from the cuff into the syringe.
12. Again aspirate the entire volume of air from the cuff and measure the volume.
13. The volume obtained this time will be lower than before because of air captured in the connecting tube.
14. Determine the volume of air lost in the connecting tubing; for example, if the first volume reading was 12.0 ml and the second volume reading was 10.0 ml, then 2.0 ml was captured in the tubing.
15. Reinject the original plus the lost volume of air into the cuff.
16. Rotate the stopcock to allow the pressure to be measured.
17. The second pressure should be noted and represents the actual intracuff pressure and volume.
18. Attempt to maintain the intracuff pressure at the lowest level necessary for an effective seal. A pressure of 17 mm Hg or less is desirable. **Note:* Compensation for volume lost in connecting tubing may be required when significant lengths of tubing are used in the system.

Exercise E: Addition and Removal of Mechanical Deadspace

1. Obtain a small section (about 50.0 ml) of large-bore aerosol tubing.
2. Fill the tubing with sterile water and empty into a beaker calibrated in metric units of volume.
3. Observe and record the volume of tubing used.
4. Attach the tubing between the T-tube (or ventilator connector) and the endotracheal tube in order to add mechanical deadspace (Fig. 34-5).
5. Because the addition of mechanical deadspace may produce rebreathing of carbon dioxide and significantly increase the work of breathing, it is imperative to differentiate clearly between mechanical deadspace and reservoir tubing added to a T-tube system.

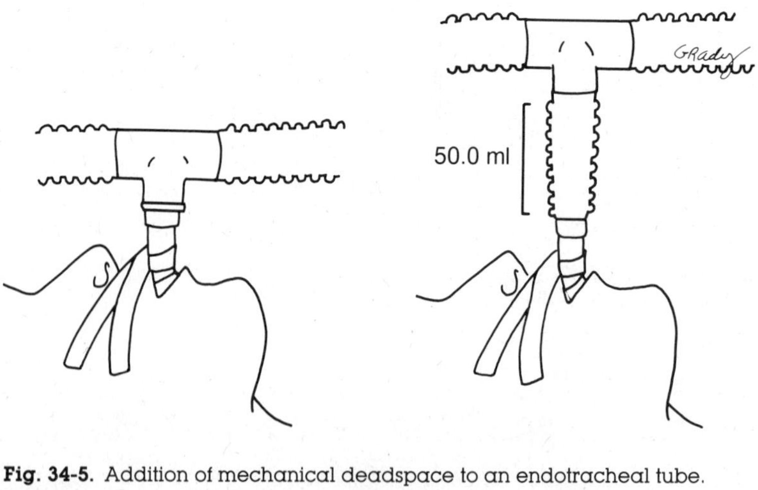

Fig. 34-5. Addition of mechanical deadspace to an endotracheal tube. Note that mechanical deadspace tubing is added between the endotracheal tube and the "T" tube connections.

Exercise F: Stabilization of Artificial Airways

1. Obtain a connector used to stabilize an artificial airway.
2. Attach the connector around the endotracheal tube and connect the endotracheal tube to a mechanical ventilator breathing circuit (Fig. 34-6).
3. Verify that the connection is secure and that the suction port is locked (if applicable).

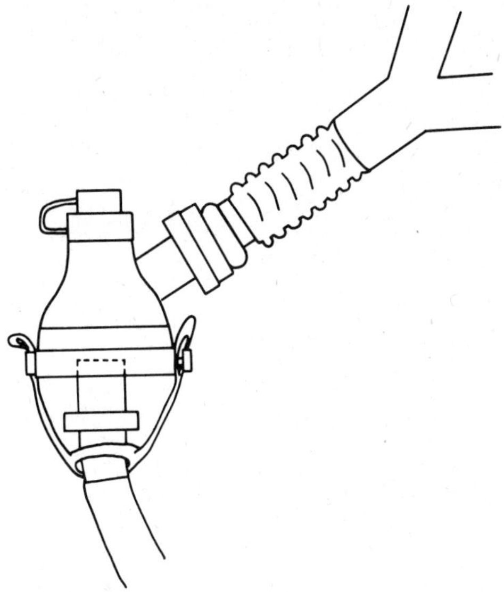

Fig. 34-6. Endotracheal tube adapter to prevent accidental disconnection and to allow suctioning.

Exercise G: Determination of "Unknown"

1. Your instructor will provide you with an intubated mannequin or will maintain an endotracheal tube in a simulated trachea (glass test tube). Your instructor will determine the cuff volume and pressure.
2. Using the apparatus provided, determine the cuff volume and pressure in the cuff of the artificial airway. Record your results on the laboratory report.

RECOMMENDED READING

Applebaum EL, Bruce DL: Tracheal Intubation. Philadelphia, WB Saunders, 1976

Burton GG, Hodgkin JE: Respiratory Care. A Guide to Clinical Practice, 2nd ed. Philadelphia, JB Lippincott, 1984

Kacmarek RM, Dimas S, Mack C: Essentials of Respiratory Therapy, 2nd ed. Chicago, Year Book Medical Publishers, 1985

Shapiro BA, Harrison RA, Kacmarek RM, Cane RD: Clinical Applications of Respiratory Care, 3rd ed. Chicago, Year Book Medical Publishers, 1985

Laboratory Performance Evaluation (#34)

Topic: Artificial Airway Maintenance

Student ____________________ Course ____________________

Date ____________________ Section ____________________

Performance Elements	Acceptable	Unacceptable	Not Applicable	Comments
1. Airway humidification: **A.** Provides prescribed $F_{I_{O_2}}$ and adequate humidification				
2. Tracheobronchial aspiration: **A.** Provides preoxygenation **B.** Maintains sterile technique **C.** Suctions for 15 seconds or less				
3. Evaluation of patient after suctioning: **A.** Auscultates **B.** Monitors ECG, pulse **C.** Checks color				
4. Saline lavage: **A.** Hyperinflates and oxygenates before and after lavage and suction				
5. Medication administration by means of the following: **A.** Ventilator circuit **B.** IPPB nebulizer **C.** Micronebulizer				
6. Monitoring of cuff volume and pressure: **A.** Maintains minimal leak **B.** Auscultates neck during inspiration **C.** Measures and records cuff pressure and volume				

Knowledge of Procedure

☐ Good; student is knowledgeable about rationale and theory related to procedure

☐ Fair; student has adequate understanding of rationale and theory related to procedure

☐ Poor; student has inadequate understanding of rationale and theory related to procedure

Performance Deficiencies (check those that apply)

☐ Excessive time needed to complete procedure

☐ Broke aseptic or sterile technique

☐ Gross inaccuracy noted

☐ Technique may be harmful to patient

☐ Incorrect dosage or gas concentration

☐ Incorrect equipment assembly/use

☐ Unable to answer questions correctly about rationale and/or theory related to procedure

☐ Other ______

Evaluation Summary

☐ Satisfactory performance

☐ Unsatisfactory performance

Recommendations of Evaluator

☐ Skills may be applied/observed in clinical setting

☐ Specific evaluation deficiencies require correction

☐ Complete re-evaluation required

☐ Additional laboratory practice required

Signatures:

Evaluator ______ Date ______

Student ______ Date ______

Laboratory Report

Student ______________________ Acceptable ______________________

Date ______________________ Unacceptable ______________________

Course ______________________

Topic: Artificial Airway Maintenance

Data or Measurements

Exercise G: Determination of "Unknown" Cuff Volume and Pressure

Initial cuff volume (ml) ______________________

Initial cuff pressure (mm Hg) ______________________

Second cuff volume (ml) ______________________

Second cuff pressure (mm Hg) ______________________

Scenario: Once again you are assigned to the medical intensive care unit. The patients you are responsible for include the following: a tracheostomized patient in bedspace #1; a nasally intubated patient who is on a mechanical ventilator in bedspace #2; and a patient who had open-heart surgery yesterday is in bedspace #3. He is orally intubated and, if all goes well, should be extubated later today. Please answer the following questions:

1. Why must additional humidity be provided when an artificial airway is used?

2. Why is suctioning frequently necessary when an artificial airway is used?

3. What volume of saline may be used for tracheal lavage?

4. Why is hyperinflation and oxygenation performed before, during, and after tracheal lavage and suctioning?

5. What is the difference between a reservoir and mechanical deadspace in a T-tube system?

6. Why may the initial cuff volume and pressure measurements be inaccurate when using a sphygmomanometer with extensive rubber tubing?

7. Describe in detail the system you would use to provide adequate humidity to the patient in bedspace #1 (equipment and so forth).

8. After consultation, it has been determined that the patient in bedspace #2 would benefit from an additional 150 ml of mechanical deadspace. Please describe the method used to accomplish this.

9. All of these patients require frequent suctioning, especially the patient in bedspace #2 who needs tracheal lavage and suctioning. Please describe in detail the suctioning and lavage technique you would use.

10. The measured endotracheal tube cuff pressure of the patient in bedspace #2 is 60 mm Hg. Knowing this, what would you do?

11. All of these patients have a physician's order for 0.5 ml of isoetharine with 4 to 5 ml of normal saline every 4 hours. Please discuss the equipment and methods used to carry out these orders.

chapter 35

Endotracheal tube extubation

INTRODUCTION

The procedure of removing a nasal or oral endotracheal tube is referred to as extubation. An artificial airway may be needed to (1) relieve airway obstruction, (2) protect the airway, (3) facilitate suction, and (4) maintain mechanical ventilation. It is important to realize that an endotracheal tube may be inserted for reasons other than mechanical ventilation and that discontinuance of mechanical ventilation may not necessarily mean that an endotracheal tube should be removed. In essence, extubation is performed when the need no longer exists for an endotracheal tube.

Before removing an endotracheal tube, the airway should be thoroughly suctioned and evaluated for the presence (or absence) of airway reflexes. Both the gag and cough reflexes are vital functions that may protect the lower respiratory tract against aspiration when an endotracheal tube is removed. Both reflexes may be easily tested by stimulating the trachea (or carina) and oropharynx with a suction catheter before extubation. When the gag or cough reflexes are obtunded or absent, the tube should not be removed.

Two methods of extubation have been described. After suctioning and cuff deflation, one method involves simultaneous hyperinflation with a manual bag as the tube is removed. The rationale for hyperinflation during extubation is to minimize blood gas changes and to provide a large gas volume for a cough following tube removal. A second method involves the insertion of a suction catheter within the endotracheal tube with the application of suction as the tube is removed. The rationale for this technique is to remove secretions pooled above the cuff as the tube is removed. Because the application of suction during extubation may (1) cause lung deflation and hypoxemia, (2) induce a vagal response, and (3) traumatize the tracheal mucosa, the authors recommend hyperinflation during extubation. The purpose of this chapter is to introduce you to the procedure of endotracheal tube extubation.

OBJECTIVES

After completing this chapter, you should be able to do the following:

1. *Understand the procedure of endotracheal tube extubation.*
2. *Verify the presence of intact airway reflexes before extubation.*
3. *Examine the chest after extubation.*
4. *Administer postextubation therapy.*

EQUIPMENT NEEDED

- ☐ Oxygen source and flowmeter
- ☐ Manual ventilation bag
- ☐ Suction source and catheters
- ☐ Adult intubation mannequin
- ☐ Oral airway
- ☐ Magill forceps
- ☐ Nasal decongestant, topical anesthetic gel
- ☐ Stylet
- ☐ Syringe
- ☐ Laryngoscope blade
- ☐ Tape
- ☐ Jet nebulizer
- ☐ Aerosol tubing
- ☐ Aerosol mask

ACTIVITIES

Exercise A: Equipment Assembly and Function Check

1. Assemble the needed equipment and check the functions of the following:
   - A. Bag-valve-mask unit and oxygen flow
   - B. Endotracheal tube cuff
   - C. Laryngoscope blade light bulb
   - D. Suction catheter patency and pressure
2. Verify that all of the equipment needed for intubation is readily available before removing an endotracheal tube, since immediate reintubation may be required.

Exercise B: Airway Reflex Evaluation

1. Before extubation, the trachea should be suctioned using sterile technique.
2. During the suctioning procedure, advance the catheter until it meets resistance near the carina.
3. Verify the presence of a cough reflex (Fig. 35-1).
4. After suctioning the trachea, suction the oropharynx.
5. Verify the presence of a gag reflex (Fig. 35-2).

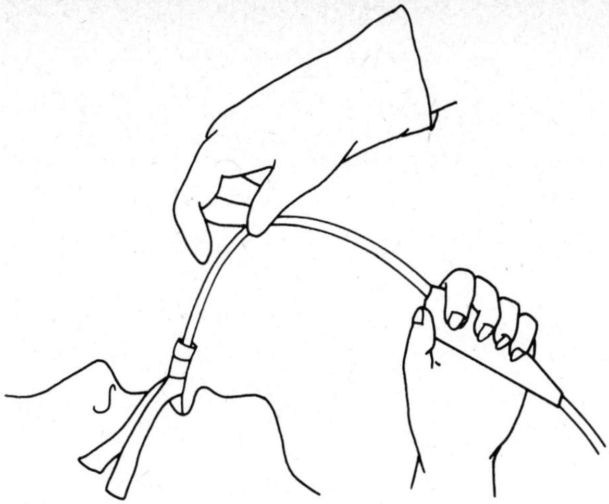

Fig. 35-1. Evaluation of airway reflexes during endotracheal suction.

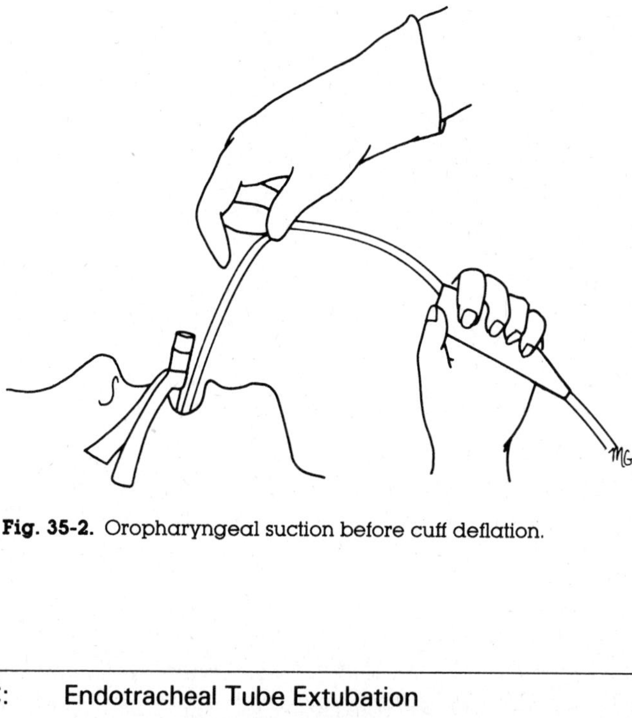

Fig. 35-2. Oropharyngeal suction before cuff deflation.

Exercise C: Endotracheal Tube Extubation

1. Explain the procedure to the patient.
2. Using the manual ventilation bag, preoxygenate and ventilate with 100% oxygen.
3. Prepare postextubation apparatus (usually an aerosol mask and nebulizer). The apparatus should be functional *before* tube removal for immediate application.
4. Remove the tape that secures the endotracheal tube.
5. Give a maximum breath with the manual bag.
6. Deflate the endotracheal tube cuff with a syringe (Fig. 35-3).
7. Request that the patient inhale while simultaneously compressing the manual bag and removing the tube. Attempt to remove the tube in one gentle, continuous motion (Fig. 35-4).
8. Immediately administer oxygen and aerosol therapy.

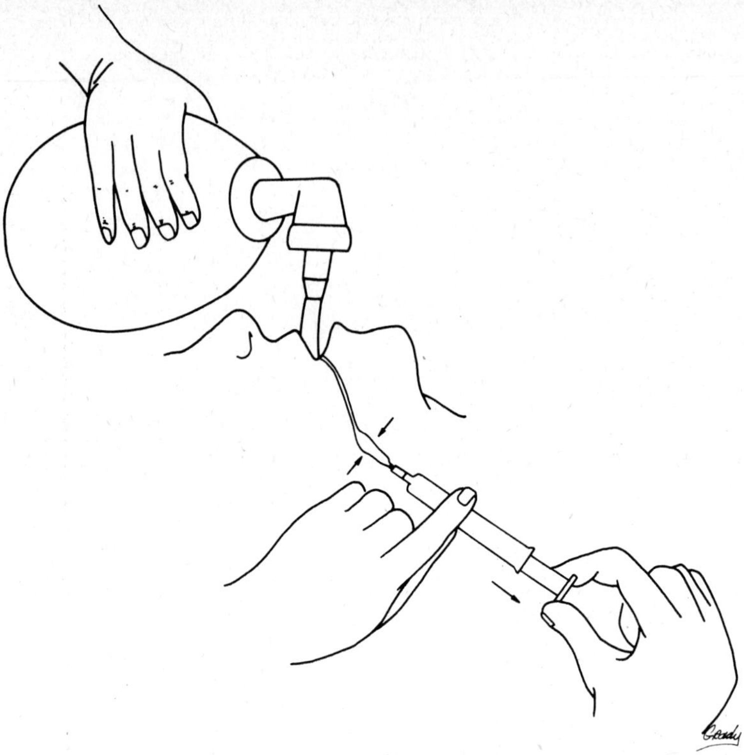

Fig. 35-3. Cuff deflation.

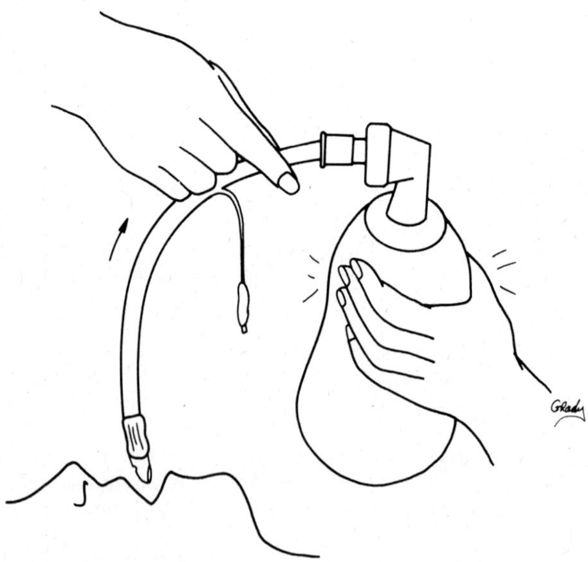

Fig. 35-4. Removal of endotracheal tube during a manual breath.

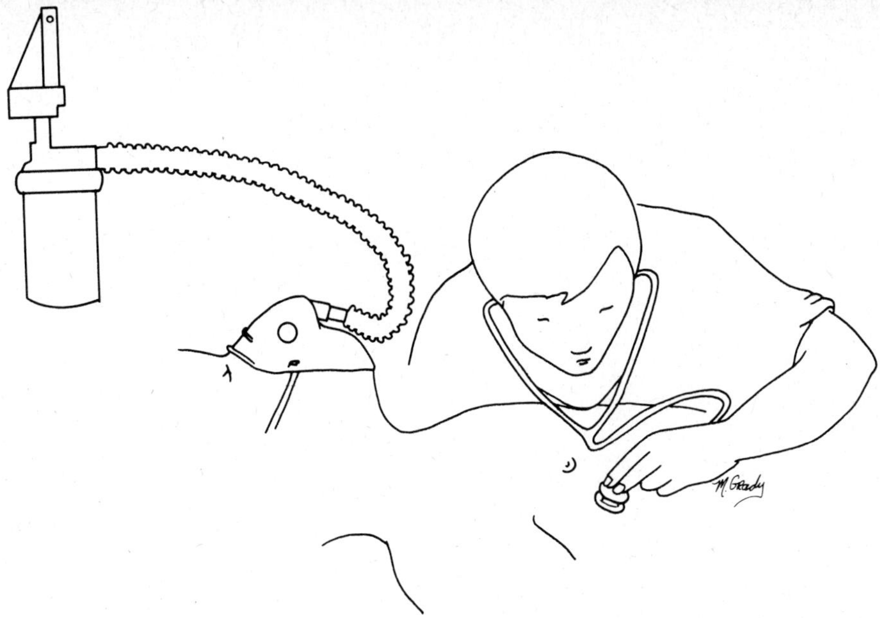

Fig. 35-5. Postextubation evaluation.

Exercise D: Postextubation Evaluation

1. Evalute the airway for signs of obstruction, stridor, or distress.
2. Encourage coughing and deep breathing.
3. Auscultate the chest (Fig. 35-5).
4. Remain with the patient until stability in ventilation and airway patency is established.
5. Review the entire sequence of steps in endotracheal tube extubation (Fig. 36-6).

RECOMMENDED READING

Applebaum EL, Bruce DL: Tracheal Intubation. Philadelphia, WB Saunders, 1976

Burton GG, Hodgkin JE: Respiratory Care. A Guide to Clinical Practice, 2nd ed. Philadelphia, JP Lippincott, 1984

Shapiro BA, Harrison RA, Kacmarek RM, Cane RD: Clinical Application of Respiratory Care, 3rd ed. Chicago, Year Book Medical Publishers, 1985

Spearman CB, Sheldon RL: Egan's Fundamentals of Respiratory Therapy, 4th ed. St Louis, CV Mosby, 1982

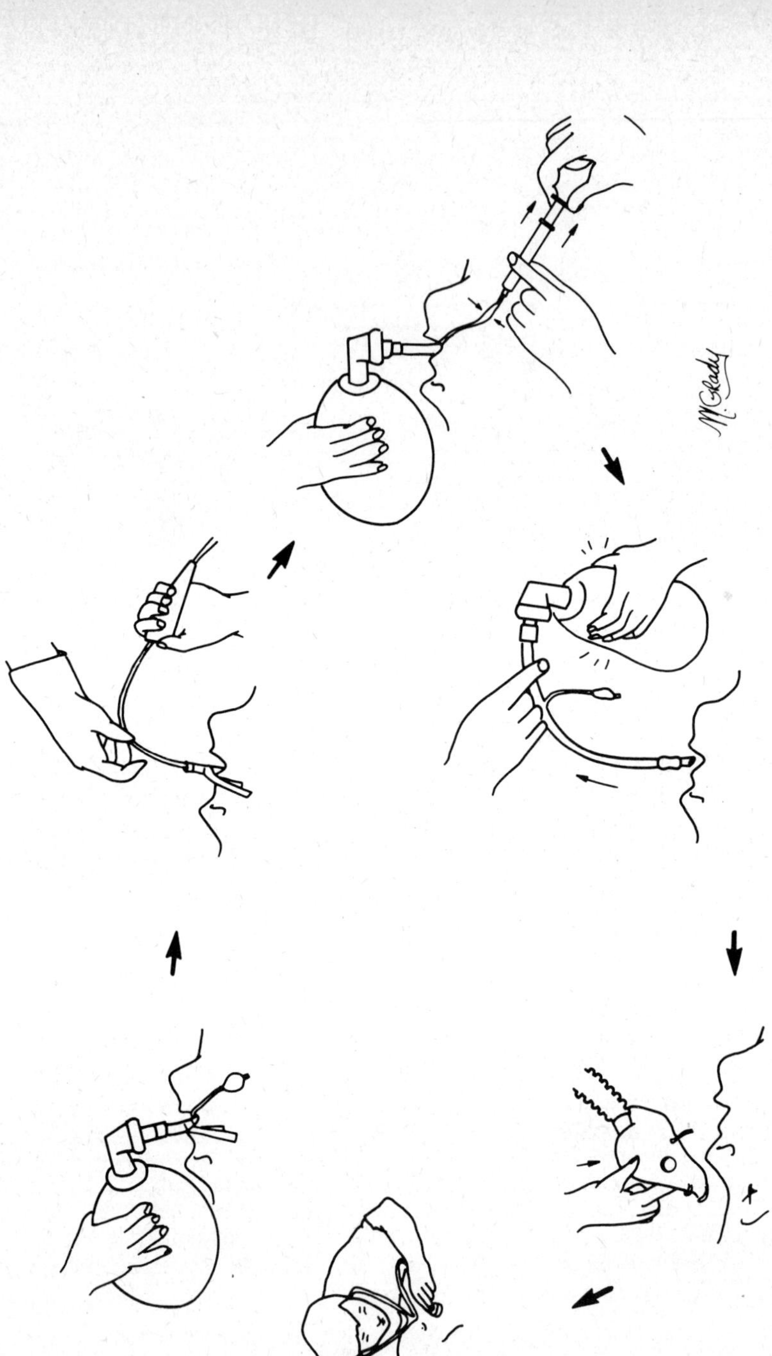

Fig. 35-6. Sequence of steps in endotracheal tube extubation.

Laboratory Performance Evaluation (#35)

Topic: Endotracheal Tube Extubation

Student ______________________ Course ______________________

Date ______________________ Section ______________________

Performance Elements	Acceptable	Unacceptable	Not Applicable	Comments
1. Verifies the order				
2. Assembles needed materials (all materials for intubations)				
3. Checks functioning of equipment				
4. Identifies self and simulated patient				
5. Explains the procedure to the patient. Washes hands.				
6. Preoxygenates with 100% oxygen and ventilates				
7. Suctions trachea, then the oropharynx and nasopharynx				
8. Evaluates airway reflexes				
9. Deflates cuff using a syringe				
10. Provides maximum inspiration by means of a manual bag				
11. Removes endotracheal tube				
12. Administers oxygen and aerosol. Evaluates airway by observation and auscultation				

Knowledge of Procedure

- ☐ Good; student is knowledgeable about rationale and theory related to procedure
- ☐ Fair; student has adequate understanding of rationale and theory related to procedure
- ☐ Poor; student has inadequate understanding of rationale and theory related to procedure

Performance Deficiencies (check those that apply)

- ☐ Excessive time needed to complete procedure
- ☐ Broke aseptic or sterile technique
- ☐ Gross inaccuracy noted
- ☐ Technique may be harmful to patient
- ☐ Incorrect dosage or gas concentration
- ☐ Incorrect equipment assembly/use
- ☐ Unable to answer questions correctly about rationale and/or theory related to procedure
- ☐ Other ______________________________

Evaluation Summary

- ☐ Satisfactory performance
- ☐ Unsatisfactory performance

Recommendations of Evaluator

- ☐ Skills may be applied/observed in clinical setting
- ☐ Specific evaluation deficiencies require correction
- ☐ Complete re-evaluation required
- ☐ Additional laboratory practice required

Signatures:

Evaluator ______________________ Date ______________________

Student ______________________ Date ______________________

Laboratory Report

Student ______________________ Acceptable ______________________

Date ______________________ Unacceptable ______________________

Course ______________________

Topic: Endotracheal Tube Extubation

Scenario: You are paged to the recovery room and asked to evaluate an elderly female patient for extubation. The patient has a confirmed diagnosis of cerebral vascular accident (CVA) and is spontaneously breathing through a 7.5 mm ID endotracheal tube.

1. Before extubating the patient with a recent history of CVA (stroke), you note no cough response during suctioning. In the event that physician orders were written to extubate the patient, briefly describe what you would do.

2. Immediately after extubation, severe inspiratory stridor is noted. Describe the actions you would take.

3. How may airway patency and ventilatory stability be determined?

4. What postextubation therapy would you recommend for
   A. hoarseness?

   B. stridor and glottic edema?

chapter 36

Weaning and replacement of a tracheostomy tube

INTRODUCTION

In general, the indications for a tracheostomy tube are similar to those for endotracheal intubation. A tracheostomy tube, however, is usually indicated for long-term airway care. As is the case with endotracheal tube extubation, a tracheostomy tube may be "weaned" or removed when the need for its placement no longer exists. Several brands of tracheostomy tube weaning devices are commercially available.

Two types of devices that facilitate weaning from a tracheostomy tube are the fenestrated tube and the tracheal button. The fenestrated tube has a window or hole cut into the outer cannula. With the inner cannula in place, the fenestrated tube functions similarly to other conventional tracheostomy tubes. With a fenestrated tracheostomy tube, however, air may be breathed through the upper airway when (1) the cuff is deflated, (2) the inner cannula is removed, and (3) the opening or patient end of the outer cannula is "corked." A tracheal button is a short, Teflon, tubelike appliance that maintains the patency of the tracheostomy stoma. With the tracheal button, air may be breathed through the upper airway when the opening is corked. Removal of the cork allows for gas flow through the tube and may allow suctioning.

In clinical practice, a patent, functional tracheostomy tube rarely requires replacement; however, certain conditions such as a ruptured cuff or acute obstruction may necessitate the replacement of a tracheostomy tube. Because of the risk of bleeding and tissue trauma, tracheostomy tubes should be replaced only by a surgeon within 3 postoperative days from the time of a tracheotomy. Beyond this time, it is reasonable for respiratory care personnel to replace tracheostomy tubes. The purpose of this chapter is to introduce you to tracheostomy tube care, weaning, and replacement.

OBJECTIVES

After completing this chapter, you should be able to do the following:

1. *Identify the components of a fenestrated tracheostomy tube and tracheal button.*

2. *Describe patient positioning and stabilization before tracheostomy tube replacement.*
3. *Understand the functions of an obturator and inner cannula in a tracheostomy tube.*
4. *Understand the use of a "tube changer" guide when replacing a tracheostomy tube.*
5. *Explain the routine care and cleaning of a tracheostomy tube.*
6. *Replace a tracheostomy tube in a simulated patient.*

EQUIPMENT NEEDED

- ☐ Oxygen source and flowmeter
- ☐ Manual ventilation bag
- ☐ Suction source and catheters
- ☐ Adult intubation mannequin
- ☐ Oral airway
- ☐ Magill forceps
- ☐ Nasal decongestant, topical anesthetic gel
- ☐ Stylet
- ☐ Syringe
- ☐ Laryngoscope blade
- ☐ Tape
- ☐ Trachea model
- ☐ Two tracheostomy tubes with inner cannulas and obturator
- ☐ Fenestrated tracheostomy tube
- ☐ Tracheal button
- ☐ Tracheostomy tube cleaning kit
- ☐ Sterile gloves

ACTIVITIES

Exercise A: Identification of Tracheostomy Weaning Devices

1. Your instructor will provide you with a fenestrated tracheostomy tube and tracheal button.
2. Examine a tracheal button (Fig. 36-1).
3. Identify the following components:
   - A. Inner cannula
   - B. Outer cannula
   - C. Cork
   - D. Probe (not shown)
   - E. Spacers (not shown)
4. Using a model of an adult trachea, determine the distance from the anterior tracheal wall to the skin with the probe. Record the measurement on the laboratory report.
5. Using spacers, adjust the length of the tracheal button to conform to the measured distance from the anterior tracheal wall to the skin.
6. Practice the insertion of the inner cannula into the outer cannula. Lock the inner cannula into the outer cannula.
7. Examine a fenestrated tracheostomy tube (Fig. 36-2).
8. Identify the following components of a fenestrated tracheostomy tube:
   - A. Inner cannula
   - B. Outer cannula

C. Cuff
D. Pilot balloon
E. Fenestration
F. Flanges

9. Practice the insertion and removal of the inner cannula into the outer cannula. Trace the flow of air through the fenestration with the inner cannula removed.

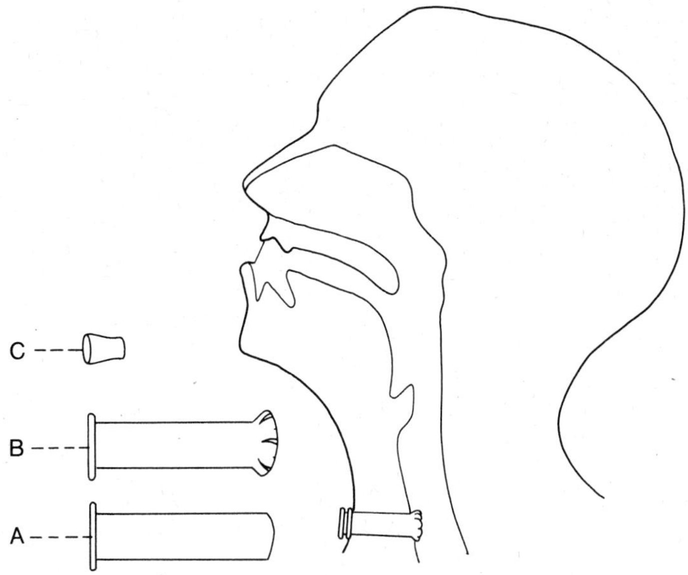

Fig. 36-1. Tracheostomy button components and position.

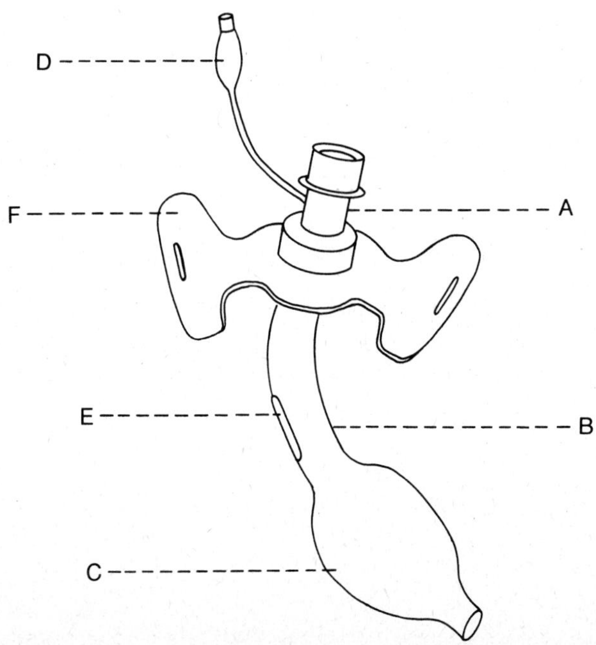

Fig. 36-2. Fenestrated tracheostomy tube components.

Exercise B: Subject Stabilization and Preparation for Tracheostomy Tube Replacement

1. Your instructor will provide you with an adult mannequin having a tracheostomy tube in place.
2. Prepare the subject for the replacement of the tracheostomy tube by explaining the procedure and stabilizing the neck. The neck may be stabilized by hyperextension and by placement of a small cushion beneath the shoulders and neck (Fig. 36-3).
3. To prevent dissection of the tracheal stoma beneath the fascia, avoid turning the head from side to side.
4. Wash your hands.
5. Prepare the necessary equipment. Verify that a sterile suction catheter, sterile gloves, saline, manual bag and mask, syringe, and the spare tracheostomy tube are easily retrievable.
6. Using aseptic technique, prepare a small volume of sterile saline. The cuff of the tracheostomy tube replacement may be checked by inflation of the pilot balloon. Immerse the cuff of the tracheostomy tube into the sterile saline. Verify that no leaks exist (Fig. 36-4). The presence of bubbles may indicate a cuff leak.
7. Suction the tracheostomy tube and oropharynx.
8. Using the manual bag, ensure adequate ventilation and oxygeneration.
9. Lubricate the tip of the replacement tracheostomy tube with sterile lubricant.

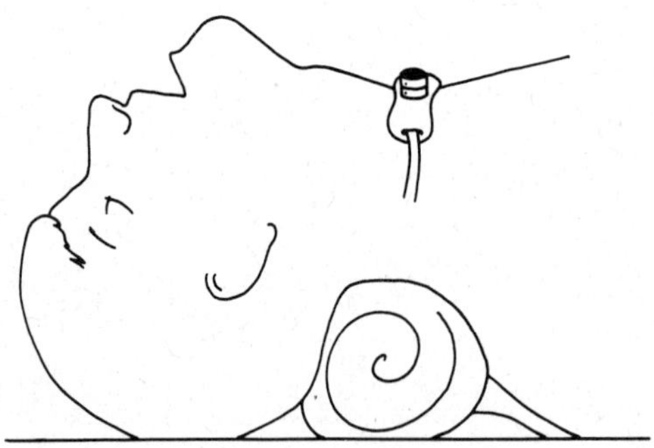

Fig. 36-3. Stabilization of head and neck before tracheostomy tube removal.

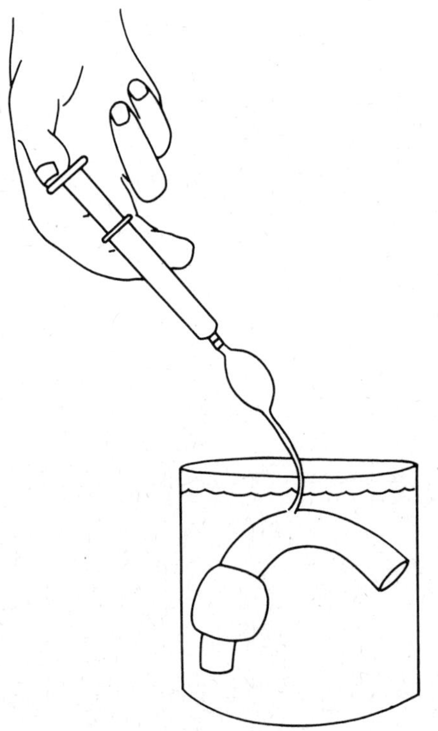

Fig. 36-4. Evaluation of cuff for leaks.

Exercise C: Tracheostomy Tube Extubation

1. When removing a tracheostomy tube for the purpose of replacing the tube, modification of a sterile suction catheter may maintain the location of the stoma.

2. Using a pair of scissors, cut off the thumb port and suction tubing adapter from the catheter, or use a commercial "tube changer."
3. Put on sterile gloves.
4. Using aseptic technique, insert the modified suction catheter proximal to the tip of the tracheostomy tube. Avoid contact with the carina or tracheal wall, which may induce coughing.
5. Deflate the tracheostomy tube cuff.
6. While maintaining the catheter within the tracheal stoma, gently remove the existing tracheostomy tube.
7. Thread the catheter into the lumen of the replacement tracheostomy tube. Be certain that the catheter is first threaded through the distal or cuff end of the tube.
8. Using the catheter as a guide, gently advance the tip of the tracheostomy tube through the stoma. Carefully advance the tube into position.
9. Inflate the cuff and remove the catheter guide.
10. Connect a manual bag to the tracheostomy tube. Check for the presence of bilateral breath sounds and lung inflation.
11. Review the steps for the replacement of a tracheostomy tube (Fig. 36-5).

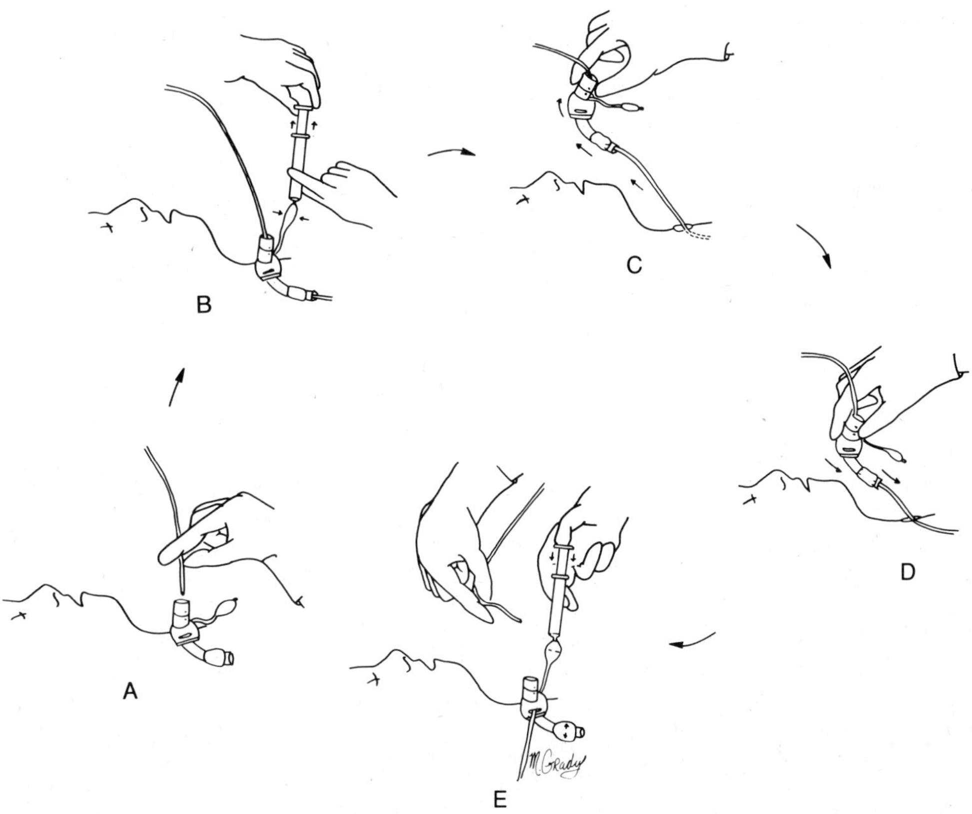

Fig. 36-5. **A.** Insertion of modified catheter to act as a guide into stoma. **B.** Tracheostomy tube cuff deflation. **C.** Removal of tracheostomy tube around catheter guide. **D.** Insertion of new tracheostomy tube around catheter guide. **E.** Cuff inflation and removal of catheter guide.

Exercise D: Tracheostomy Tube Intubation

1. After subject preparation and stabilization, a tracheostomy tube may also be inserted using the obturator.

2. Put on sterile gloves. Assume that the subject has had a tracheostomy tube removed and requires insertion of a new tube.
3. Remove the inner cannula from a tracheostomy tube. Insert the obturator into the outer cannula.
4. Lubricate the tip of the obturator and tube with sterile, water-soluble lubricant.
5. Gently advance the obturator and tube into the stoma.
6. After proper placement, stabilize the outer cannula while removing the obturator.
7. Stabilize the outer cannula while inserting the inner cannula (if applicable). Be certain to lock the inner cannula.
8. Inflate the cuff.
9. Verify tube position by auscultation during manual ventilation.
10. Fasten the ties to the flanges on the tracheostomy tube. Secure the ties. Apply a bib if necessary.
11. Review the steps for tracheostomy tube intubation in Figure 36-6.

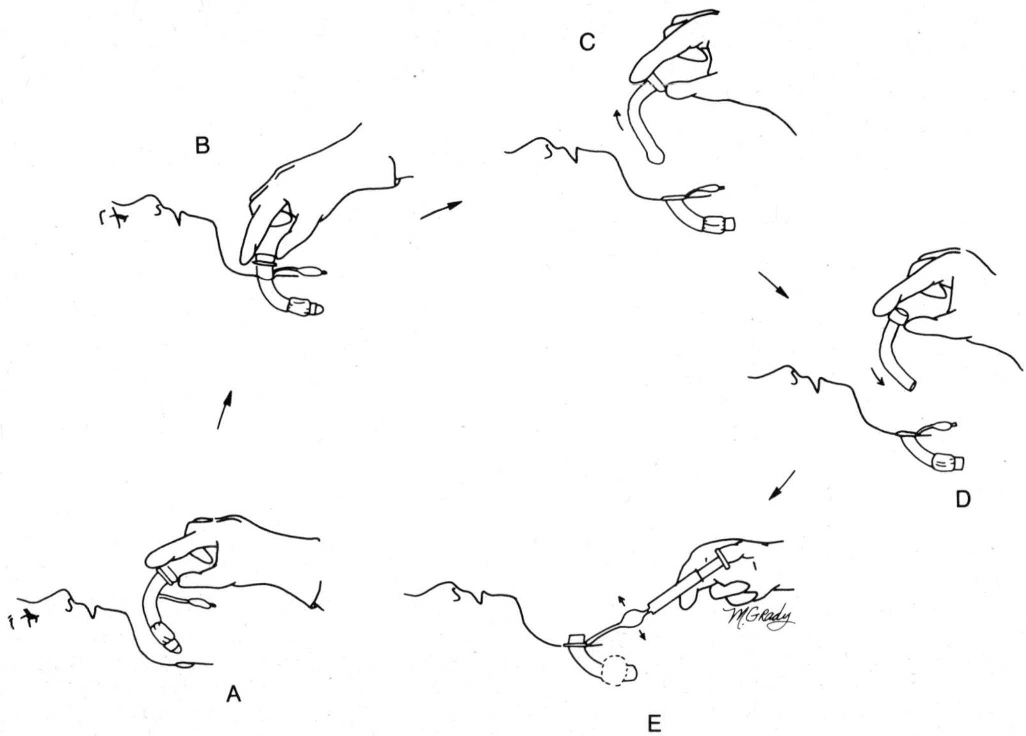

Fig. 36-6. A. Insertion of a tracheostomy tube with an obturator. **B.** Tracheostomy tube with obturator in position. **C.** Removal of obturator. **D.** Insertion of inner cannula. **E.** Cuff inflation.

Exercise E: Tracheostomy Tube Care

1. Your instructor will provide you with an adult mannequin having a two-cannula tracheostomy tube in place.
2. Approach the simulated patient and explain the procedure.
3. Wash your hands.
4. Assemble the needed equipment for tracheostomy tube care. The equipment should include the following:
   A. Suction catheters and sterile gloves
   B. 2% hydrogen peroxide solution

C. Sterile saline
D. Tracheostomy care kit
E. Sterile 4″ × 4″ gauze

5. Stabilize the head and neck by placing a cushion beneath the neck and shoulders.
6. Suction the tracheostomy tube, if necessary.
7. Place a sterile drape under the tracheostomy tube.
8. Prepare a solution of saline and one of hydrogen peroxide.
9. Put on sterile gloves.
10. Remove and discard the soiled tracheostomy dressing bib.
11. Unlock and remove the inner cannula. Place the inner cannula in a solution of hydrogen peroxide.
12. Clean the inner cannula with a sterile brush or pipe cleaner. Be certain that mucus plugs are removed from the lumen of the inner cannula.

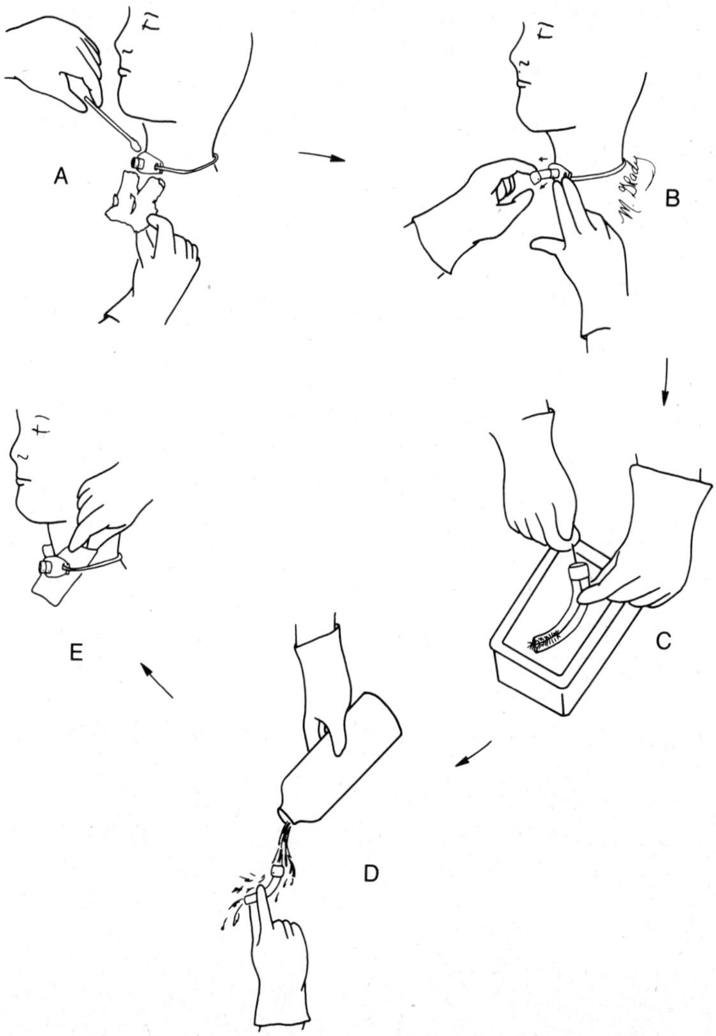

Fig. 36-7. A. Removal of soiled dressing and tube cleaning with hydrogen peroxide. **B.** Removal of inner cannula. **C.** Cleaning of inner cannula. **D.** Rinsing of inner cannula with sterile water. **E.** Replacement of dressing and ties.

13. Rinse the inner cannula in sterile saline.
14. The skin, stoma site, outer cannula, and flanges may be cleaned with 4″ × 4″ gauze pads that have been soaked in sterile hydrogen peroxide or a sterile swab. Do not use the hydrogen peroxide previously used in cleaning the inner cannula. Dry the inner cannula thoroughly.
15. If necessary, suction the outer cannula. Avoid removal of the inner cannula for prolonged periods, since secretions may form in the outer cannula.
16. Reinsert the inner cannula. Lock the inner cannula in place.
17. Replace the tracheostomy tube bib and ties as needed.
18. Review the steps in tracheostomy tube care in Figure 36-7. *Note:* Sterile gloves should be worn when contact with a tracheostomy tube is necessary.

RECOMMENDED READING

Applebaum EL, Bruce DL: Tracheal Intubation. Philadelphia, WB Saunders, 1976

Blodgett D: Manual of Respiratory Care Procedures. Philadelphia, JB Lippincott, 1980

Burton GG, Hodgkin JE: Respiratory Care. A Guide to Clinical Practice, 2nd ed. Philadelphia, JP Lippincott, 1984

McPherson SP, Spearman CB: Respiratory Therapy Equipment, 3rd ed. St Louis, CV Mosby, 1985

Shapiro BA, Harrison RA, Kacmarek RM, Cane RD: Clinical Application of Respiratory Care, 3rd ed. Chicago, Year Book Medical Publishers, 1985

Spearman CB, Sheldon RL: Egan's Fundamentals of Respiratory Therapy, 4th ed. St Louis, CV Mosby, 1982

Laboratory Performance Evaluation (#36)

Topic: Weaning and Replacement of a Tracheostomy Tube

Student ______________________ Course ______________________

Date ______________________ Section ______________________

Performance Elements	Acceptable	Unacceptable	Not Applicable	Comments
1. Explains procedure				
2. Washes hands				
3. Stabilizes head and neck				
4. Assembles equipment				
5. Puts on sterile gloves				
6. Checks tube cuff				
7. Inserts tube changer				
8. Deflates cuff				
9. Removes existing tube				
10. Maintains stoma position				
11. Inserts new tube				
12. Maintains aseptic technique				
13. Inflates cuff				
14. Checks tube placement				

Knowledge of Procedure

- ☐ Good; student is knowledgeable about rationale and theory related to procedure
- ☐ Fair; student has adequate understanding of rationale and theory related to procedure
- ☐ Poor; student has inadequate understanding of rationale and theory related to procedure

Performance Deficiencies (check those that apply)

- ☐ Excessive time needed to complete procedure
- ☐ Broke aseptic or sterile technique
- ☐ Gross inaccuracy noted
- ☐ Technique may be harmful to patient
- ☐ Incorrect dosage or gas concentration
- ☐ Incorrect equipment assembly/use
- ☐ Unable to answer questions correctly about rationale and/or theory related to procedure
- ☐ Other ______________________________

Evaluation Summary

- ☐ Satisfactory performance
- ☐ Unsatisfactory performance

Recommendations of Evaluator

- ☐ Skills may be applied/observed in clinical setting
- ☐ Specific evaluation deficiencies require correction
- ☐ Complete re-evaluation required
- ☐ Additional laboratory practice required

Signatures:

Evaluator ______________________ Date ______________________

Student ______________________ Date ______________________

Laboratory Report

Student ______________________ Acceptable ______________________

Date ______________________ Unacceptable ______________________

Course ______________________

Topic: Weaning and Replacement of a Tracheostomy Tube

Data or Measurements

Distance from anterior tracheal wall to skin (mm) ______________________

Scenario: The patient is a teenage auto accident victim who suffered multiple facial traumas and a head injury 3 weeks ago. Two weeks ago, the oral endotracheal tube was replaced with a cuffed tracheostomy tube. Until this past week, she has been comatose. Now, she seems to be emerging from her coma. This change in neurologic status combined with respiratory and cardiovascular stability has made weaning her from the tracheostomy tube quite feasible. The initial plan of action is to remove the existing tracheostomy tube and replace it with a fenestrated tracheostomy tube which, at a future date, will be replaced with a tracheal button. Please respond to the following questions:

1. Before removing a tracheostomy tube, describe the positioning of the head and neck.

2. After insertion of a fenestrated tracheostomy tube, what three things must be done to allow breathing through the upper airway?

3. What is the purpose of a tracheal button?

4. What may occur if a fenestrated tracheostomy tube is "corked" while the inner cannula remains in the outer cannula and the cuff is inflated in a spontaneously breathing patient?

5. What postoperative period of time is recommended before changing a tracheostomy tube? Why?

6. What is the function of a modified suction catheter or "tube changer" when replacing a tracheostomy tube?

7. Briefly describe the function of the following:
   A. An obturator

   B. Flanges

   C. Probe (used with a tracheal button)

   D. Spacers (for use with a tracheal button)

8. What three hazards are associated with changing a tracheostomy tube?

9. Other than when the patient is being mechanicaly ventilated, when should the tracheostomy tube cuff be inflated?

10. Why is it advisable to have endotracheal intubation equipment on hand when replacing a tracheostomy tube?

chapter 37

Mechanical ventilator preparation

INTRODUCTION

Before initiating mechanical ventilation, you need a thorough knowledge of the ventilator and the ventilator circuit. You also need to perform quality assurance measures. There are numerous types of ventilators on the market today. All types must be checked before patient use to assure patient safety. The quality assurance exercises described herein will ensure that a ventilator is ready for patient use. The purpose of this chapter is to introduce you to mechanical ventilators and quality assurance measures that will result in patient safety.

OBJECTIVES

After completing this chapter, you should be able to do the following:

1. *Dissassemble the breathing circuit for an adult volume ventilator (i.e., Bennett MA-1, Bear 1).*
2. *Locate and identify the parts of the adult ventilator circuit.*
3. *Use appropriate nomenclature when referring to the breathing circuit components.*
4. *Identify and implement the appropriate controls and alarms of the adult mechanical ventilator pertinent to testing the assembled circuit for leaks.*
5. *Test the assembled circuit for leaks and other malfunctions.*
6. *Change a ventilator breathing circuit with circuit detachment for three inspiratory cycles or less.*

EQUIPMENT NEEDED

☐ Volume-cycled ventilator
☐ Tubing circuit
☐ Spirometer
☐ Lung simulator or mannequin

- ☐ 50 psi oxygen and air source
- ☐ Watch with a second hand
- ☐ Sterile gauze or glove
- ☐ Oxygen analyzer

Exercise A: Identification of an Adult Ventilator Breathing Circuit

1. Your instructor will assemble and connect a breathing circuit to an adult volume-cycled ventilator (Fig. 37-1).
2. Identify the following parts as you trace the gas flow from the ventilator.
   - A. Tube from the ventilator to the humidifier
   - B. Large-reservoir humidifier
   - C. Humidifier inlet
   - D. Humidifier outlet
   - E. Large-bore inspiratory tubing
   - F. Medication nebulizer
   - G. Small-bore medication nebulizer tubing
   - H. Patient connection Wye
   - I. Swivel adapter
   - J. Temperature monitoring device
   - K. Large-bore exhalation tubing
   - L. Exhalation valve

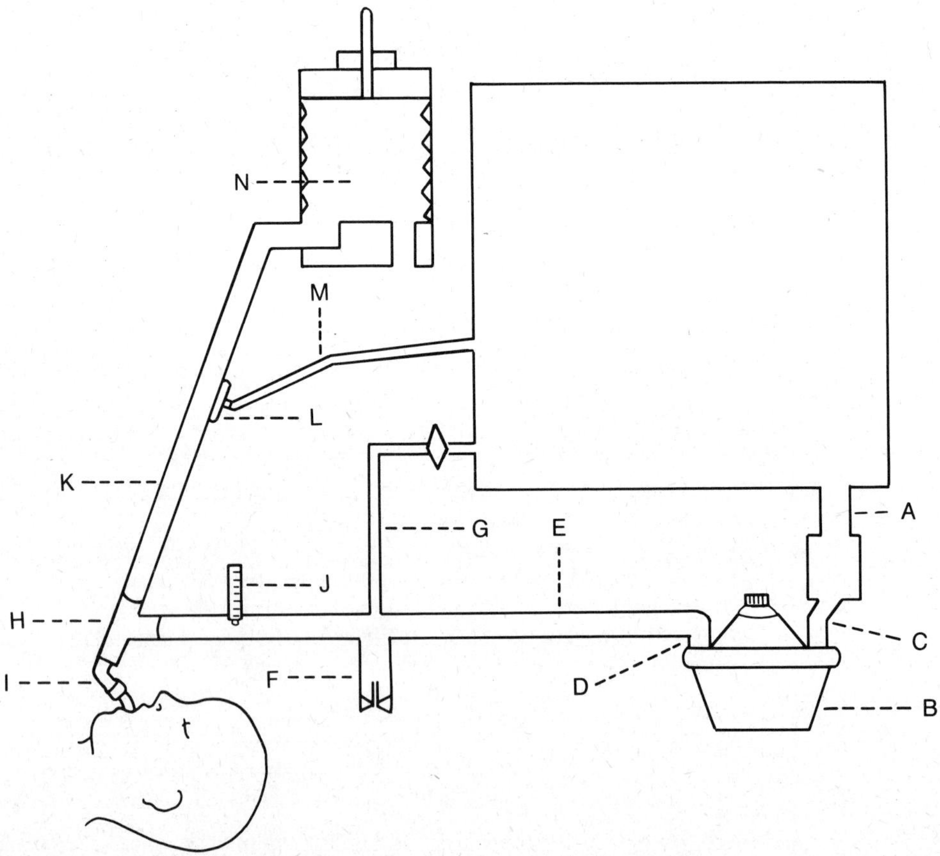

Fig. 37-1. Major components of a typical adult ventilator breathing circuit.

M. Small-bore exhalation tubing

N. Expiratory volume-measuring device (*i.e.*, spirometer)

You may also see proximal airway pressure tubing, water traps, and bacteria filters. Your ventilator circuit may not contain all the above-mentioned items.

Exercise B: Disassembly and Reassembly of an Adult Ventilator Breathing Circuit

1. Disassemble the circuit completely.
2. Reassemble the circuit, connecting it to the ventilator using the adjustable flex arm for support. Tighten all connections. Make sure the humidifier is filled with sterile water (Fig. 37-2).
3. Connect ventilator to electrical source and 50 psi oxygen, or both air and oxygen.

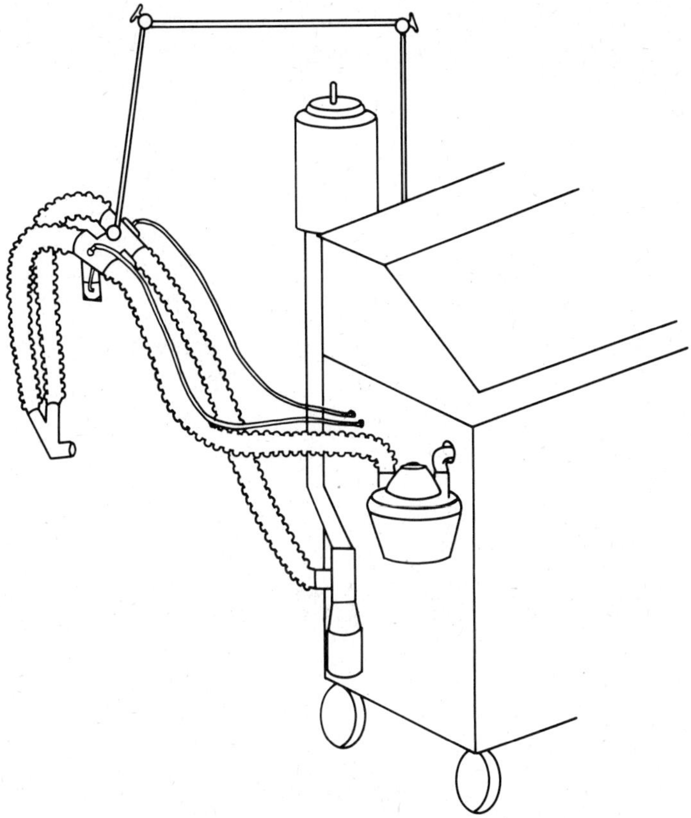

Fig. 37-2. Assembled breathing circuit supported by ventilator flex arm.

Exercise C: Location of Ventilator Controls, Monitoring Devices, and Alarms

1. Locate the following controls: sensitivity, peak flow, power on/off, pressure limit, tidal volume (V_T), rate, sigh pressure limit, sigh volume, sighs/hour, $F_{I_{O_2}}$, expiratory resistance, PEEP, manual breath, humidity temperature, medication nebulizer on/off, inflation hold or inspiratory pause, and mode selection conrol.
2. Locate the following monitoring devices and visual indicators: pressure manometer, temperature read-out device, spirometer, digital rate indicator, alarm lights, digital I:E indicator, mode indicator, and so on. You may not find all of these

monitoring devices and visual indicators on your ventilator. On your laboratory report, note which of the above are available on the ventilator you are using.

3. Locate the following alarm controls: low exhaled volume, low inspiratory pressure, high rate, low PEEP, apneic period, low oxygen, and so on. You may not find all of these on the ventilator you are using. On your laboratory report, note which of the above are available on the ventilator you are using.

Exercise D: Performance of a Leak Test

1. Set all controls off except:
   A. Flow rate or peak flow—20 liters/minute
   B. Tidal volume—500 ml
   C. Pressure limit—maximum
2. Occlude patient wye using the thumb of your gloved hand or sterile gauze (Fig. 37-3).
3. Turn the power on and press the manual breath button.
4. The pressure gauge should reach 80 cm H_2O or greater.
5. If the manometer needle does not reach 80 cm H_2O or greater, a leak may be present in the breathing circuit. Check all of your connections, and be certain that the humidifier is assembled and attached properly. *Note:* The use of a ventilator circuit containing leaks may be hazardous or *fatal* to an actual patient requiring ventilation.

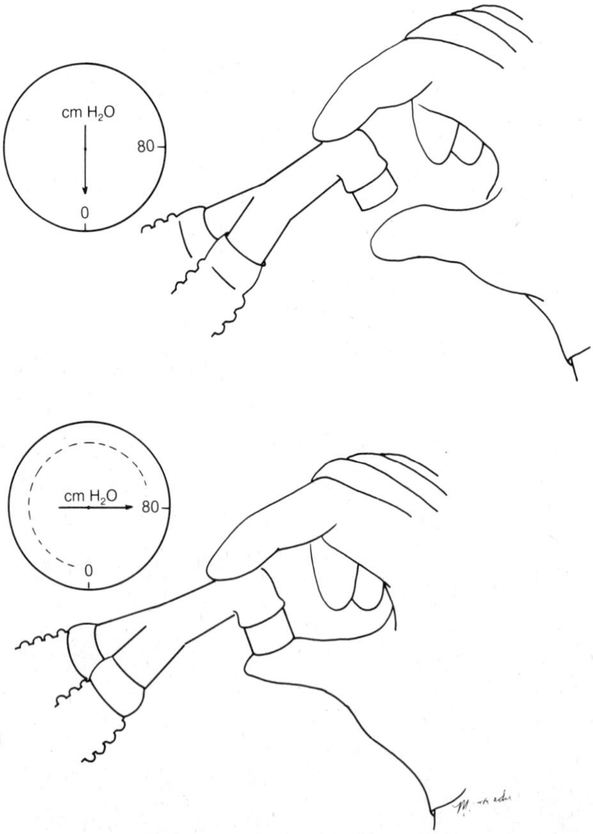

Fig. 37-3. Occlusion of circuit with sterile glove for detection of gas leak during inspiratory phase or a "leak test."

Exercise E: Assessment of the Operation of the Ventilator Controls

1. Set the following controls:
   A. Peak flow—40 liters/minute
   B. Tidal volume—500 ml
   C. Pressure limit—40 cm H_2O
   D. Rate—12 breaths/minute
   E. Sigh volume—750 ml
   F. $F_{I_{O_2}}$—0.40
2. Turn the ventilator power on.
3. Monitor the normal pressure limit.
   A. Occlude patient wye using the palm of your hand and sterile gauze.
   B. Observe the manometer; it should stop at 40 cm H_2O. An audible alarm should be heard and a pressure limit light illuminated.
   C. Adjust the pressure limit control to 40 cm H_2O, if necessary.
4. Monitor sigh pressure limit.
   A. Press manual sigh button while occluding the patient wye.
   B. Observe manometer, sigh light, pressure light, and audible alarm.
5. Connect test lung or intubated mannequin. Note pressure reading on the manometer; it should be less than 40 cm H_2O.
6. Measure exhaled tidal volume (V_T).
   A. Attach a spirometer to the exhalation port.
   B. Allow the ventilator to cycle several times.
   C. Measure the exhaled volume; adjust to 500 ml.
7. Analyze the oxygen concentration.
   A. Calibrate the oxygen analyzer (see previous laboratory exercises).
   B. Connect the oxygen analyzer "T" into the inspiratory line of the ventilation circuit (Fig. 37-4).
   C. Wait for the analyzer to stabilize.
   D. If the analyzer does not read 0.40, adjust the oxygen control on the ventilator until the analyzer reads 0.40.
8. Leave all controls set as they are above.

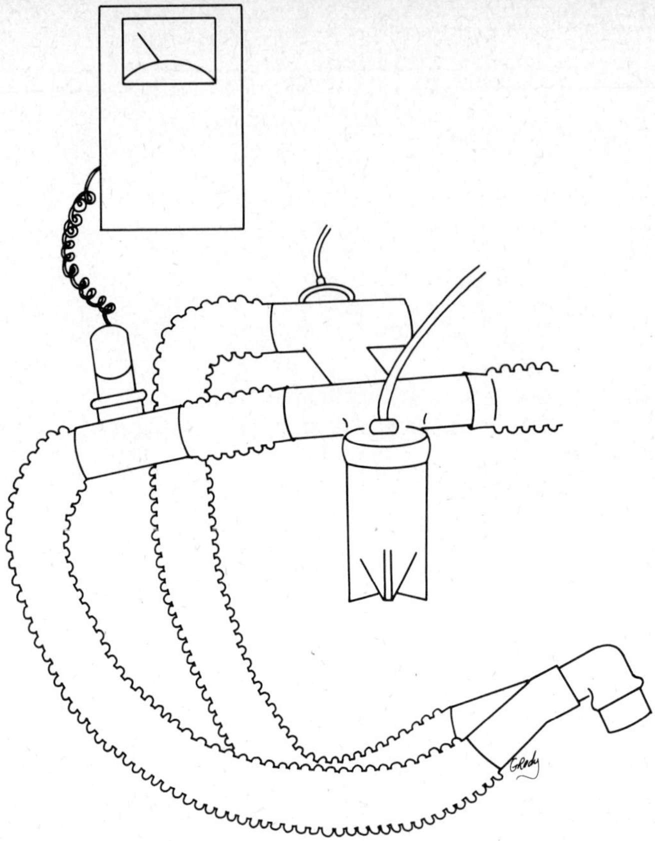

Fig. 37-4. Analysis of oxygen concentration using an adapter in the inspiratory line of a ventilator breathing circuit.

Exercise F: Replacement of the Ventilator Breathing Circuit

Assume that a paralyzed patient on a mechanical ventilator requires replacement of the breathing circuit without a significant interruption (three breaths or less) in ventilation.

1. Assemble a clean breathing circuit.
2. Unbolt the used manifold from the support arm.
3. Attach the clean manifold to the support arm.
4. Shut off the spirometer and low-pressure or low-volume alarms.
5. Loosen (but do not remove) all hoses and tubes to be changed.
6. Remove the used spirometer hose and water trap or the large-bore exhalation tubing from the manifold to the ventilator.
7. Attach the clean spirometer hose and water trap or the large-bore exhalation tubing.
8. Turn off the nebulizer if it is on and remove the used small-bore medication nebulizer tubing.
9. Attach the clean nebulizer tubing.
10. Remove the tubing from the ventilator to the cascade humidifier. Remove the tubing from the cascade to the manifold and attach it to the ventilator outlet port. This will allow the ventilator to function while you change the cascade humidifier (Fig. 37-5).

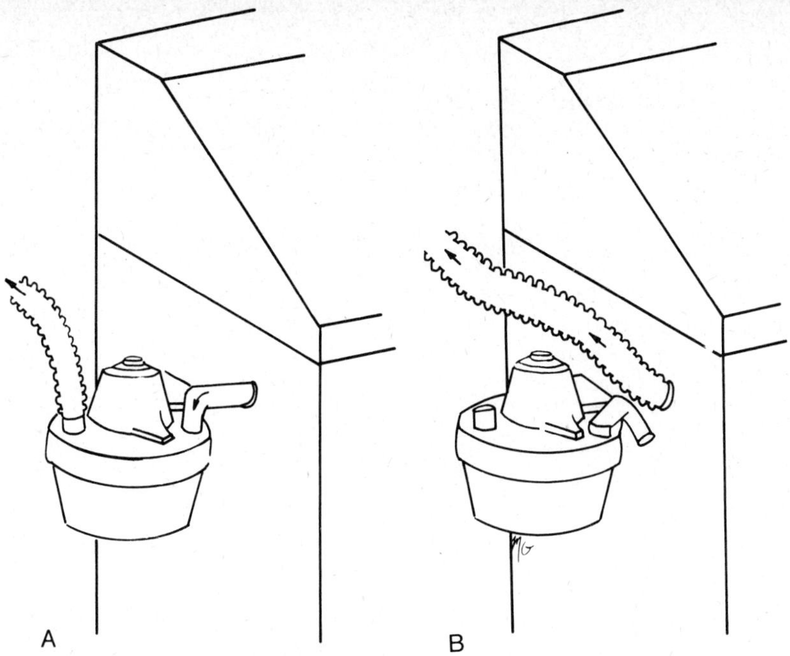

Fig. 3-5. Bypass of the humidifier during continuous ventilation by *(A)* disconnection of humidifier inlet tube and *(B)* connection of humidifier outlet tube directly to gas outlet on ventilator.

11. Remove the used cascade humidifier.
12. Attach the clean cascade humidifier and fill it with the sterile distilled water. Set the humidifier temperature, if necessary.
13. Attach the clean cascade humidifier outlet hose to the cascade humidifier outlet port.
14. You now have 20 seconds to perform five steps (work as fast as possible).
    A. Remove the patient wye from the patient's airway.
    B. Remove the used small-bore exhalation tubing and attach the new exhalation tubing.
    C. Remove the used hose from the ventilator to the humidifier and replace it with a clean one.
    D. Check that the entire circuit has no pressure leaks by occluding the outlet port at the clean patient wye. The manometer should read 40 cm H_2O.
    E. Attach the patient to the clean circuit at the patient wye.
15. Reactivate the alarms from step #3.
16. Recheck the operation of the ventilator.
17. Repeat the leak test after reconnection of the patient to the ventilator. Ensure that the pressure exceeds 80 cm H_2O.

Exercise G: Determination of "Unknown"

1. Your laboratory instructor will provide you with a ventilator in operation.
2. Record all the control settings on your laboratory report.
3. Record the alarm settings on your laboratory report and also indicate if all alarms were set appropriately.

RECOMMENDED READING

Blodgett DE: Manual of Respiratory Care Procedures. Philadelphia, JB Lippincott, 1980

Rattenborg C: Clinical Use of Mechanical Ventilation. Chicago, Year Book Medical Publishers, 1981

Laboratory Performance Evaluation (#37)

Topic: Mechanical Ventilation Preparation

Student ______________________ Course ______________________

Date ______________________ Section ______________________

Performance Elements	Acceptable	Unacceptable	Not Applicable	Comments
1. Obtains appropriate equipment and supplies				
2. Washes hands				
3. Properly assembles CMV breathing circuit				
4. Attaches breathing circuit to ventilator				
5. Performs "leak test"				
6. Locates the following: A. Ventilator controls B. Ventilator monitors C. Ventilator alarms				
7. Sets prescribed ventilator controls				
8. Activates the ventilator				
9. Attaches the "activated ventilator" to a simulated patient or test lung				
10. Assesses the function of ventilator's controls, monitors, and alarms				

Performance Elements	Acceptable	Unacceptable	Not Applicable	Comments
11. Exchanges (changes out) unused breathing circuit for "in use" breathing circuit				
12. Accomplishes breathing circuit "change out" in fewer than three inspiratory cycles				
13. Checks new breathing circuit for leaks				
14. Reactivates alarms and monitors				

Knowledge of Procedure

- ☐ Good; student is knowledgeable about rationale and theory related to procedure
- ☐ Fair; student has adequate understanding of rationale and theory related to procedure
- ☐ Poor; student has inadequate understanding of rationale and theory related to procedure

Performance Deficiencies (check those that apply)

- ☐ Excessive time needed to complete procedure
- ☐ Broke aseptic or sterile technique
- ☐ Gross inaccuracy noted
- ☐ Technique may be harmful to patient
- ☐ Incorrect dosage or gas concentration
- ☐ Incorrect equipment assembly/use
- ☐ Unable to answer questions correctly about rationale and/or theory related to procedure
- ☐ Other ______________________

Evaluation Summary

- ☐ Satisfactory performance
- ☐ Unsatisfactory performance

Recommendations of Evaluator

- ☐ Skills may be applied/observed in clinical setting
- ☐ Specific evaluation deficiencies require correction
- ☐ Complete re-evaluation required
- ☐ Additional laboratory practice required

Signatures:

Evaluator ______________________ Date ______________________

Student ______________________ Date ______________________

Laboratory Report

Student ______________________ Acceptable ______________________

Date ______________________ Unacceptable ______________________

Course ______________________

Topic: Mechanical Ventilation Preparation

Data or Measurements

1. What is the name of the ventilator(s) you are using for this laboratory?

2. List the monitoring devices and visual indicators located on the ventilator(s) you are using.

3. List the alarm controls located on the ventilator(s) you are using.

4. The normal pressure reading while ventilating the test lung is ______________________.

5. Record all the control settings from the unknown exercise of your laboratory.

6. Record all the alarm settings from the unknown exercise of your laboratory.

7. Were the alarms set appropriately? If not, indicate which alarms were not and how they would be corrected.

Scenario: Today, you have been assigned, for the first time, to one of the critical care units. You know that your first task after rounds will be "changing out" the breathing circuits of the patients who are being sustained by mechanical ventilators. You have mentally rehearsed the procedure many times. You also know that your supervisor will be carefully observing your every move, since prolonged interruptions in continuous ventilation may be dangerous to your assigned patients. Please address the following questions and requests:

1. List the components of the breathing circuit.

2. Describe how you changed the circuit.

3. How much time was necessary to change the ventilator circuit?

4. What are the possible consequences if more than a few breaths are "missed" by a paralyzed, apneic, or unstable patient when replacing a breathing circuit?

5. If a patient is breathing spontaneously or assisting a ventilator, how may you ensure adequate ventilation when replacing the breathing circuit?

6. Briefly describe the procedure for checking gas leaks on a ventilator circuit.

chapter 38

Initiation of adult mechanical ventilation

INTRODUCTION

A life-threatening situation may exist before the initiation of mechanical ventilation. The indications for mechanical ventilation are numerous; however, there are standard guidelines for initial ventilator settings that can be used regardless of the indications. The initial ventilator settings described in this chapter are standard guidelines that may result in a safe method of ventilation. In the clinical setting, an arterial blood gas sample is obtained and analyzed shortly after ventilation is initiated in order to readjust the ventilator and optimize the settings. The purpose of this chapter is to introduce you to the initiation of mechanical ventilation.

OBJECTIVES

After completing this chapter, you should be able to do the following:

1. *Demonstrate familiarity with the power source(s), gas sources(s), alarms, monitors, and controls of the adult mechanical ventilator provided by your instructor.*
2. *Select, given a hypothetical situation, appropriate control settings for the mechanical ventilator.*
3. *Interface the adult mechanical ventilation system with a test lung or mannequin.*
4. *Initiate mechanical ventilation when given appropriate background information for a simulated adult patient.*
5. *Demonstrate an ability to determine the effectiveness of the system by observing lung inflation, the manometer, alarms, and monitors.*

EQUIPMENT NEEDED

☐ Adult mechanical ventilator
☐ Adult breathing circuit

- ☐ Spirometer or other measuring device(s)
- ☐ Test lung or intubated mannequin
- ☐ Watch or clock with a second hand

ACTIVITIES

Exercise A: Functional Analysis of Ventilator Controls, Monitors, and Alarms

Your instructor will provide you with an appropriate operator's manual or alternative instructional materials. Before beginning this exercise, it is imperative that you become thoroughly familiar with the operation of the provided mechanical ventilator. Figures 38-1 through 38-12 will help familiarize you with the ventilator you are using.

1. Assemble, then attach, an adult breathing circuit to the ventilator.
2. Connect the gas source and activate the power source.
3. Perform a leak test.
4. Check the function of all available alarms on your ventilator. *Note:* Inactive or inoperable alarms during continuous ventilation may be harmful or *fatal* to a patient.
5. On the laboratory report, list all the alarms and the purpose of each.
6. On the laboratory report, list each monitor present on the ventilator (*i.e.*, visual indicators, pressure manometers, temperature indicators, and so on).
7. Describe, on the laboratory report, the purpose of each monitor.
8. On the laboratory report, list each control available for this ventilator. Describe the purpose of each control.
9. Your instructor will assign a mechanical ventilator to you. Locate the diagram of the assigned ventilator, and turn in the completed form with your laboratory report.

Directions: Using the diagram (Fig. 38-1), identify the controls, alarms, and monitors that correspond to the appropriate letter in the diagram. Briefly describe the purpose of each control, alarm, and monitor. Detach this page and turn it in with your laboratory report.

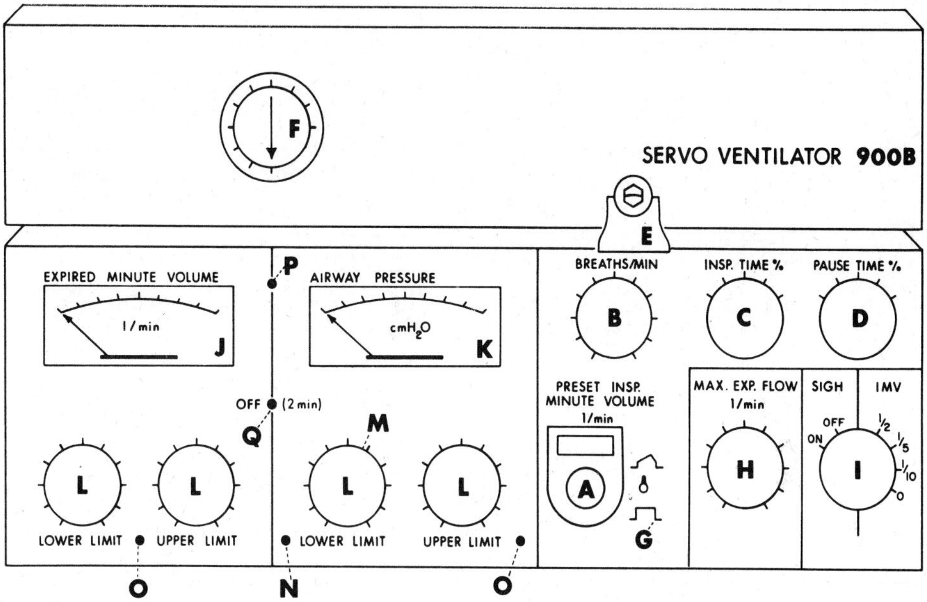

Fig. 38-1. Servo 900 B ventilator control panel. *(Reproduced with permission from Burton GG, Hodgkin JE: Respiratory Care. A Guide to Clinical Practice, 2nd ed. Philadelphia, JB Lippincott, 1984)*

VENTILATOR BRAND AND MODEL ______________________________

A. ______________________________

B. ______________________________

C. ______________________________

D. ______________________________

E. ______________________________

F. ______________________________

G. ______________________________

H. ______________________________

I. ______________________________

J. ______________________________

K. ______________________________

L. ______________________________

M. ______________________________

N. ______________________________

O. ______________________________

P. ______________________________

Q. ______________________________

Directions: Using the diagram (Fig. 38-2), identify the controls, alarms, and monitors that correspond to the appropriate letter in the diagram. Briefly describe the purpose of each control, alarm, and monitor. Detach this page and turn it in with your laboratory report.

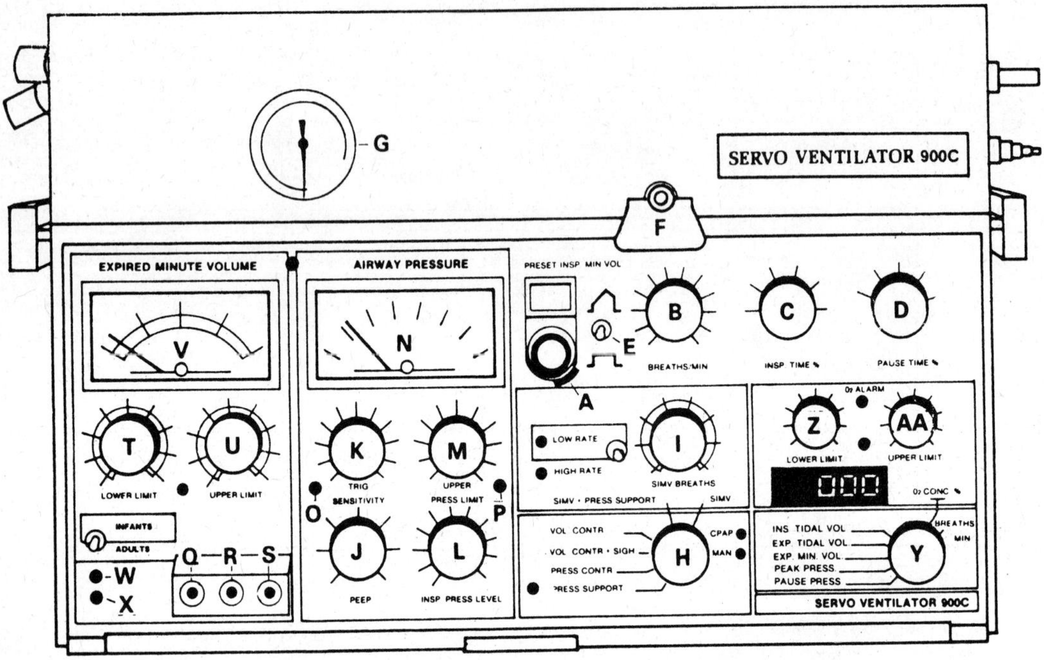

Fig. 38-2. Servo 900 C ventilator control panel. *(Reproduced with permission from Burton GG, Hodgkin JE: Respiratory Care. A Guide to Clinical Practice, 2nd ed. Philadelphia, JB Lippincott, 1984)*

VENTILATOR BRAND AND MODEL ____________________

A. ________	J. ________	S. ________
B. ________	K. ________	T. ________
C. ________	L. ________	U. ________
D. ________	M. ________	V. ________
E. ________	N. ________	W. ________
F. ________	O. ________	X. ________
G. ________	P. ________	Y. ________
H. ________	Q. ________	Z. ________
I. ________	R. ________	AA. ________

Directions: Using the diagram (Fig. 38-3), identify the controls, alarms, and monitors that correspond to the appropriate letter in the diagram. Briefly describe the purpose of each control, alarm, and monitor. Detach this page and turn it in with your laboratory report.

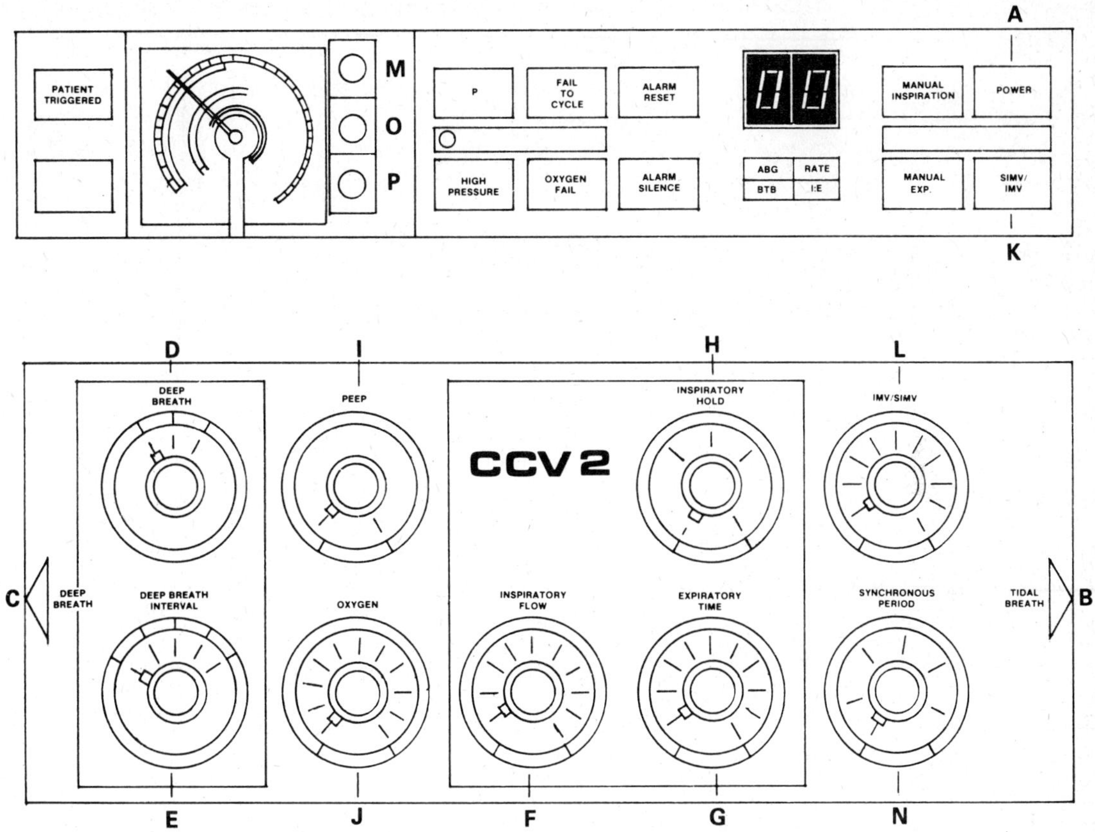

Fig. 38-3. Ohio CCV 2 ventilator. *(Reproduced with permission from Burton GG, Hodgkin JE: Respiratory Care. A Guide to Clinical Practice, 2nd ed. Philadelphia, JB Lippincott, 1984)*

VENTILATOR BRAND AND MODEL ____________________

A. ____________________

B. ____________________

C. ____________________

D. ____________________

E. ____________________

F. ____________________

G. ____________________

H. ____________________

I. ____________________

J. ____________________

K. ____________________

L. ____________________

M. ____________________

N. ____________________

O. ____________________

P. ____________________

Directions: Using the diagram (Fig. 38-4), identify the controls, alarms, and monitors that correspond to the appropriate letter in the diagram. Briefly describe the purpose of each control, alarm, and monitor. Detach this page and turn it in with your laboratory report.

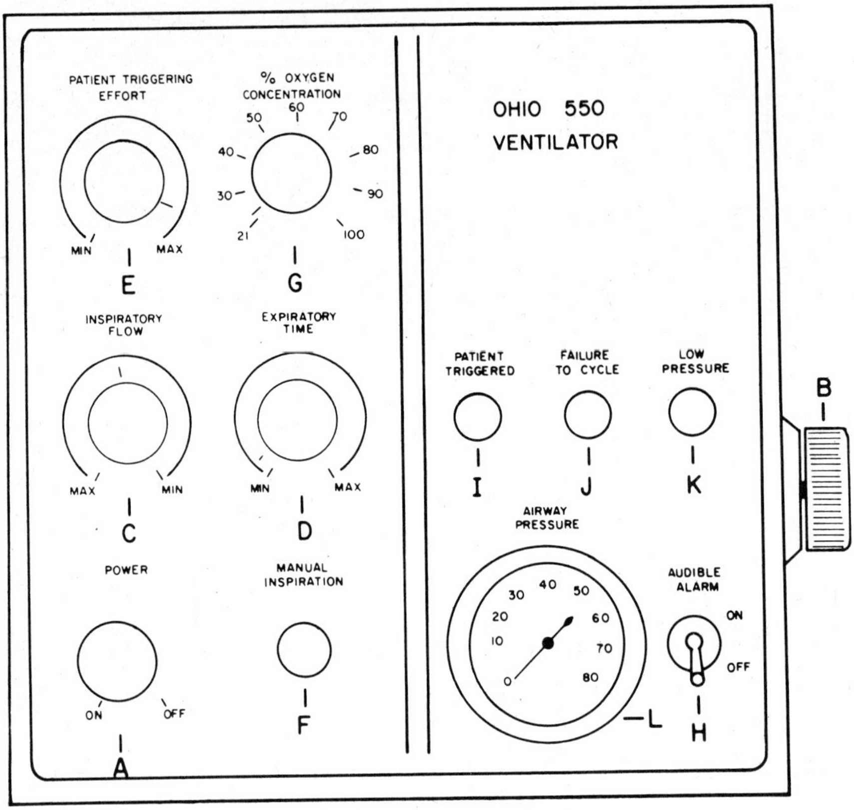

Fig. 38-4. Ohio 550 ventilator. *(Reproduced with permission from Burton GG, Hodgkin JE: Respiratory Care. A Guide to Clinical Practice, 2nd ed. Philadelphia, JB Lippincott, 1984)*

VENTILATOR BRAND AND MODEL ______________________________

A.	____________________	G.	____________________
B.	____________________	H.	____________________
C.	____________________	I.	____________________
D.	____________________	J.	____________________
E.	____________________	K.	____________________
F.	____________________	L.	____________________

Directions: Using the diagram (Fig. 38-5), identify the controls, alarms, and monitors that correspond to the appropriate letter in the diagram. Briefly describe the purpose of each control, alarm, and monitor. Detach this page and turn it in with your laboratory report.

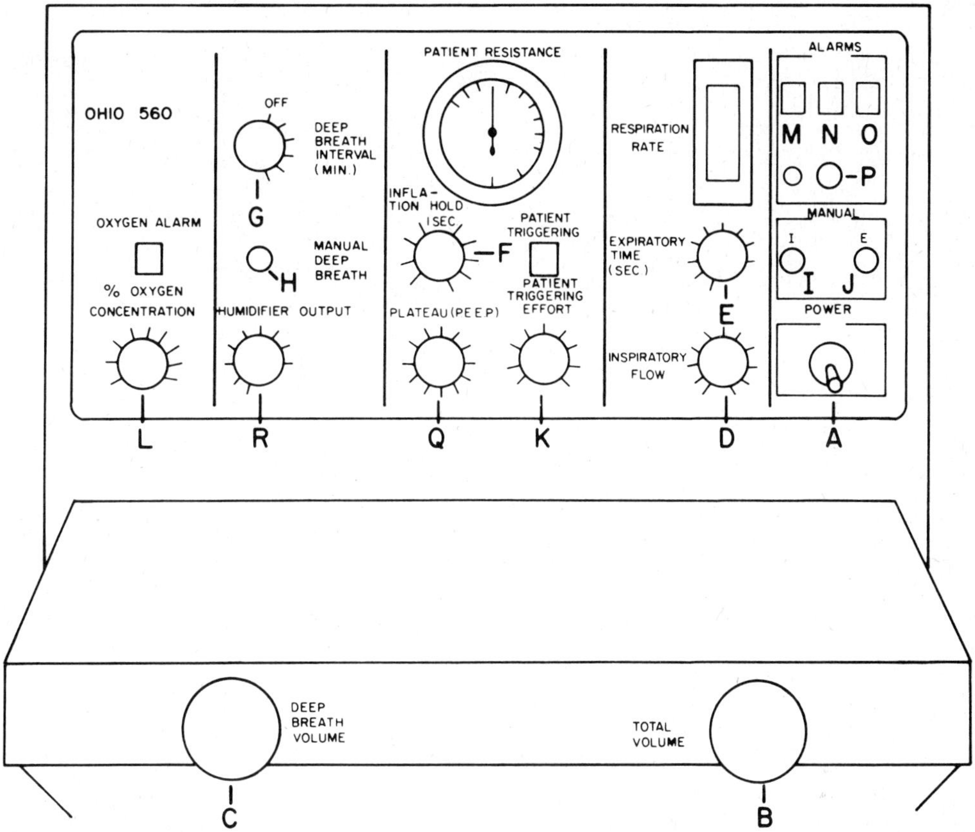

Fig. 38-5. Ohio 560 ventilator. *(Reproduced with permission from Burton GG, Hodgkin JE: Respiratory Care. A Guide to Clinical Practice, 2nd ed. Philadelphia, JB Lippincott, 1984)*

VENTILATOR BRAND AND MODEL ______________________

A. ____________ H. ____________ O. ____________

B. ____________ I. ____________ P. ____________

C. ____________ J. ____________ Q. ____________

D. ____________ K. ____________ R. ____________

E. ____________ L. ____________

F. ____________ M. ____________

G. ____________ N. ____________

Directions: Using the diagram (Fig. 38-6), identify the controls, alarms, and monitors that correspond to the appropriate letter in the diagram. Briefly describe the purpose of each control, alarm, and monitor. Detach this page and turn it in with your laboratory report.

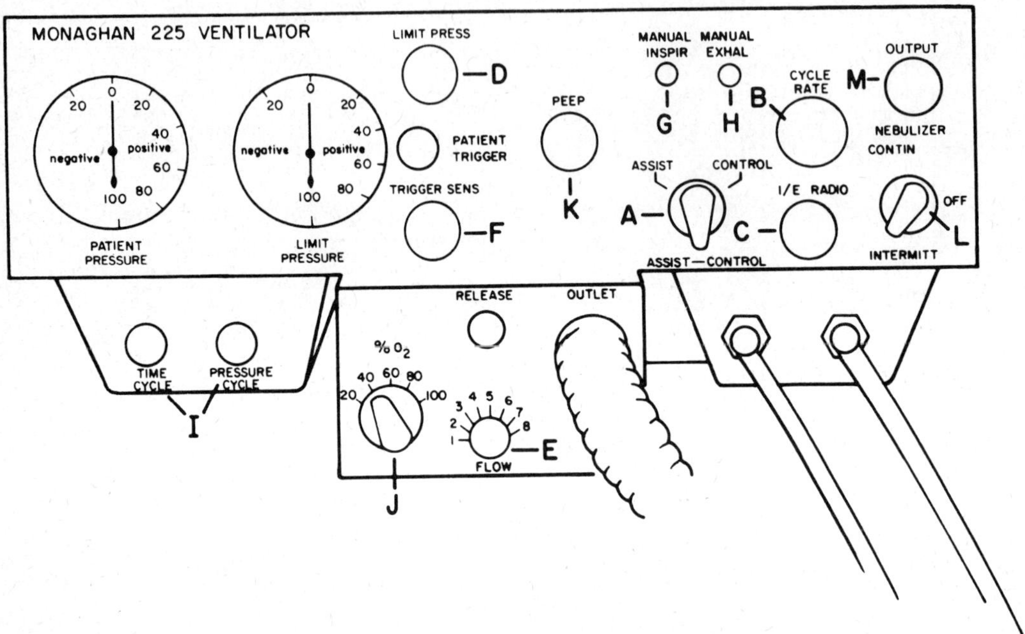

Fig. 38-6. Monaghan 225 ventilator. *(Reproduced with permission from Burton GG, Hodgkin JE: Respiratory Care. A Guide to Clinical Practice, 2nd ed. Philadelphia, JB Lippincott, 1984)*

VENTILATOR BRAND AND MODEL ____________________

A. ____________________

B. ____________________

C. ____________________

D. ____________________

E. ____________________

F. ____________________

G. ____________________

H. ____________________

I. ____________________

J. ____________________

K. ____________________

L. ____________________

M. ____________________

N. ____________________

Directions: Using the diagram (Fig. 38-7), identify the controls, alarms, and monitors that correspond to the appropriate letter in the diagram. Briefly describe the purpose of each control, alarm, and monitor. Detach this page and turn it in with your laboratory report.

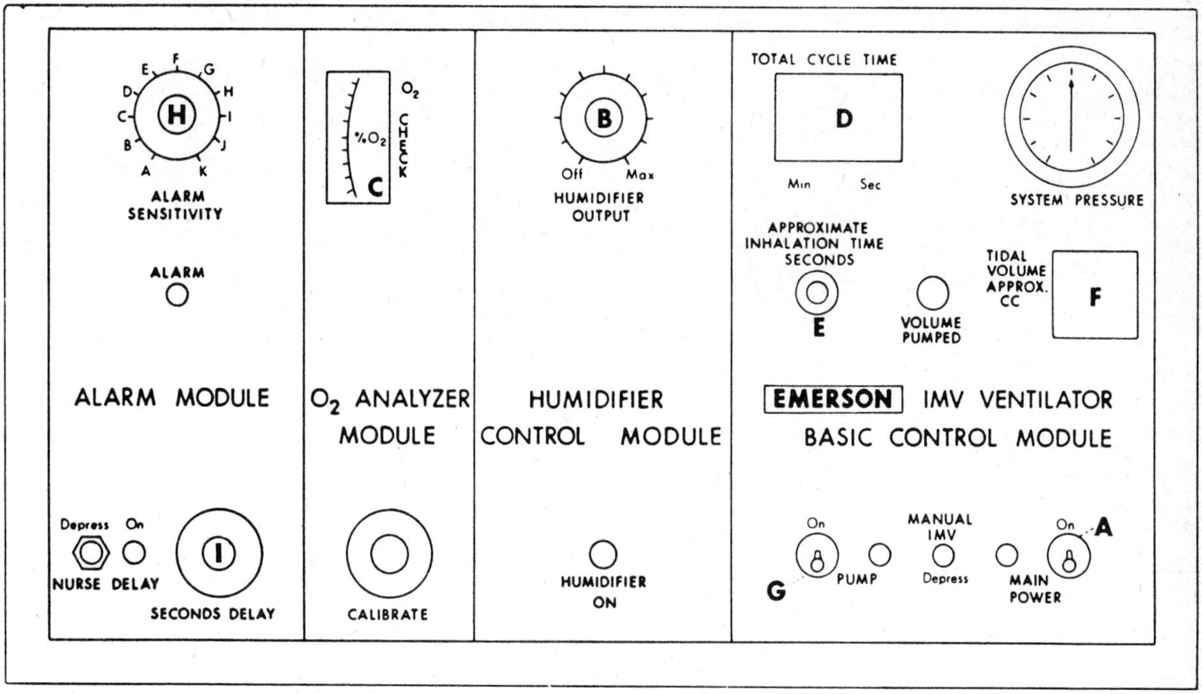

Fig. 38-7. Emerson IMV ventilator. *(Reproduced with permission from Burton GG, Hodgkin JE: Respiratory Care. A Guide to Clinical Practice, 2nd ed. Philadelphia, JB Lippincott, 1984)*

VENTILATOR BRAND AND MODEL ______________________________

A. ______________________ F. ______________________

B. ______________________ G. ______________________

C. ______________________ H. ______________________

D. ______________________ I. ______________________

E. ______________________

Directions: Using the diagram (Fig. 38-8), identify the controls, alarms, and monitors that correspond to the appropriate letter in the diagram. Briefly describe the purpose of each control, alarm, and monitor. Detach this page and turn it in with your laboratory report.

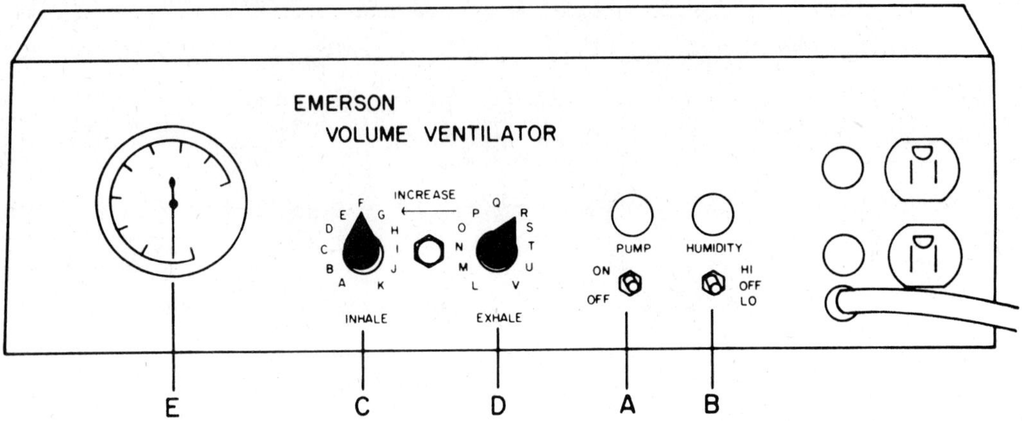

Fig. 38-8. Emerson 3 PV volume ventilator. *(Reproduced with permission from Burton GG, Hodgkin JE: Respiratory Care. A Guide to Clinical Practice, 2nd ed. Philadelphia, JB Lippincott, 1984)*

VENTILATOR BRAND AND MODEL ____________________

A. ____________________

B. ____________________

C. ____________________

D. ____________________

E. ____________________

Directions: Using the diagram (Fig. 38-9), identify the controls, alarms, and monitors that correspond to the appropriate letter in the diagram. Briefly describe the purpose of each control, alarm, and monitor. Detach this page and turn it in with your laboratory report.

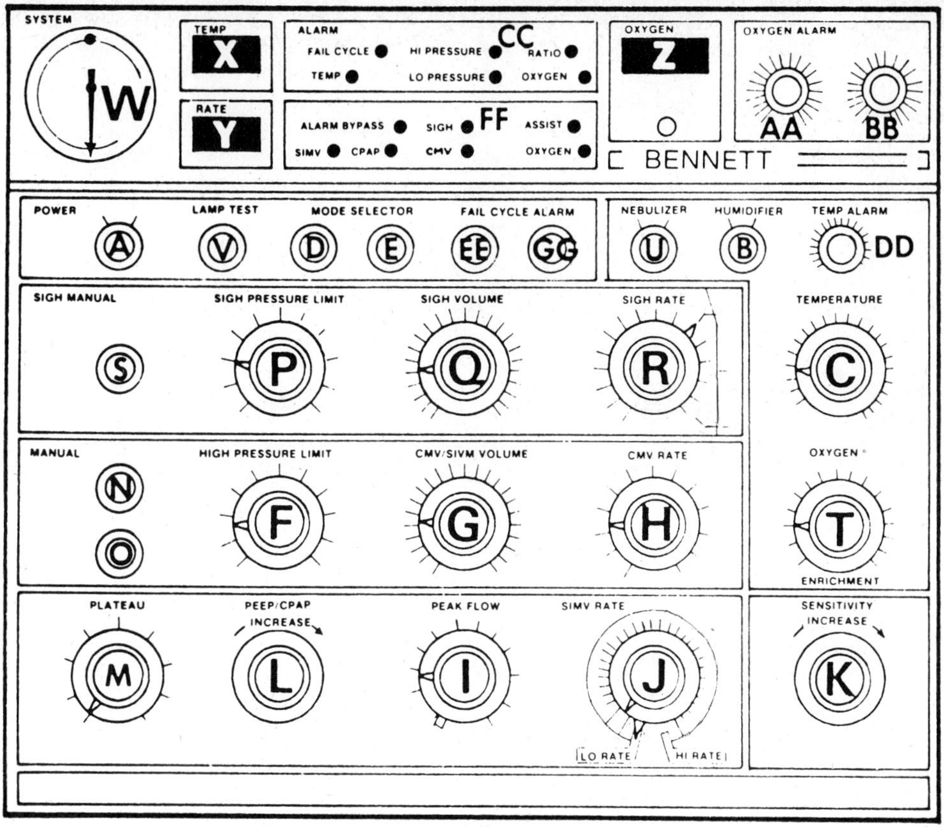

Fig. 38-9. Bennett M:A-2 ventilator. *(Reproduced with permission from Burton GG, Hodgkin JE: Respiratory Care. A Guide to Clinical Practice, 2nd ed. Philadelphia, JB Lippincott, 1984)*

VENTILATOR BRAND AND MODEL ______________________

A. ______________________

B. ______________________

C. ______________________

D. ______________________

E. ______________________

F. ______________________

G. ______________________

H. ______________________

I. ______________________

J. ______________________

K. ______________________

L. ______________________

M. ______________________

N. ______________________

O. ______________________

P. ______________________

Q. ______________________

R. ______________________

S. ______________________

T. ______________________

U. ______________________

V. ______________________

W. ______________________

X. ______________________

Y. ______________________

Z. ______________________

AA. ______________________

BB. ______________________

CC. ______________________

DD. ______________________

EE. ______________________

FF. ______________________

GG. ______________________

Directions: Using the diagram (Fig. 38-10), identify the controls, alarms, and monitors that correspond to the appropriate letter in the diagram. Briefly describe the purpose of each control, alarm, and monitor. Detach this page and turn it in with your laboratory report.

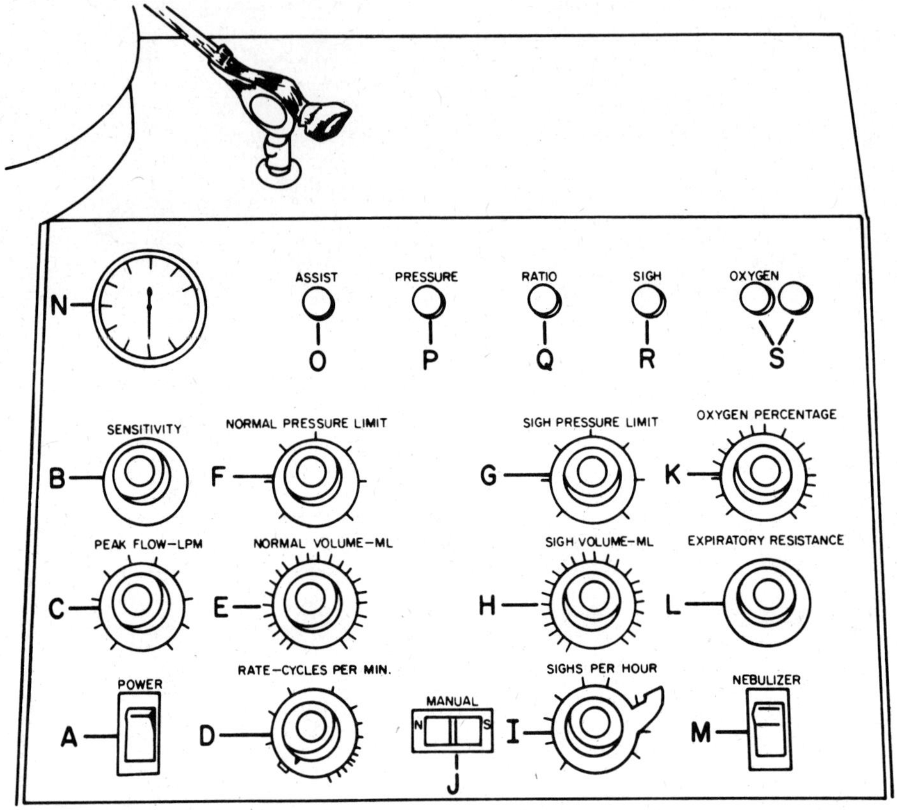

Fig. 38-10. Bennett MA-1 ventilator. *(Reproduced with permission from Burton GG, Hodgkin JE: Respiratory Care. A Guide to Clinical Practice, 2nd ed. Philadelphia, JB Lippincott, 1984)*

VENTILATOR BRAND AND MODEL ____________________

A. ____________

B. ____________

C. ____________

D. ____________

E. ____________

F. ____________

G. ____________

H. ____________

I. ____________

J. ____________

K. ____________

L. ____________

M. ____________

N. ____________

O. ____________

P. ____________

Q. ____________

R. ____________

S. ____________

Directions: Using the diagram (Fig. 38-11), identify the controls, alarms, and monitors that correspond to the appropriate letter in the diagram. Briefly describe the purpose of each control, alarm, and monitor. Detach this page and turn it in with your laboratory report.

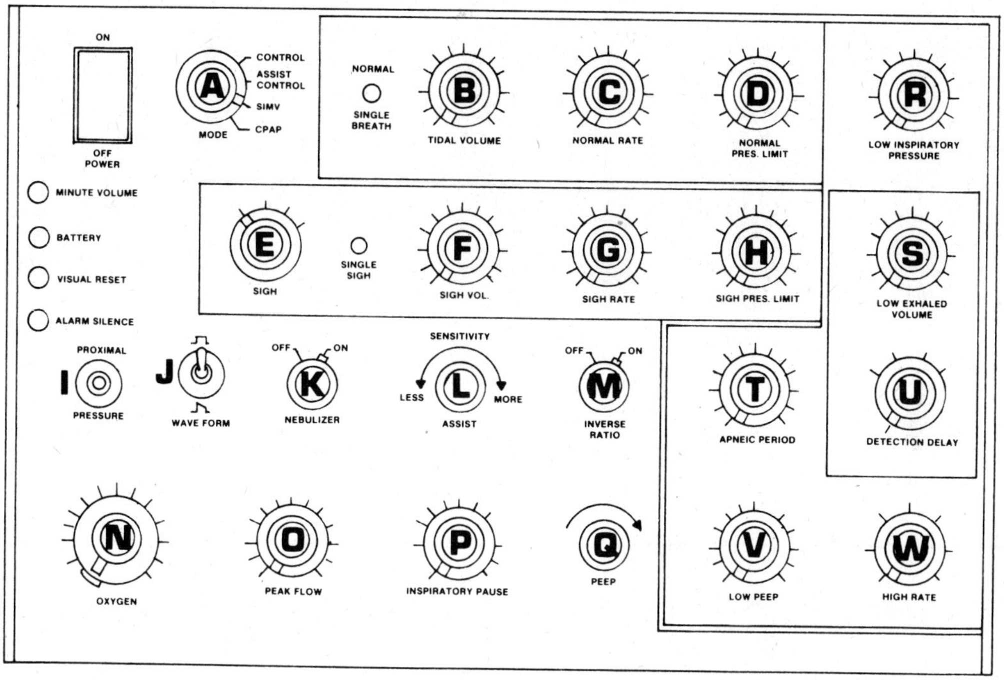

Fig. 38-11. Bourns Bear 2 ventilator. *(Reproduced with permission from Burton GG, Hodgkin JE: Respiratory Care. A Guide to Clinical Practice, 2nd ed. Philadelphia, JB Lippincott, 1984)*

VENTILATOR BRAND AND MODEL ______________________________

A. ____________________

B. ____________________

C. ____________________

D. ____________________

E. ____________________

F. ____________________

G. ____________________

H. ____________________

I. ____________________

J. ____________________

K. ____________________

L. ____________________

M. ____________________

N. ____________________

O. ____________________

P. ____________________

Q. ____________________

R. ____________________

S. ____________________

T. ____________________

U. ____________________

V. ____________________

W. ____________________

Directions: Using the diagram (Fig. 38-12), identify the controls, alarms, and monitors that correspond to the appropriate letter in the diagram. Briefly describe the purpose of each control, alarm, and monitor. Detach this page and turn it in with your laboratory report.

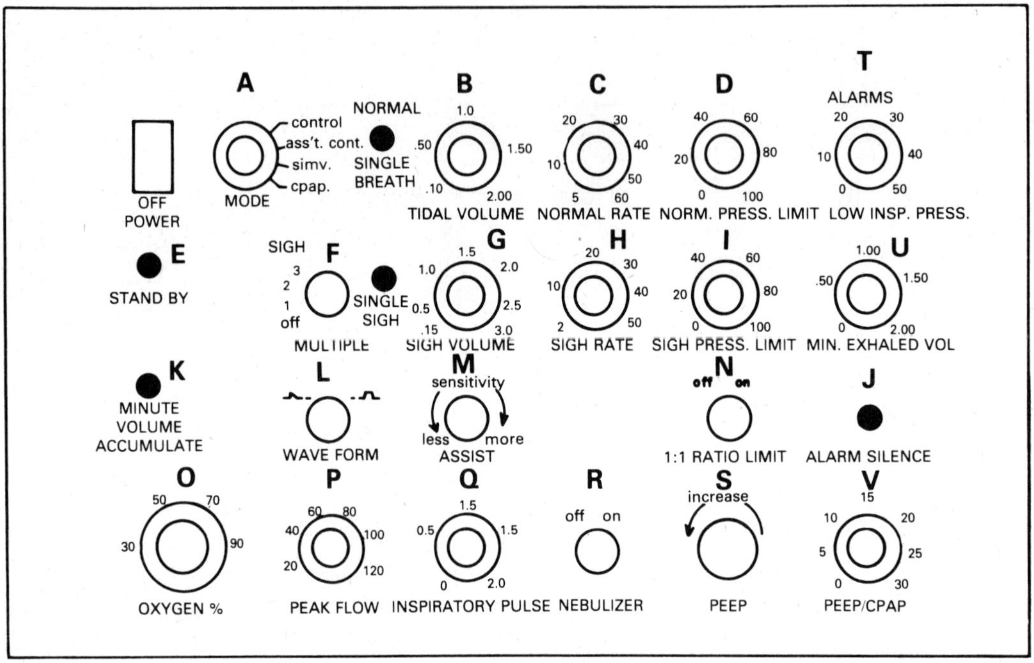

Fig. 38-12. Bourns Bear 1 ventilator. *(Reproduced with permission from Burton GG, Hodgkin JE: Respiratory Care. A Guide to Clinical Practice, 2nd ed. Philadelphia, JB Lippincott, 1984)*

VENTILATOR BRAND AND MODEL ______________________________

A. ____________________ J. ____________________ S. ____________________

B. ____________________ K. ____________________ T. ____________________

C. ____________________ L. ____________________ U. ____________________

D. ____________________ M. ____________________ V. ____________________

E. ____________________ N. ____________________

F. ____________________ O. ____________________

G. ____________________ P. ____________________

H. ____________________ Q. ____________________

I. ____________________ R. ____________________

Exercise B: Determination and Adjustment of Initial Ventilator Settings

1. The initial tidal volume (VT) is determined by multiplying the ideal body weight in kilograms (kg) by 10 ml to 15 ml. Assume your subject weighs 150 lb. Adjust the ventilator to deliver the appropriate tidal volume.
2. Adjust the rate of the ventilator to deliver 12 breaths/minute. Select the IMV or SIMV mode. *Note:* For adults an initial rate of 2 to 12 breaths/minute may be used depending on the degree of ventilatory support needed.
3. Confirm the rate by timing it for 60 seconds.
4. Set the sigh volume by multiplying the VT times 1.5. Set the sigh rate at 6 to 9 sighs/hour.
5. Set the FI_{O_2} control to deliver 100% oxygen.
6. Adjust the other controls as follows: PEEP 0, flowrate 40 to 60 liters/minute. *Note:* The flowrate may be adjusted to achieve the desired I:E ratio depending on the VT and the rate used.
7. These guidelines may be used to initiate ventilation until an arterial blood gas sample is drawn. After the blood gas analysis, rate or VT is adjusted according to the Pa_{CO_2} and pH of arterial blood. The FI_{O_2} or PEEP level may be adjusted according to the Pa_{O_2} and cardiopulmonary status.

Exercise C: Connection of System to a Test Lung or Intubated Mannequin

1. Activate the power and connect the ventilator to a test lung or intubated patient.
2. Set the pressure limit at 10 to 15 cm H_2O above the average peak pressure achieved during the tidal volume breaths.
3. If applicable, readjust the initial inspiratory flowrate to obtain a 1:3 I:E ratio.
4. On your laboratory report, document the flowrate necessary to obtain a 1:3 I:E ratio.
5. If applicable, adjust the sigh pressure limit 10 to 15 cm H_2O pressure above the pressure required to deliver the sigh volume.
6. If applicable, adjust any low pressure limits to 10 to 15 cm H_2O below the average peak pressure: The low pressure limit should also be set to 2 to 3 cm H_2O above the CPAP or PEEP pressure.
7. Adjust humidifier and gas temperature controls until 35° to 37°C is reached.
8. If applicable, adjust the apnea alarm 10 seconds greater than the seconds between each breath, that is, 12 breaths/minute = 1 breath every 6 seconds. Apnea interval = 6 seconds + 10 seconds = 16 seconds.

Exercise D: Evaluation of System and Verification of Settings

1. Using a spirometer, measure the expired VT.
2. Record the measured expired VT on the laboratory report.
3. Document the following observations on your laboratory report: peak pressure manometer reading and all pressure limits.

Exercise E: Determination of "Unknown"

Your instructor will provide you with a hypothetical situation in which an apneic adult has been intubated and requires full ventilatory support.

1. Determine the initial ventilator settings.
2. Ventilate the mannequin or test lung.
3. Evaluate the effectiveness of your ventilation.
4. Record on your laboratory report the situation you were given, including the simulated patient's body weight in kilograms, the tidal volume, rate, and FI_{O_2} delivered.

5. Record on the laboratory report your initial settings and the results of your evaluation on the effectiveness of your ventilation.

RECOMMENDED READING

Burton GG, Hodgkin JE: Respiratory Care. A Guide to Clinical Practice, 2nd ed. Philadelphia, JB Lippincott, 1984

McPherson SP: Respiratory Therapy Equipment, 3rd ed. St.Louis, CV Mosby, 1985

Shapiro BA, Harrison RA, Kacmarek RM, Cane RD: Clinical Application of Respiratory Care, 3rd ed. Chicago, Year Book Medical Publishers, 1985

Laboratory Performance Evaluation (#38)

Topic: Initiation of Adult Mechanical Ventilation

Student ______________________ Course ______________________

Date ______________________ Section ______________________

Performance Elements	Acceptable	Unacceptable	Not Applicable	Comments
1. Obtains appropriate equipment and supplies				
2. Washes hands				
3. Prepares ventilator for use with simulated patient A. Assembles and attaches appropriate breathing circuit correctly B. Performs "leak test" C. Assesses function of ventilator controls, alarms, monitors				
4. Confirms order for CMV				
5. Determines appropriate initial ventilator settings for simulated patient				
6. Activates ventilator properly A. Controls B. Alarms C. Monitors				
7. Attaches CMV breathing circuit to simulated patient				
8. Adjusts (for the simulated patient situation) the following properly: A. Ventilator alarms B. Ventilator controls C. Ventilator monitors				
9. Evaluates and verifies ventilator settings				

Performance Elements	Acceptable	Unacceptable	Not Applicable	Comments
10. Responds appropriately to changes in simulation status				
11. Determines "unknown"				

Knowledge of Procedure

- ☐ Good; student is knowledgeable about rationale and theory related to procedure
- ☐ Fair; student has adequate understanding of rationale and theory related to procedure
- ☐ Poor; student has inadequate understanding of rationale and theory related to procedure

Performance Deficiencies (check those that apply)

- ☐ Excessive time needed to complete procedure
- ☐ Broke aseptic or sterile technique
- ☐ Gross inaccuracy noted
- ☐ Technique may be harmful to patient
- ☐ Incorrect dosage or gas concentration
- ☐ Incorrect equipment assembly/use
- ☐ Unable to answer questions correctly about rationale and/or theory related to procedure
- ☐ Other ______________________

Evaluation Summary

- ☐ Satisfactory performance
- ☐ Unsatisfactory performance

Recommendations of Evaluator
☐ Skills may be applied/observed in clinical setting
☐ Specific evaluation deficiencies require correction
☐ Complete re-evaluation required
☐ Additional laboratory practice required

Signatures:

Evaluator ______________________ Date ______________________

Student ______________________ Date ______________________

Laboratory Report

Student ______________________ Acceptable ______________________

Date ______________________ Unacceptable ______________________

Course ______________________

Topic: Initiation of Adult Mechanical Ventilation

Data and Measurements

Name of Ventilator ______________________

Model ______________________

1. <u>Alarms</u>

2. <u>Monitors</u>

3. <u>Controls</u>

4. From Exercise D, record the following:

   A. Measured exhaled V_T ______________________

   B. Peak pressure ______________________

   C. Pressure limit ______________________

   D. Sigh pressure limit ______________________

   E. Low pressure limit ______________________

5. Record below the unknown situation given to you by your instructor.

   A. Situation you were given:

B. Initial ventilator settings:

C. Results of your evaluation of effectiveness.

Scenario: A shoot-out between rival gangs had the following outcome: a 350 lb male victim of a gunshot wound to the head is being returned from surgery to the intensive care unit.

1. Specifically, what mechanical ventilator have you chosen to place him on?

2. What tidal volume will you use?

3. What I:E ratio?

4. What FI_{O_2}?

Another victim of the same shoot-out is a 160 lb man who suffered gunshot wounds to the chest and abdomen. He will be arriving on the unit with chest tubes and abdominal drains in place.

5. Again, what specific ventilator have you chosen to place this patient on?

6. What I:E ratio will be used?

7. What tidal volume will be used?

8. What FI_{O_2} will you begin with?

9. Please discuss the alarms systems of the ventilators you have chosen.

10. Using the ventilator assigned by your instructor, what control(s) allow adjustment of the following settings: Name of ventilator: ______________________________

A. VT

B. Rate

C. I:E ratio

D. FI_{O_2}

E. Pressure limit

11. Classify the assigned ventilator according to the following:

A. Power

B. Cycling (ending inspiration)

C. Positive/negative pressure or force

D. Circuits (single or double)

E. Drive

F. Mechanism(s) to start inspiration

chapter 39

Mechanical ventilator mode modification

INTRODUCTION

Mechanical ventilators can be operated in many different ways. The different ways in which ventilation may be provided by a ventilator are referred to as modes of operation, or simply modes. Each different mode may affect the patient's ventilation. One patient may benefit from a particular mode more than another patient. It is important for you to learn all the modes, what the function of each mode is, and how each mode affects ventilation. The purpose of this chapter is to introduce you to the most common ventilator modes.

OBJECTIVES

After completing this chapter, you should be able to do the following:

1. *Identify and describe the function of all available inspiratory and expiratory modes on the ventilator provided by your instructor.*
2. *Initiate ventilation in all available modes.*
3. *Identify and describe the function of any and all expiratory modes.*
4. *Identify and describe the function of any and all mode combinations.*

EQUIPMENT NEEDED

- ☐ Adult mechanical ventilator
- ☐ Adult breathing circuit
- ☐ Watch or clock with second hand
- ☐ Intubated mannequin or test lung

ACTIVITIES

Exercise A: Identification and Operation of the Assist, Control, and Assist/Control Modes

Your instructor will provide you with an appropriate operator's manual or alternative learning materials.

1. Assemble and attach an adult breathing circuit to the ventilator.
2. Connect the gas source and activate the power source.
3. Perform a leak test, then attach the system to a test lung or intubated mannequin.
4. Set the following ventilator controls: VT 500 ml, flowrate 40 liters/minute, an I:E ratio of 1 : 2, FI_{O_2} 0.40, and pressure limit of 50 cm H_2O. Set the number of breaths at 8 breaths/minute. Adjust the sensitivity control one half turn or halfway between the most and least sensitive setting.
5. Turn the mode selection to control. In the control mode, patient effort will not cycle the ventilator into the inspiratory phase.
6. Count the number of breaths delivered by the mechanical ventilator for 1 full minute.
7. Document on your laboratory report the timed rate you obtained.
8. Adjust the ventilator to the "assist only" mode. Do not change any other controls. Count for 1 minute the number of breaths delivered by the ventilator.
9. Record on your laboratory report the number of breaths delivered during 1 minute's time in the "assist only" mode.
10. Set the ventilator to the assist/control mode. Document the number of breaths delivered in 1 minute's time.
11. Vigorously compress the test lung so that the ventilator cycles into inspiration. If this does not occur, increase the sensitivity setting. Document the amount of negative pressure required for initiation of a ventilator breath. The ideal value is −2 cm H_2O.

Exercise B: Identification and Operation of Intermittent Mandatory Ventilation (IMV) or Synchronized Intermittent Mandatory Ventilation (SIMV)

1. Change the mode selection to IMV or SIMV. All other settings should remain the same.
2. Time the breath rate for 60 seconds. Document the number of breaths delivered in the IMV or SIMV mode on your laboratory report.
3. In the clinical setting the patient would be able to obtain a spontaneous volume of gas in between mandatory breaths in either the IMV or SIMV mode.

Exercise C: Identificaton of Inspiratory Hold or Inspiratory Pause Mode

1. Locate the inspiratory hold or inspiratory pause control.
2. Activate the inspiratory hold mode so that peak inspiration is sustained for 1 second.
3. If the ventilator provided by your laboratory instructor *does not* have an inspiratory hold control, an inspiratory hold maneuver may be obtained by completely occluding the exhalation valve line at the point of peak inspiration during a machine generated breath (Fig. 39-1).
4. Observe the manometer function while performing the inspiratory hold maneuver.
5. Record your observations on the laboratory report.

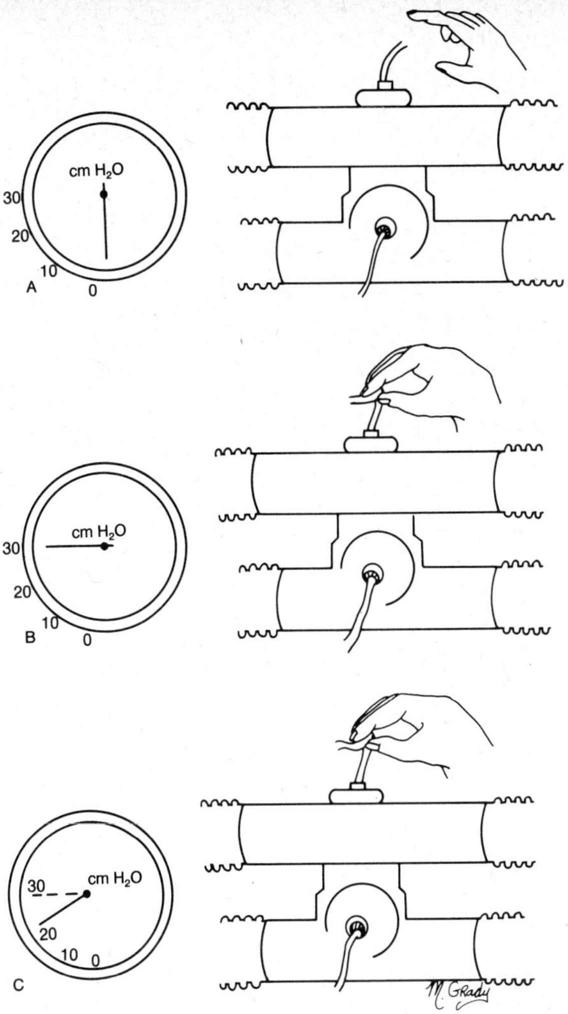

Fig. 39-1. Occlusion of expiratory valve line to produce a "plateau" pressure or inspiratory hold maneuver. **A.** *Before peak inspiration.* **B.** *Occlusion of line at peak inspiration.* **C.** *Production of plateau pressure during inspiratory pause.*

Exercise D: Identification and Operation of Expiratory Retard Mode

1. If applicable, identify the expiratory resistance or expiratory retard control on the ventilator.
2. Activate the expiratory resistance or retard control in accordance with the operator's manual or directions provided by your laboratory instructor.
3. Set the expiratory resistance so that exhalation occurs over approximately 2 seconds' duration.
4. On your laboratory report, briefly describe the effect of expiratory resistance on lung deflation.

Exercise E: Identification and Operation of Positive End-Expiratory Pressure

1. Locate the positive end-expiratory pressure (PEEP) control on your ventilator.
2. Activate the PEEP control mode to deliver a sample pressure of + 8 cm H_2O pressure.
3. Observe the manometer and test lung for several ventilatory cycles.
4. Record your observations on the laboratory report.

Exercise F: Identification and Operation of Combined Modes

Complete Exercises A through E before attempting Exercise F.

1. Adjust the ventilator to provide the modes to accommodate the following situation: a 60 kg man who is apneic.
   - **A.** IMV, rate 8, with 6 cm H_2O PEEP; FI_{O_2} 0.40.
   - **B.** IMV, rate 12; FI_{O_2} 0.60.
   - **C.** Control, rate 16, PEEP + 10 cm H_2O; FI_{O_2} 0.80.
   - **D.** Assist/control, inflation hold 1.0 second; PEEP 0; and FI_{O_2} 0.80.

Exercise G: Determination of "Unknown"

1. Your instructor will provide you with a ventilator operating in one or more of the modes described in these exercises.
2. On your laboratory report, identify the "unknown" mode(s).

RECOMMENDED READING

Burton GG, Hodgkin JE: Respiratory Care, 2nd ed. Philadelphia, JB Lippincott, 1984

Shapiro BA, Harrison RA, Kacmarek RM, Cane RD: Clinical Application of Respiratory Care, 3rd ed. Chicago, Year Book Medical Publishers, 1985

Spearman CB, Sheldon RL, and Egan DE: Egan's Fundamentals of Respiratory Care, 4th ed. St. Louis, CV Mosby, 1982

Laboratory Performance Evaluation (#39)

Topic: Mechanical Ventilation Mode Modification

Student ______________________ Course ______________________

Date ______________________ Section ______________________

Performance Elements	Acceptable	Unacceptable	Not Applicable	Comments
1. Washes hands				
2. Prepares ventilator for use with simulated patient: A. Assembles and attaches appropriate breathing circuit B. Performs "leak test" C. Assesses function of ventilator's controls, alarms, monitors				
3. Confirms order for CMV				
4. Initiates CMV for simulated patient situation				
5. Identifies, selects, and operates prescribed patient cycling modes: A. Assist only B. Assist/control C. Control only				
6. Identifies, selects, and operates IMV/SIMV mode				
7. Identifies, selects, and operates the inspiratory hold/pause mode				
8. Identifies, selects, and operates the following expiratory modes: A. Retard B. Positive end-expiratory pressure (PEEP)				

Performance Elements	Acceptable	Unacceptable	Not Applicable	Comments
9. Adjusts and operates combined modes prescribed for patient simulation				
10. Determines "unknowns"				

Knowledge of Procedure

☐ Good; student is knowledgeable about rationale and theory related to procedure

☐ Fair; student has adequate understanding of rationale and theory related to procedure

☐ Poor; student has inadequate understanding of rationale and theory related to procedure

Performance Deficiencies (check those that apply)

☐ Excessive time needed to complete procedure

☐ Broke aseptic or sterile technique

☐ Gross inaccuracy noted

☐ Technique may be harmful to patient

☐ Incorrect dosage or gas concentration

☐ Incorrect equipment assembly/use

☐ Unable to answer questions correctly about rationale and/or theory related to procedure

☐ Other ____________________

Evaluation Summary

☐ Satisfactory performance

☐ Unsatisfactory performance

Recommendations of Evaluator

- ☐ Skills may be applied/observed in clinical setting
- ☐ Specific evaluation deficiencies require correction
- ☐ Complete re-evaluation required
- ☐ Additional laboratory practice required

Signatures:

Evaluator ______________________ Date ______________________

Student ______________________ Date ______________________

Laboratory Report

Student ______________________ Acceptable ______________________

Date ______________________ Unacceptable ______________________

Course ______________________

Topic: Mechanical Ventilator Mode Modification

Data or Measurements

1. Rate in control mode ______________________

2. Rate in assist mode ______________________

3. Rate in assist/control mode ______________________

4. Negative pressure required to initiate inspiration in the assist/control mode ____________

5. Rate in IMV or SIMV mode ______________________
6. How was the ventilator manometer affected by an inspiratory hold maneuver?

7. Briefly explain the effect of expiratory resistance or expiratory retard on lung deflation. Was exhalation complete or were the lungs deflated at end-exhalation?

8. How did the application of 8 cm H_2O PEEP affect
   A. manometer function during inspiration and expiration?

   B. lung deflation?

9. Record below the modes from the determination of the "unknown" section of this laboratory exercise.

Scenario: The aftereffects of the last holiday weekend are continuing to be felt. The gunshot wound to the head, for instance, has become combative to the extent that paralysis is indicated to ventilate him effectively. Knowing the above, you would make sure the ventilator is set in the **1)** __________ mode.

The gunshot wound of the chest, on the other hand, is manifesting signs and symptoms of adult respiratory distress syndrome and would probably benefit from PEEP.

2. Please describe, for the specific ventilator you have chosen, the method used to initiate 5 cm H_2O PEEP.

3. How did you determine when you obtained 5 cm H_2O?

You have been asked what could be done to prolong the expiratory phase of a COPD patient on the medical intensive care unit. It is hoped that prolonging the expiratory phase of his breathing cycle will physiologically simulate his own "pursed-lip" breathing and therefore facilitate his weaning from the mechanical ventilator.

4. What mode modification would you use to accomplish the aforementioned?

5. How would the mode modification used to prolong expiration affect the I:E ratio?

6. Could the expiratory phase be altered by adjustment of the inspiratory flowrate control?

7. Which alarms, if any, would need resetting in this mode?

8. How does IMV or SIMV differ from control mode?

9. How does PEEP compare with zero end-expiratory pressure (ZEEP)?

10. At what specific point in the ventilatory cycle should PEEP pressure be monitored?

11. If a ventilator is operating in the assist-control mode in which the sensitivity has been adjusted to allow inspiration to begin when -2 cm H_2O is generated, how much negative pressure must be generated to trigger a breath if + 5 cm H_2O is added without readjustment of the sensitivity control?

chapter 40

Monitoring and maintenance of continuous mechanical ventilation

INTRODUCTION

Patients who are receiving mechanical ventilation must be monitored frequently. The mechanical ventilator must also be monitored at regular intervals to ensure proper operation. It is the respiratory care practitioner's responsibility to monitor the patient/ventilator system on a regular basis, such as every 2 hours. Monitoring is done more frequently during the initial or acute phase of ventilator commitment. The purpose of this chapter is to introduce you to ventilator monitoring and the validation of ventilator control settings.

OBJECTIVES

After completing this chapter, you should be able to do the following:

1. *Use the appropriate sequence when monitoring a simulated patient who requires continuous mechanical ventilation (i.e., assure ventilation by listening with a stethoscope and observing chest expansion* before *measurement/monitoring of the mechanical ventilator modes).*
2. *Determine the compression factor and compressed volume of the ventilator and breathing circuit.*
3. *Measure and validate the control settings of the ventilator.*
4. *Explain all symbols and terms on the monitoring log sheet.*
5. *Monitor an adult mechanical ventilator.*
6. *Determine the ventilator's functions.*
7. *Determine the "unknown."*

EQUIPMENT NEEDED

- ☐ Adult mechanical ventilator
- ☐ Watch with second hand
- ☐ Oxygen analyzer

- ☐ Stethoscope
- ☐ Complete ventilator breathing circuit
- ☐ Spirometer
- ☐ Test lung/adult mannequin
- ☐ 50 psi gas source(s)

ACTIVITIES

Exercise A: Determination of Ventilator and Breathing Circuit Compression Factor

1. Assemble a volume cycled ventilator.
2. Adjust the following settings:
   VT 200 ml
   Flowrate 40 liters/minute
   Pressure limit maximum
   Frequency 10/minute
   All other controls off or minimum
3. Occlude the patient wye and measure the expiratory volume. Also, note the maximum or peak pressure.
4. Calculate the *compression factor* using the following formula:

$$\text{Compression factor (CF)} = \frac{\text{Expiratory volume}}{\text{Maximum or peak pressure}}$$

   Example: When the tidal volume is 200 ml, a peak pressure of 65 cm H_2O is generated. What is the compression factor?

$$CF = \frac{200 \text{ ml}}{65 \text{ cm } H_2O}$$

$$CF = 3.08 \text{ ml/cm } H_2O$$

5. Record the CF you obtained on the laboratory report provided. The normal CF is 3 to 5 ml/cm H_2O for an adult ventilator breathing circuit.

Exercise B: Observational Assurance of Adequate Ventilation Before Ventilator Monitoring

1. Your instructor will provide you with a volume ventilator that has been connected to a test lung or mannequin that is operational. Observe inflation/deflation of the test lung or rise and fall of the mannequin's chest.
2. In the clinical setting with an actual patient, auscultation is also performed using a stethoscope.
3. Review the suggested sequence for monitoring a patient who requires continuous mechanical ventilation (Fig. 40-1).

Exercise C: Measurement and Validation of Ventilator Control Settings

1. Measure the exhaled tidal volume (VT) by attaching a spirometer to the expired gas side of the breathing circuit distal to the exhalation valve (Fig. 40-2). Record this volume on the attached ventilator monitoring record.
2. Observe the peak or maximum inspiratory pressure. Record this on the monitoring log.
3. Using the compression factor, determine the actual tidal volume delivered to the patient by subtracting the compressed volume from the exhaled VT. For example, determine the actual tidal volume delivered if the set VT is 1000 ml, the peak pressure is 40 cm H_2O, and the CF is 3.08 ml/cm H_2O.

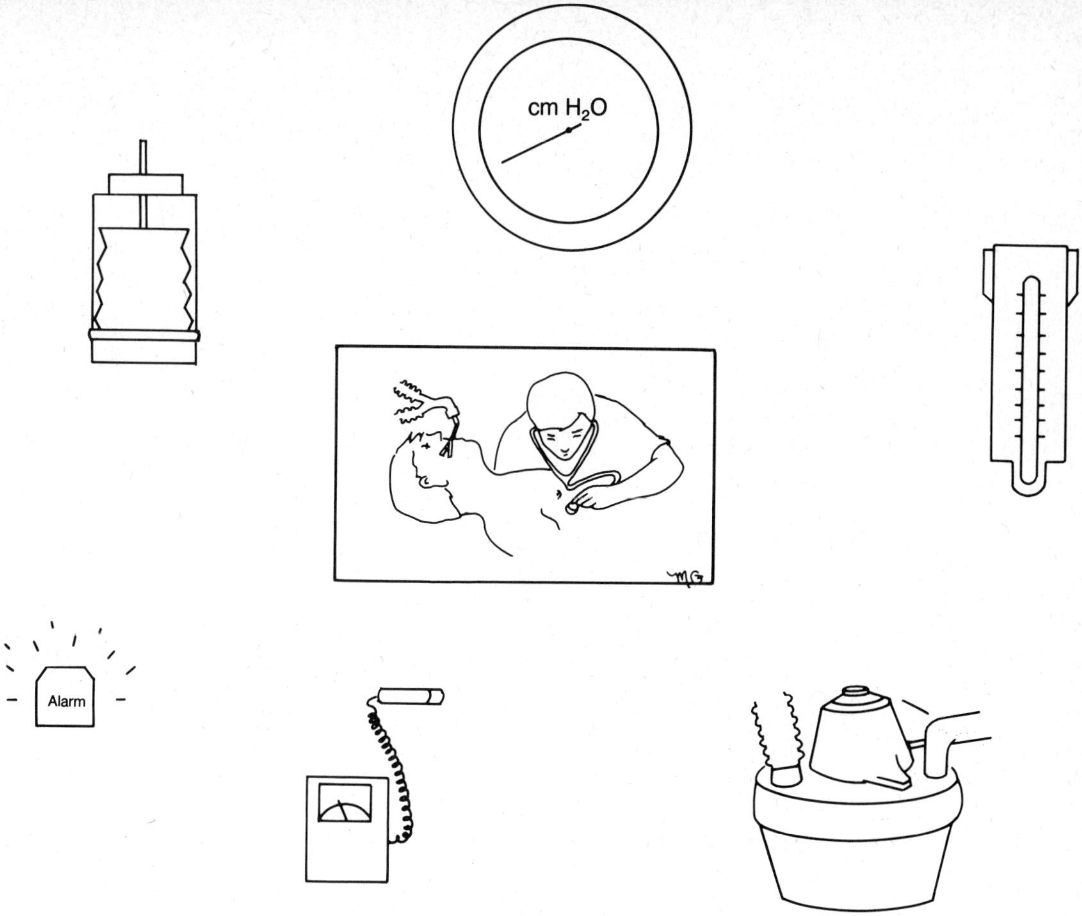

Fig. 40-1. Sequence for monitoring mechanical ventilator: The patient comes first, not the machine.

A. First, multiply the compression factor by the peak pressure, which will give you the compressed volume, that is,

$$\text{Compressed volume} = \text{CF} \times \text{Peak pressure}$$
$$= 3.08 \text{ ml/cm } H_2O \times 40 \text{ cm } H_2O = 123.20 \text{ ml.}$$

B. Then, subtract the compressed volume from the measured exhaled V_T, which will give you the actual tidal volume delivered to the patient, that is,

$$\begin{array}{l} \text{Measured exhaled } V_T \\ \underline{-\text{Compressed volume}} \\ \text{Actual } V_T \end{array}$$

$$\begin{array}{lr} \text{Example:} & 1000 \text{ ml} \\ & \underline{-\ 123.2 \text{ ml}} \\ \text{Actual } V_T = & 876.80 \text{ ml} \end{array}$$

4. Record the above information on your laboratory report and on the laboratory report ventilator monitoring log.
5. Using a watch or clock with a second hand, measure the ventilator rate for 60 seconds.

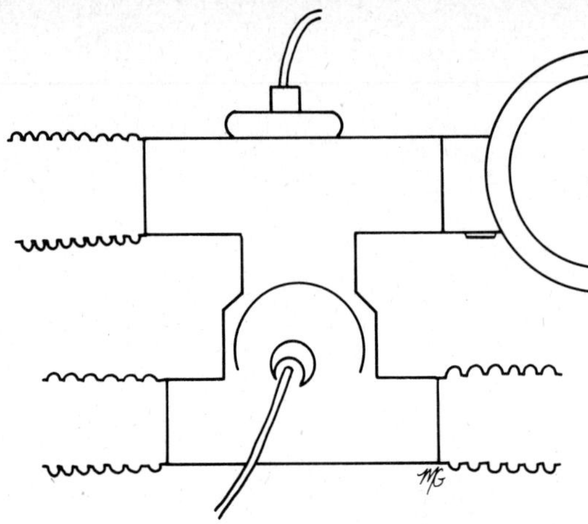

Fig. 40-2. Measurement of expired tidal volume during mechanical ventilation by connection of a spirometer distal to the exhalation valve.

6. Analyze the fraction of inspired oxygen.
7. Record all information obtained on the ventilator monitoring record.

Exercise D: Monitoring the Ventilator Modes and Functions

1. Determine which mode or combination of modes the ventilator is being operated in, that is, assist, control, assist/control, PEEP, IMV, inflation hold, sigh volume, and so forth.
2. Record your determinations on the ventilator monitoring record.
3. Observe the peak pressure, PEEP, and sigh pressure (Fig. 40-3).
4. Disconnect the ventilator from the test lung or mannequin and test the pressure limits. Do this by occluding the patient wye and observing the peak pressure during a normal breath and, if applicable, a sigh breath.
5. Observe the flowrate and its effect on the I : E ratio.
6. Observe the proximal airway gas temperature (if possible). Compare your observation with the set temperature.
7. Observe the values set on all alarms. Determine the appropriateness of these settings.
8. Record all findings on the ventilator monitoring record.

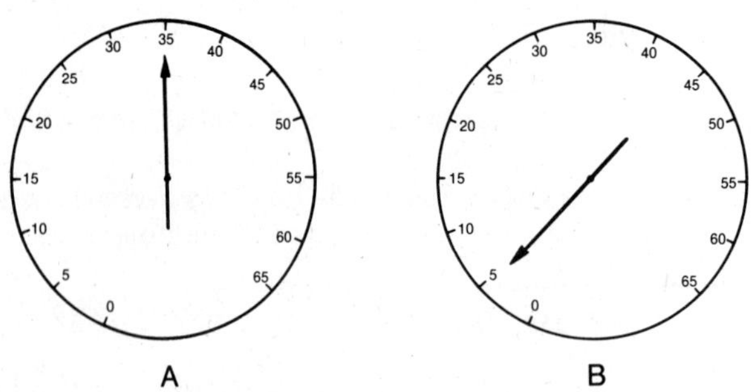

Fig. 40-3. Example of pressure at peak inspiration (35 cm H_2O) and at end expiration (+5 cm H_2O).

Exercise E: Determination of "Unknown"

Complete Exercises A through D before attempting Exercise E.

1. Your laboratory instructor will provide you with a ventilator that has been connected to a test lung or mannequin and a ventilator log sheet. You are to assume that the ventilator has been operating indefinitely. You are to carry out routine monitoring.

2. Use the Respiratory Care Ventilator Monitoring Record to record the information obtained (Fig. 40-4).

7

FORM
M4203
09-84

DUKE UNIVERSITY MEDICAL CENTER

Respiratory Care Ventilator Monitoring Record

Date: ____________ Type of Ventilator: ____________

Unit/Room #: ____________ Ventilator Name: ____________

Equipment Change: Tube size/Route: ____/____ cm Mark: ____

Circuit ____________ Age: ______ Weight: ______ Height: ______

HME ____________ Patient Diagnosis: ____________

Laerdal Bag ____________ ____________

Humidifier ____________ Isolation: ____________

Time															
FIO_2															
Mode of Ventilation															
Delivered Vt															
Exhaled Vt															
Exhaled Spontaneous Vt															
Ventilator Rate Setting															
Actual Ventilatory Rate															
Minute Volume															
Sigh Volume/Rate															
Peak Inspiratory Pressure															
CPAP or PEEP Pressure															
Mean Airway Pressure															
Pressure Support Level															
Inspiratory Time															
I:E Ratio															
HME or Heater															
Heater Setting/Temperature															
Alarms: Pressure Limit															
High/Low Pressure															
Low Exhaled Volume															
PEEP															
Apnea															
Peak Flow															
IAT Freq. Dose															
Suction / Lavage															
O_2 Calibration / Analysis															
$TCPO_2$ or $TCPCO_2$															
Site Change / Time of Site Change															
TCOM Cal. / 1 or 2 points															
Temperature / Membrane Change															
Inspiratory Flow Rate															
Notes															
Initials															

Indications for Mechanical Ventilation: ____________

Therapeutic Objectives: ____________

Indications for IAT: ____________ Therapeutic Objectives ____________

Pulmonary Mechanics		
Time		
NIFM		
VC		
$\dot{V}E$		
Spont. Vt.		
RR		
Cuff Pressure		
AVO_2		
SVO_2		
Initials		

Blood Gas Values															
Time															
ABG/CBG															
pH															
$PaCO_2$															
PaO_2															
HCO_3/BE															
SaO_2															
Hgb															
CDyn															
CSt															

Fig. 40-4. Respiratory care ventilator monitoring record.

1.
2.
3.
4.
5.
6.
7.
8.
9.
10.
11.
12.
13.
14.
15.
16.
17.
18.
19.
20.
21.
22.
23.
24.
25.
26.
27.
28.
29.
30.
31.
32.
33
34.
35.
36.
37.
38.
39.
40.

Initials	Signature	Initials	Signature

ABBREVIATIONS		SaO_2	– Arterial Oxygen Saturation
Cal.	– Calibration	PEEP	– Positive End Expiratory Pressure
CBG	– Capillary Blood Gas	CDyn	– Dynamic Compliance
ABG	– Arterial Blood Gas	CSt	– Static Compliance
AVO_2	– Arterial/Venous Oxygen Difference	TCOM	– Transcutaneous Oxygen Monitor
IAT	– Intermittant Aerosol Therapy	NIFM	– Negative Inspiratory Force Maneuver
$TCPO_2$	– Transcutaneous PO_2	HME	– Heat Moisture Exchanger
$TCPCO_2$	– Transcutaneous PCO_2	RR	– Respiratory Rate
VC	– Vital Capacity	Vt	– Tidal Volume
$\dot{V}E$	– Minute Ventilation	SVO_2	– Venous Oxygen Saturation
PaO_2	– Tension of Arterial Oxygen	$PaCO_2$	– Tension of Arterial Carbon Dioxide

RECOMMENDED READING

Blodgett D: Manual of Respiratory Care Procedures. Philadelphia, JB Lippincott, 1980

Demers RR, Pratter MR, Irwin RS: Use of the concept of ventilator compliance in the determination of static total compliance. Respir Care 26(7), July 1981

Laboratory Performance Evaluation (#40)

Topic: Monitoring and Maintenance of Continuous Mechanical Ventilation

Student ______________________ Course ______________________

Date ______________________ Section ______________________

Performance Elements	Acceptable	Unacceptable	Not Applicable	Comments
1. Obtains appropriate equipment and supplies				
2. Prepares ventilator for use with simulated patient				
3. Determines compression factor and volumes				
4. Performs bilateral chest auscultation				
5. Reviews monitoring log: A. Explains all symbols and terms B. Interprets previous entries				
6. Validates measurable ventilator settings: A. Tidal volume B. Minute volume C. Sigh volume D. FI_{O_2} E. Control rate F. I:E ratio				
7. Checks all ventilator alarms and monitors				
8. Records appropriate information in CMV monitoring log				
9. Signs or initials recorded entries				

Performance Elements	Acceptable	Unacceptable	Not Applicable	Comments
10. Suggests appropriate recommendations pertinent to obtained monitoring results				
11. Determines "unknowns"				

Knowledge of Procedure

☐ Good; student is knowledgeable about rationale and theory related to procedure

☐ Fair; student has adequate understanding of rationale and theory related to procedure

☐ Poor; student has inadequate understanding of rationale and theory related to procedure

Performance Deficiencies (check those that apply)

☐ Excessive time needed to complete procedure

☐ Broke aseptic or sterile technique

☐ Gross inaccuracy noted

☐ Technique may be harmful to patient

☐ Incorrect dosage or gas concentration

☐ Incorrect equipment assembly/use

☐ Unable to answer questions correctly about rationale and/or theory related to procedure

☐ Other ______________________________

Evaluation Summary

☐ Satisfactory performance

☐ Unsatisfactory performance

Recommendations of Evaluator

- ☐ Skills may be applied/observed in clinical setting
- ☐ Specific evaluation deficiencies require correction
- ☐ Complete re-evaluation required
- ☐ Additional laboratory practice required

Signatures:

Evaluator ______________________ Date ______________________

Student ______________________ Date ______________________

Laboratory Report

Student ______________________ Acceptable ______________________

Date ______________________ Unacceptable ______________________

Course ______________________

Topic: Routine Monitoring and Maintenance of Continuous Mechanical Ventilation

Data and Measurements

1. Record the values you obtained to calculate the compression factor.

   A. Maximum or peak pressure ______________________

   B. Expiratory volume ______________________

   C. Compression factor ______________________

2. Record the values you obtained to calculate the actual VT when the VT was set at 500 ml.

   A. Peak pressure ______________________

   B. Compressed volume ______________________

   C. Actual VT ______________________

Review Questions

1. Describe the recommended sequence of items you would monitor during mechanical ventilation (be brief).

2. In the clinical setting, how often should ventilators be monitored?

3. When monitoring, what is checked first?

4. For each ventilator setting monitored, describe the method used to validate your finding, for example, FI_{O_2}—oxygen analyzer.

	Ventilation Control	Validation Method
A.		
B.		
C.		
D.		
E.		
F.		
G.		

5. If the measured tidal volume is 200 ml, what is the compression factor if the pressure generated is
   A. 80 cm H_2O?
   B. 65 cm H_2O?
   C. 40 cm H_2O?
   D. 25 cm H_2O?
6. If the compression factor is 3.0 ml/cm H_2O and the measured tidal volume is 800 ml, what is the captured and delivered volume if the peak airway pressure is
   A. 70 cm H_2O?
   B. 60 cm H_2O?
   C. 40 cm H_2O?

chapter 41

Continuous positive airway pressure (CPAP)

INTRODUCTION

Continuous positive airway pressure (CPAP) systems are used to improve oxygenation in patients who can adequately ventilate spontaneously. CPAP systems deliver constant pressure to the airways, thereby increasing functional residual capacity, decreasing physiologic shunting, and therefore improving oxygenation. CPAP is used for infants and adults to treat hypoxia and may sometimes be used as a weaning technique. The purpose of this chapter is to introduce you to the assembly and use of various adult and infant CPAP systems.

OBJECTIVES

After completion of this chapter, you should be able to do the following:

1. *Recognize the essential components of adult and infant CPAP systems.*
2. *Identify devices used and methods of administering CPAP.*
3. *Assemble the appropriate components necessary for administering CPAP.*
4. *Monitor and obtain measurements from a functioning CPAP system.*
5. *Explain the purpose of CPAP.*

EQUIPMENT NEEDED

- ☐ 50 psi gas source
- ☐ Air/oxygen blending system
- ☐ Gas reservoir bag(s) (1 liter, 3–5 liters)
- ☐ Screw clamp(s)
- ☐ Manometer(s)
- ☐ Humidifiers
- ☐ Pressure relief valves
- ☐ Wide- and small-bore gas delivery tubing
- ☐ Nasal prongs (CPAP)

- ☐ Endotracheal tubes
- ☐ Assorted anesthesia masks
- ☐ Thermometer
- ☐ Oxygen analyzer
- ☐ One-way valves
- ☐ Adult breathing circuit
- ☐ "T" adaptor
- ☐ Adult ventilator

ACTIVITIES

Exercise A: Identification of the Components and Assembly of an Adult CPAP System

1. Refer to Figure 41-1 and identify the following components of an adult CPAP system.
   - **A.** Tubing from ventilator to "T" piece
   - **B.** One-way valves
   - **C.** Three to 5 liter reservoir bag
   - **D.** Adjustable pressure relief valve
   - **E.** Gas blending system (blender with flowmeter or air and oxygen flowmeters)
   - **F.** CPAP gas delivery line
   - **G.** Tubing from "T" piece to humidifier inlet
   - **H.** Humidifier

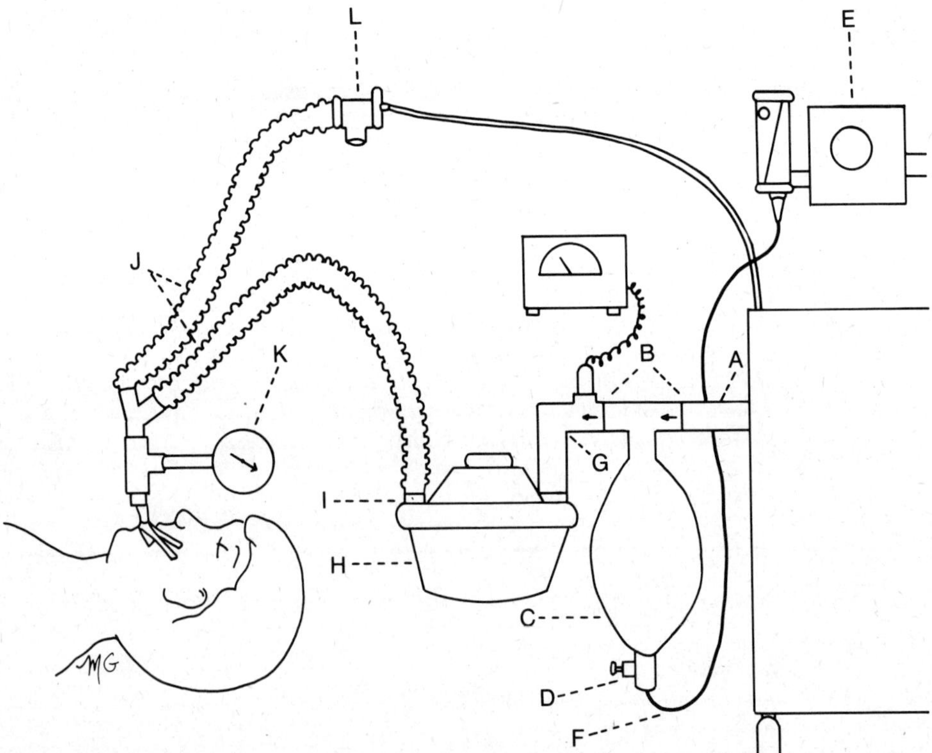

Fig. 41-1. Components of an adult CPAP system. *(Modified from McPherson SP, Spearman CB: Respiratory Therapy Equipment, 3rd ed. St Louis CV Mosby, 1985)*

I. Humidifier outlet
J. Adult breathing circuit
K. CPAP pressure manometer
L. Adult ventilator with PEEP control

2. Assemble an adult CPAP system using the components identified in Step 1.
3. Attach a gas blender or appropriate gas mixing system (air and oxygen flowmeters) to the appropriate 50 psi gas sources.
4. Connect the tubing from the gas blending system to the reservoir bag.
5. Attach the inspired gas delivery tubing of the adult breathing circuit to the *outlet* of the humidifier.
6. Attach a manometer "in line" proximal to the breathing circuit wye.
7. Connect to the expired gas side of the system an appropriate resistor (threshold or flow). *Note:* Your laboratory instructor will assist you in selecting, initiating, and adjusting the appropriate expiratory resistance. You may adjust the PEEP control on the ventilator and turn the ventilator rate to zero breaths/minute.
8. Attach a screw clamp or other adjustable pressure relief device to the distal end (nipple) of the reservoir bag.
9. Occlude the distal end of the adult breathing circuit (place hand firmly over the wye connector).
10. "Charge" the complete CPAP system by turning on the gas blender or flowmeters.
11. Adjust the pressure relief valve (screw clamp at distal end of reservoir) until a small leak is present and a sample pressure of 6 cm H_2O is maintained on the manometer.
12. Trace the flow of gas from the point of entry into the CPAP system, to its exit at the breathing circuit wye.
13. It is imperative that the reservoir bag remain inflated.
14. Connect the functioning CPAP system to a test lung or mannequin. Readjust the continuous positive airway pressure until it is maintained at 6 cm H_2O.
15. On your laboratory report, draw and label a diagram that traces the flow of gas through the adult CPAP system.

Exercise B: Identification of the Components and Assembly of an Infant CPAP System

1. Referring to Figure 41-2, identify the following components of an infant CPAP system.
2. Locate the following components:
   A. Gas mixing system or blender
   B. Oxygen analyzer in line
   C. Humidifier
   D. Reservoir "T"
   E. One-liter reservoir bag
   F. CPAP adjustment screw clamp
   G. Manometer
   H. Exhalation valve
   I. Pressure relief valve
3. Obtain a portable, flow-resistor, CPAP device such as a Carden valve (Fig. 41-3).
4. Identify the following components of a Carden valve:
   A. Gas delivery line
   B. Exhalation port
   C. Jet
   D. Manometer
   E. Patient connection
   F. Entrainment port

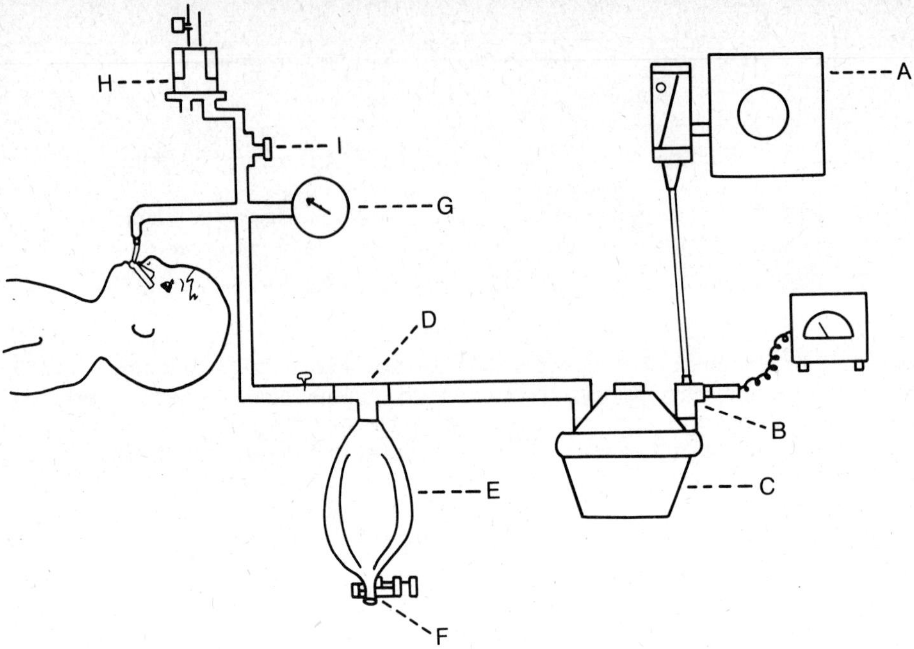

Fig. 41-2. Components of a neonatal CPAP system.

5. Observe the CPAP delivery devices that may be used to provide CPAP to a neonate (Fig. 41-4).
6. Assemble an infant CPAP system:
   A. Attach gas blending system (refer to Exercise A).
   B. Connect CPAP delivery tubing to reservoir of infant CPAP system.
   C. Attach manometer proximal to the patient connector.
   D. Connect expiratory resistor.
   E. Charge system by turning on gas flow.
   F. Occlude distal end of delivery device.

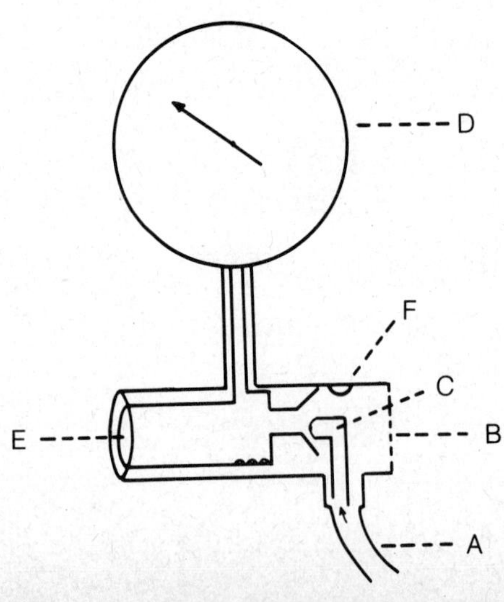

Fig. 41-3. Components of a Carden valve for delivery of CPAP.

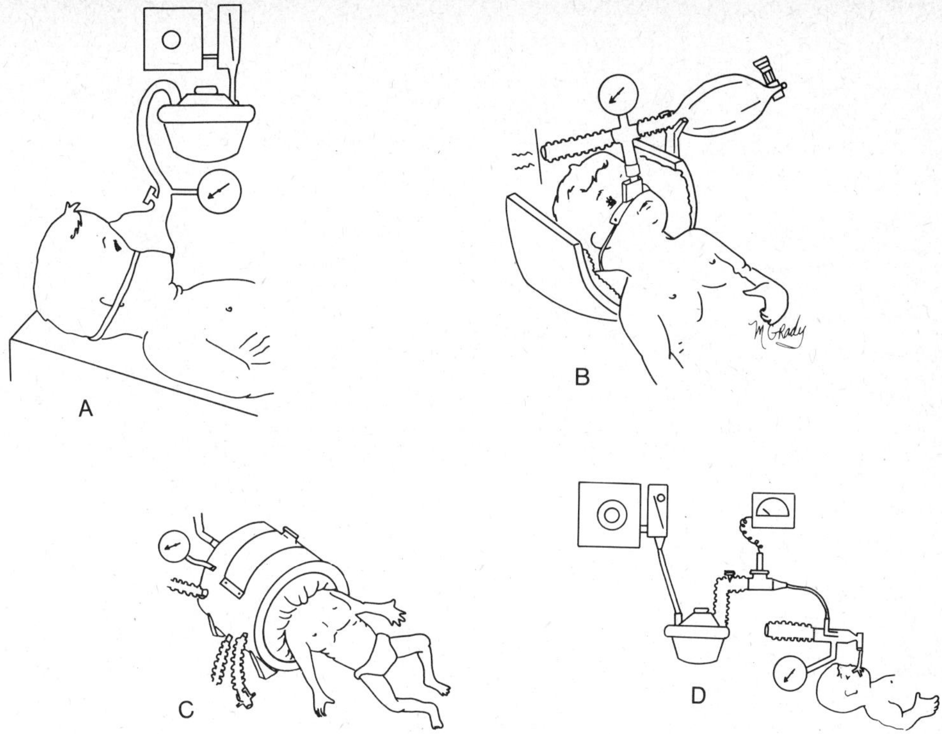

Fig. 41-4. CPAP delivery devices. A. Face mask. B. Nasal prongs. C. Head box. D. Endotracheal tube. *(Modified from Lough MD, Williams TJ, Rawson JE: Newborn Respiratory Care. Chicago, Year Book Medical Publishers, 1979)*

G. Adjust inspiratory flow and expiratory resistance until a sample pressure of 5 cm H_2O CPAP is maintained (reflected in manometer).
H. It is imperative at this point that the reservoir be checked to assure a constant flow of gas through it.
I. It is imperative that the pressure relief mechanism be checked again. To accomplish this, occlude the distal end of the inspired gas tubing and watch the manometer, being sure that excess pressure (i.e., pressure above desired CPAP) is vented to ambient.
J. Attach functioning, infant CPAP system to test lung or mannequin.
K. Compress the test lung. What happens after compression of the test lung? Why does this occur?

Exercise C: Identification and Assembly of CPAP Delivery Devices

1. Identify the adult and infant CPAP delivery devices.
2. Using one assembled adult and one assembled infant CPAP system from Exercises A and B, properly attach the devices to the appropriate mannequin.

Exercise D: Monitoring CPAP Systems

1. Measure/calculate the total flow through the CPAP systems.
2. Record the obtained results on the laboratory report.
3. Measure the delivered CPAP pressure.
4. Record the obtained results on the laboratory report.
5. Measure the pressure limit of the CPAP system.

6. Record the results obtained on your laboratory report.
7. Measure the FI_{O_2} delivered through the system.
8. Record the FI_{O_2} on the laboratory report.
9. Measure the inspired gas temperature.
10. Record the obtained results on the laboratory report.

Exercise E: Determination of "Unknown"

1. Your instructor will provide you with an activated CPAP system. You are to monitor the system's function and record your results in the column labeled "unknown" on the laboratory report.

RECOMMENDED READING

Burgess WR, Chernick V: Respiratory Therapy in Newborn Infants and Children. New York, Thieme-Stratton, 1982

Burton GG, Hodgkin JE: Respiratory Care. A Guide to Clinical Practice, 2nd ed. Philadelphia, JB Lippincott, 1984

Goldsmith JP, Karotkin EH: Assisted Ventilation of the Neonate. Philadelphia, WB Saunders, 1981

Lough MD, Williams TJ, Rawson JE: Newborn Respiratory Care. Chicago, Year Book Medical Publishers, 1979

Thibeault DW, Gregory GA: Neonatal Pulmonary Care. Menlo Park, CA, Addison–Wesley, 1981

Laboratory Performance Evaluation (#41)

Topic: Continuous Positive Airway Pressure

Student ______________________ Course ______________________

Date ______________________ Section ______________________

Performance Elements	Acceptable	Unacceptable	Not Applicable	Comments
1. Obtains appropriate equipment and supplies				
2. Identifies the CPAP system components: A. Power/gas source B. Gas reservoir/mixing system C. One-way valves D. Safety relief mechanisms E. Pressure manometers F. Gas humidification source G. CPAP pressure adjustment device				
3. Washes hands				
4. Assembles *adult* CPAP system correctly				
5. Assembles *infant* CPAP system correctly				
6. Activates CPAP system adjusting: A. Flow B. FI_{O_2} C. Prescribed CPAP pressure				
7. Using appropriate device, attaches CPAP system to simulated patient				

Performance Elements	Acceptable	Unacceptable	Not Applicable	Comments
8. Monitors and records the following: A. Total gas flowrate B. FI_{O_2} C. CPAP pressure D. CPAP pressure limit E. Gas temperature				
9. Signs or initials monitoring record				
10. Identifies "unknowns"				

Knowledge of Procedure

☐ Good; student is knowledgeable about rationale and theory related to procedure

☐ Fair; student has adequate understanding of rationale and theory related to procedure

☐ Poor; student has inadequate understanding of rationale and theory related to procedure

Performance Deficiencies (check those that apply)

☐ Excessive time needed to complete procedure

☐ Broke aseptic or sterile technique

☐ Gross inaccuracy noted

☐ Technique may be harmful to patient

☐ Incorrect dosage or gas concentration

☐ Incorrect equipment assembly/use

☐ Unable to answer questions correctly about rationale and/or theory related to procedure

☐ Other ______________________________

Evaluation Summary

☐ Satisfactory performance

☐ Unsatisfactory performance

Recommendations of Evaluator

- ☐ Skills may be applied/observed in clinical setting
- ☐ Specific evaluation deficiencies require correction
- ☐ Complete re-evaluation required
- ☐ Additional laboratory practice required

Signatures:

Evaluator ____________________ Date ____________________

Student ____________________ Date ____________________

Laboratory Report

Student ______________________ Acceptable ______________________

Date ______________________ Unacceptable ______________________

Course ______________________

Topic: Continuous Positive Airway Pressure

Data or Measurements

1. Draw and label a diagram of the adult CPAP system. Trace the flow of gas through the adult CPAP system.

2. What are four methods of attaching CPAP systems to infants?

3. Record the following information obtained from the laboratory exercises:

	Adult CPAP System	Infant CPAP System	"Unknown"
CPAP pressure	______	______	______
FI_{O_2}	______	______	______
Inspired gas temperature	______	______	______
Pressure relief level	______	______	______
Total gas flowrate	______	______	______

Scenario: You have been assigned to the intensive care nursery. Every bed space was occupied and every effort being made to wean patients from ventilators as quickly as possible. The ventilator being used by the patient in bed space #2 was needed for a transfer to a rural hospital. You have been asked to place that patient on CPAP. Please answer the following questions:

1. What is one indication for CPAP?

2. What patient requirement must be present to be a candidate for CPAP?

3. How would an inadequate total gas flow be indicated when monitoring a CPAP system?

4. What safety components should be included in all CPAP systems?

5. When a test lung or mannequin is connected to an activated CPAP system, what happens after lung compression? Based on your observation, how may CPAP affect atelectatic alveoli and the FRC within actual lungs?

6. Other than using a mechanical ventilator, how may CPAP be administered, that is, describe three devices or systems that may be used.

7. Discuss the hazards associated with CPAP administration.

You did not have to wait long before the ventilator from bed space #2 was needed for a new admission, a 1000 g premature infant who suffered from respiratory distress syndrome. It was determined that he might benefit from CPAP.

8. Discuss the method of administering CPAP by means of mechanical ventilator.

9. Compare and contrast the following: IMV, PEEP, IMV with PEEP, and CPAP.

10. Describe a situation in which adult CPAP may be useful.

11. Does adult CPAP differ from pediatric CPAP?

chapter 42

Measurement of effective dynamic compliance, effective static compliance, and airway resistance

INTRODUCTION

The stiffness or elasticity of the respiratory system is expressed in terms of compliance. Dynamic compliance is measured during air movement. Static compliance is measured under conditions of no air movement. Because air flow is absent during the measurement, static compliance may be a reflection of the pulmonary and chest wall compliance. When compliance is measured on a patient receiving mechanical ventilation, the values obtained are referred to as effective dynamic compliance and effective static compliance.

Airway resistance is the pressure gradient required to deliver a gas volume in a specific amount of time. Airway resistance can be easily calculated. The purpose of this chapter is to introduce you to the methods of determining effective dynamic compliance, effective static compliance, and airway resistance.

OBJECTIVES

At the completion of this chapter, you should be able to do the following:

1. *Determine the plateau pressure by activating the appropriate ventilator control(s).*
2. *Determine effective dynamic compliance and effective static compliance.*
3. *Determine airway resistance.*
4. *Identify the normal values for effective dynamic compliance, effective static compliance, and airway resistance.*

EQUIPMENT NEEDED

- ☐ Adult mechanical ventilator
- ☐ Adult breathing circuit
- ☐ Lung simulator or lung analog
- ☐ Spirometer or volume measuring device

ACTIVITIES

Exercise A: Measurement of Plateau Pressure

1. Your laboratory instructor will provide you with an adult ventilator that is ready for use.
2. Adjust the following ventilator controls:
   VT—500 ml
   Rate—15/minute
   Flowrate—40 liters/minute
   Pressure limit—maximum
   All other controls off or minimum
3. Connect the breathing circuit wye to a lung simulator. Activate the ventilator power.
4. Obtain a plateau pressure measurement by setting the inspiratory hold or inspiratory pause control for 1 second hold or pause. Observe the pressure manometer. The pressure manometer needle will reach a peak pressure, then stabilize to a pressure less than the peak. The pressure at which the needle stabilizes is called plateau pressure (see Fig. 39-1).
5. Record the plateau pressure you obtained using the inspiratory hold or pause control in your laboratory report.
6. Return the inspiratory hold to zero.
7. Obtain a plateau pressure measurement by occluding the expiratory line at peak inspiration. Occlude the expiratory line for about 1 second. Record the plateau pressure you obtained on your laboratory report.

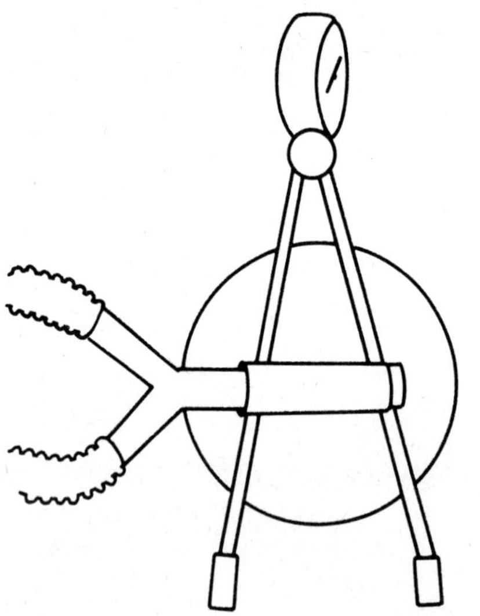

Fig. 42-1. Connection of ventilator circuit to a lung simulator.

Exercise B: Determination of Effective Dynamic Compliance (Cdyn)

1. Leave the ventilator set as in Exercise A.
2. Determine the compression factor of the ventilator and breathing circuit (see Chap. 40). Use the following formula:

$$\text{Compression factor (CF)} = \frac{\text{Expiratory volume}}{\text{Peak pressure}}$$

3. Attach the ventilator wye to a test lung and note the peak pressure.
4. Calculate the effective dynamic compliance using the following formula, and report the value on your laboratory report.

$$\text{Cdyn} = \frac{\text{V}_\text{T} - (\text{CF} \times (\text{peak pressure} - \text{PEEP}))}{\text{Peak pressure} - \text{PEEP}}$$

that is,

$$\text{Cdyn} = \frac{500 \text{ ml} - (3.5 \text{ ml/cm } H_2O\ (30 \text{ cm } H_2O - 0 \text{ cm } H_2O))}{30 \text{ cm } H_2O - 0 \text{ cm } H_2O}$$

$$= \frac{500 - (105)}{30}$$

$$= \frac{395}{30}$$

$$= 13.17 \text{ ml/cm } H_2O$$

5. Add 10 cm H_2O PEEP to the ventilator settings. Leave all other settings unchanged. Calculate the new Cdyn and record the value obtained on your laboratory report.
6. The normal range for effective Cdyn is 50 to 100 ml/cm H_2O.

Exercise C: Determination of Effective Static Compliance (Cst)

1. Using the same ventilator settings as above, obtain a plateau pressure measurement.
2. Calculate the Cst by using the following formula, and record all the values you obtain on your laboratory report.

$$\text{Cst} = \frac{\text{V}_\text{T} - (\text{CF} \times (\text{peak pressure} - \text{PEEP}))}{\text{Plateau pressure} - \text{PEEP}}$$

3. The normal range for effective Cst is 50 to 100 ml/cm H_2O. The actual value is usually higher than effective Cdyn in adults.

Exercise D: Determination of Airway Resistance (Raw)

1. Using the values you obtained above and the flowrate setting (in liters/second), you can calculate Raw.
2. Convert the flowrate from liters/minute to liters/second by using the following formula:

$$\text{Liters/second} = \frac{\text{Liters/minute}}{60 \text{ seconds}}$$

3. Report the flowrate in liters/second on your laboratory report.
4. Calculate the Raw by using the following formula:

$$\text{Raw} = \frac{\text{Peak pressure} - \text{Plateau pressure}}{\text{Flow (liters/second)}}$$

5. Report the Raw you obtained on your laboratory report.
6. The normal value for Raw is 0.5 to 5.0 cm H_2O/liter/second.

Exercise E: Determination of "Unknown"

1. Your instructor will change the compliance and airway resistance on the lung simulator and the ventilator settings.
2. Calculate the unknown Cdyn, Cst, and Raw. You may use the compression factor from Exercise B.
3. Note the results on your laboratory report.

RECOMMENDED READING

Burton GG, Hodgkin JE: Respiratory Care. A Guide to Clinical Practice, 2nd ed. Philadelphia, JB Lippincott, 1984

Demers RR et al: Use of the concept of ventilator compliance in determination of static total compliance. Respir. Care 26 : 7, July 1981

Kacmarek RM, Dimas S, Mack C: Essentials of Respiratory Therapy, 2nd ed. Chicago, Year Book Medical Publishers, 1985

Spearman CB, Sheldon RL: Egan's Fundamentals of Respiratory Therapy, 4th ed. St Louis, CV Mosby, 1982

Laboratory Performance Evaluation (#42)

Topic: Measurement of Effective Dynamic Compliance, Effective Static Compliance, and Airway Resistance

Student ______________________ Course ______________________

Date ______________________ Section ______________________

Performance Elements	Acceptable	Unacceptable	Not Applicable	Comments
1. Obtains necessary equipment and supplies				
2. Prepares an adult ventilator for use with lung simulator or lung analog				
3. Adjusts ventilator controls to conform to prescribed A. VT B. Rate C. Flowrate D. Pressure limit				
4. Attaches breathing circuit to lung simulator or analog				
5. Activates ventilator				
6. Obtains correct peak inspiratory pressure				
7. Determines effective dynamic compliance (Cdyn)				
8. Obtains correct plateau pressure				
9. Obtains correct effective static compliance (Cst)				
10. Calculates liters per second of flow				

Performance Elements	Acceptable	Unacceptable	Not Applicable	Comments
11. Calculates airway resistance (Raw)				
12. Records results (correct symbols/terms)				
13. Determines "unknowns"				

Knowledge of Procedure

- ☐ Good; student is knowledgeable about rationale and theory related to procedure
- ☐ Fair; student has adequate understanding of rationale and theory related to procedure
- ☐ Poor; student has inadequate understanding of rationale and theory related to procedure

Performance Deficiencies (check those that apply)

- ☐ Excessive time needed to complete procedure
- ☐ Broke aseptic or sterile technique
- ☐ Gross inaccuracy noted
- ☐ Technique may be harmful to patient
- ☐ Incorrect dosage or gas concentration
- ☐ Incorrect equipment assembly/use
- ☐ Unable to answer questions correctly about rationale and/or theory related to procedure
- ☐ Other ______________________________

Evaluation Summary

- ☐ Satisfactory performance
- ☐ Unsatisfactory performance

Recommendations of Evaluator

- ☐ Skills may be applied/observed in clinical setting
- ☐ Specific evaluation deficiencies require correction
- ☐ Complete re-evaluation required
- ☐ Additional laboratory practice required

Signatures:

Evaluator ______________________ Date ______________________

Student ______________________ Date ______________________

Laboratory Report

Student ______________________ Acceptable ______________________

Date ______________________ Unacceptable ______________________

Course ______________________

Topic: Measurement of Effective Dynamic Compliance, Effective Static Compliance, and Airway Resistance

Data or Measurements

1. Plateau pressure obtained by using the inspiratory hold or pause control. ____________
2. Plateau pressure obtained by occluding the exhalation line. ____________
3. Ventilator and breathing circuit compression factor. ____________
4. Dynamic compliance from Exercise B:

   Without PEEP ______________________

   With 10 cm H_2O PEEP ______________________
5. From Exercise C:

   A. VT ______________ D. PEEP ______________

   B. CF ______________ E. Plateau pressure ______________

   C. Peak pressure ______________ F. Cst ______________
6. Flowrate (liters/second) ______________________
7. Raw ______________________
8. Determination of Unknown:

   Cdyn ______________________

   Cst ______________________

   Raw ______________________

Scenario: You are continuing to experience the aftereffects of the gang war. The patient with the gunshot wound to the chest who was rushed to the operating room has become increasingly difficult to manage. His arterial blood gas values have been deteriorating while his lung compliance is decreasing. You have been asked to do compliance and resistance studies to determine whether any particular combination of ventilator settings will better oxygenate and ventilate him. Please respond to the following questions:

1. What are the normal values for the following:
   Effective Cdyn? ____________________

   Effective Cst? ____________________

   Effective Raw ____________________

2. Mathematically, how would high flowrates affect Raw values?

3. Which ventilator control affects airway resistance more than others?

4. What accounts for the difference between dynamic compliance and static compliance?

5. Please describe, step-by-step, the method used to obtain static compliance.

6. Is there any relation between endotracheal tube size and airway resistance? Why?

7. What are two possible causes of a decrease or an increase in static compliance?

chapter 43

Positive end-expiratory pressure

INTRODUCTION

Positive end-expiratory pressure (PEEP) produces positive pressure during exhalation. PEEP is most commonly applied during mechanical ventilation; however, PEEP can be applied during spontaneous breathing with the use of some special apparatus. When PEEP is applied during spontaneous breathing, it can be referred to as spontaneous PEEP (SPEEP). PEEP and SPEEP are primarily used to increase functional residual capacity, and therefore decrease physiologic shunting and improve oxygenation. The purpose of this chapter is to introduce you to SPEEP, PEEP, and BEST PEEP.

OBJECTIVES

At the completion of this chapter, you should be able to do the following:

1. *Identify various techniques used to deliver PEEP.*
2. *Assemble and activate PEEP.*
3. *Identify various amounts of PEEP.*
4. *Demonstrate the effects of PEEP on peak pressure.*
5. *Demonstrate a method of determining BEST PEEP.*

EQUIPMENT NEEDED

- ☐ Threshold resistor PEEP apparatus
- ☐ Orificial resistor PEEP apparatus
- ☐ Flow resistor PEEP apparatus
- ☐ Mechanical ventilator
- ☐ Lung simulator or lung analog
- ☐ 50 psi gas source(s)
- ☐ Manometer(s)
- ☐ Flowmeter
- ☐ Intubated mannequin

☐ Oxygen delivery tubing
☐ Adult breathing circuit

ACTIVITIES

Exercise A: Identification and Assembly of Spontaneous PEEP Apparatus

1. Using the materials provided by your instructor, identify the mechanism(s) used to deliver PEEP (Fig. 43-1).
2. On your laboratory report, diagram the flow through a threshold resistor, an orificial resistor, and a flow resistor as they are used to administer PEEP.

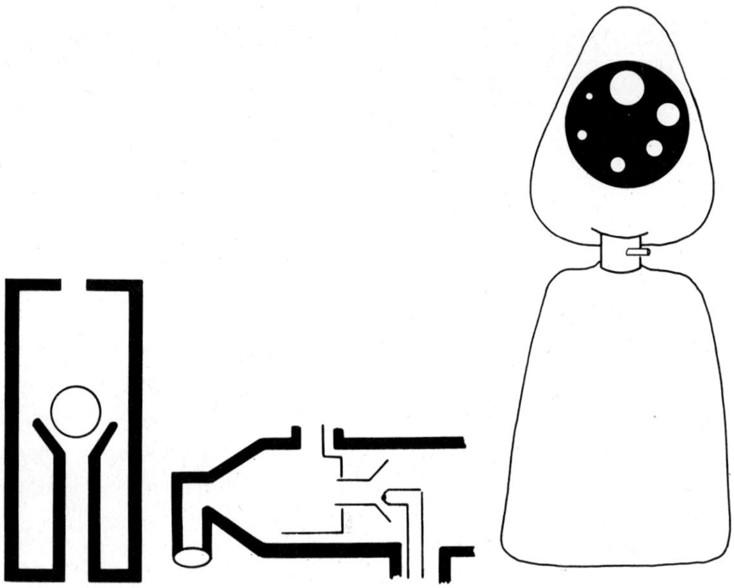

Fig. 43-1. Apparatus used to produce PEEP. **A.** Example of threshold resistor. **B.** Example of flow resistor. **C.** Example of orificial resistor. *(Modified from Kacmarek RM et al: Technical aspects of positive end expiratory pressure (PEEP): Part II: PEEP with positive pressure ventilation. Resp Care 27:1490, 1982)*

Exercise B: Activation and Monitoring of PEEP

1. Locate the PEEP control on the mechanical ventilator provided by your instructor.
2. Activate the ventilator and perform a leak test.
3. Set the following controls on the ventilator:
   Flowrate or peak flow—40 liters/minute
   Tidal volume (VT)—500 ml
   Pressure limit—50 cm H_2O
   Rate—12 breaths/minute
   Sigh volume—750 ml
   Sigh pressure limit—60 cm H_2O
   FI_{O_2}—0.40
   Sigh rate—9/hour
4. Attach the patient wye of the breathing circuit to the lung simulator.
5. Using the appropriate control, set the PEEP at 10 cm H_2O end-expiratory pressure.

Exercise C: Determination of PEEP Effect on Ventilator Function

1. Use the ventilator settings from the previous exercise and activate the ventilator.
2. Monitor the peak pressure and record your results on the laboratory report.
3. Decrease the PEEP from 10 cm H_2O to 5 cm H_2O. Monitor the peak pressure and record the results on your laboratory report.
4. Further decrease the PEEP by 3 cm H_2O.
5. Record the peak pressure now being obtained on your laboratory report.
6. Reduce the PEEP to zero and record the peak pressure on your laboratory report.

Exercise D: Determination of BEST PEEP

1. The BEST PEEP level is determined by calculation of effective static compliance (Cst) at different levels of PEEP. The highest PEEP level used before a decrease in compliance (lower numerical value) is the BEST PEEP.
2. Determine the ventilator and breathing circuit compression factor.
3. Set the following controls:
   VT—500 ml
   Flowrate—30 liters/minute
   Rate—15/minute
   Pressure limit—maximum
   All other controls off or minimum
4. Set the other lung simulator at normal compliance and airway resistance (Raw). Connect ventilator wye to lung simulator. Activate ventilator power.
5. Determine the effective static compliance at 3, 6, 9, and 12 cm H_2O PEEP. Use the following formula:

$$\text{Cst} = \frac{\text{VT} - \text{Compressed volume}}{\text{Plateau pressure} - \text{PEEP}}$$

VT = Exhaled VT as indicated on a volume measuring device or spirometer

Compressed volume = Compression factor (CF) × Peak pressure

   Pressure plateau is determined by occluding the exhalation line at peak inspiration and reading the pressure at which the pressure manometer needle stabilizes. Indicate the Cst obtained for each level of PEEP on your laboratory report.
6. Chart the values obtained on Graph #1 found in your laboratory report. Indicate the BEST PEEP level by circling it.
7. Leave the ventilator settings the same and decrease the compliance on the lung simulator. Repeat the PEEP trial as you did in Step 5. Chart your results and complete Graph #2. Again, circle the BEST PEEP level.
8. Now increase the Raw on the lung analog. Leave all the ventilator and lung simulator settings the same. Repeat the procedure in Step 5 charting your results on Graph #3 on your laboratory report.

Exercise E: Determination of "Unknown"

1. Your instructor will set a PEEP level using the PEEP control on the ventilator. The ventilator is operational and connected to the lung simulator.
2. On your laboratory report, indicate the level of PEEP by observing the pressure manometer.

RECOMMENDED READING

Burton GG, Hodgkin JE: Respiratory Care. A Guide to Clinical Practice, 2nd ed. Philadelphia, JB Lippincott, 1984

Kacmarek RM, Dimas S, Mack C: Essentials of Respiratory Therapy, 2nd ed. Chicago, Year Book Medical Publishers, 1985

Spearman CB, Sheldon RL: Egan's Fundamentals of Respiratory Therapy, 4th ed. St Louis, CV Mosby, 1982

Laboratory Performance Evaluation (#43)

Topic: Positive End-Expiratory Pressure

Student ______________________ Course ______________________

Date ______________________ Section ______________________

Performance Elements	Acceptable	Unacceptable	Not Applicable	Comments
1. Obtains appropriate equipment and supplies				
2. Identifies the following PEEP apparatus: A. Threshold resistor B. Orificial resistor C. Flow resistor				
3. Washes hands				
4. Assembles a PEEP apparatus for use with a simulated spontaneously breathing patient				
5. Adjusts the PEEP for delivery of a prescribed amount of pressure				
6. Initiates a prescribed amount of PEEP for a simulated patient receiving CMV				
7. Records procedure and results in appropriate areas of CMV monitoring log				
8. Determines best PEEP				
9. Signs or initials CMV monitoring log				

Performance Elements	Acceptable	Unacceptable	Not Applicable	Comments
10. Determines BEST PEEP for a CMV simulation				
11. Determines "unknowns"				

Knowledge of Procedure

- ☐ Good; student is knowledgeable about rationale and theory related to procedure
- ☐ Fair; student has adequate understanding of rationale and theory related to procedure
- ☐ Poor; student has inadequate understanding of rationale and theory related to procedure

Performance Deficiencies (check those that apply)

- ☐ Excessive time needed to complete procedure
- ☐ Broke aseptic or sterile technique
- ☐ Gross inaccuracy noted
- ☐ Technique may be harmful to patient
- ☐ Incorrect dosage or gas concentration
- ☐ Incorrect equipment assembly/use
- ☐ Unable to answer questions correctly about rationale and/or theory related to procedure
- ☐ Other ______________________________

Evaluation Summary

- ☐ Satisfactory performance
- ☐ Unsatisfactory performance

Recommendations of Evaluator

- ☐ Skills may be applied/observed in clinical setting
- ☐ Specific evaluation deficiencies require correction
- ☐ Complete re-evaluation required
- ☐ Additional laboratory practice required

Signatures:

Evaluator ______________________ Date ______________________

Student ______________________ Date ______________________

Laboratory Report

Student ______________________ Acceptable ______________________

Date ______________________ Unacceptable ______________________

Course ______________________

Topic: Positive End-Expiratory Pressure

Data and Measurements:

1. Record the peak pressures obtained in Exercise C:

PEEP (cm H_2O)	Peak Pressure
A. +10	
B. +5	
C. +2	
D. 0	

2. Record the static compliance levels obtained in Exercise D. Determine BEST PEEP level with the lung simulator set at normal compliance and normal airway resistance. Circle BEST PEEP level on the graph below:

	Static Compliance Level
PEEP 3 cm H_2O	________________
PEEP 6 cm H_2O	________________
PEEP 9 cm H_2O	________________
PEEP 12 cm H_2O	________________

Graph #1

3. Repeat the above with the lung simulator set on a decreased compliance setting.

	Static Compliance Level
PEEP 3 cm H_2O	
PEEP 6 cm H_2O	
PEEP 9 cm H_2O	
PEEP 12 cm H_2O	

Graph #2

4. Determine effective PEEP level with lung simulator set on a decreased compliance and increased Raw.

	Static Compliance Level
PEEP 3 cm H_2O	
PEEP 6 cm H_2O	
PEEP 9 cm H_2O	
PEEP 12 cm H_2O	

Graph #3

5. What level of PEEP did you observe in the "unknown" section of this laboratory?

6. Diagram of flow through
   A. Threshold resistor

   B. Flow resistor

   C. Orificial resistor

Scenario: You are assigned to the trauma unit. A male victim of a flail chest is intubated and receiving continuous mechanical ventilation. Currently, he is receiving 25 cm H_2O PEEP and an FI_{O_2} of 0.70. His arterial blood gas results have improved. Because of the improvement, you have been asked to accomplish the following: begin decreasing the FI_{O_2} and the level of PEEP. Please answer the following questions:

1. Which would you decrease first, the FI_{O_2}, the level of PEEP, or the level of PEEP and FI_{O_2} simultaneously?

2. By what increments would you decrease the FI_{O_2}?

3. Would determination of BEST PEEP be appropriate for this situation?

4. Please describe, step-by-step, the method used to determine BEST PEEP.

5. By what increments will you change the level of PEEP when determining BEST PEEP?

6. Diagram pressure waveforms at PEEP levels of

   A. 10 cm H_2O

   B. 5 cm H_2O

7. How is peak pressure affected as PEEP is decreased? Be specific.

chapter 44

Initiation of infant mechanical ventilation with a volume-limited ventilator

INTRODUCTION

The infant who requires mechanical ventilation is uniquely different from the adult and requires a mechanical ventilator that is specifically designed for infants. A volume-limited infant ventilator is one that terminates inspiration when a present tidal volume has been delivered. The tidal volumes delivered to infants are very small relative to adult tidal volumes, and inaccuracies can be detrimental. Therefore, the volume that is compressed or captured in the ventilator and breathing circuit and never reaches the infant must be carefully calculated. This chapter introduces you to the use of volume-limited ventilators specifically designed for infants.

OBJECTIVES

After completing this chapter, you should be able to do the following:

1. *Assemble an infant volume-limited ventilator and assess the proper function before patient use.*
2. *Determine the initial ventilator settings given a patient situation.*
3. *Monitor the infant ventilator system during operation.*
4. *Determine the compressed volume, compression factor, and tidal volume.*

EQUIPMENT NEEDED

- ☐ Volume-limited infant ventilator (*i.e.*, Bourns LS 104-150)
- ☐ Infant breathing circuit
- ☐ Infant test lung
- ☐ 50 psi gas source
- ☐ Watch with a second hand
- ☐ Sterile gauze or glove
- ☐ Oxygen analyzer

ACTIVITIES

Exercise A: Assembly of Infant Breathing Circuit and Determination of Compression Factor

1. You will be provided with an infant volume-limited ventilator with a patient breathing circuit attached (Fig. 44-1). Identify the following components:
   A. Gas mixing system for IMV gas
   B. Small-bore tubing to IMV setup
   C. 1-liter reservoir bag
   D. Tubing to ventilator inlet
   E. Bacteria filter
   F. Tubing to humidifier
   G. Humidifier
   H. Tubing from ventilator to patient
   I. Inspiratory water trap
   J. Patient connection
   K. Expiratory water trap
   L. Tubing from patient to ventilator
   M. Expiratory valve
2. Assemble an infant breathing circuit as shown in Figure 44-1.
3. Fill humidifier with sterile water and activate heater element to 35° to 37°C (if applicable).
4. Connect gas sources to ventilator.
5. Connect electrical power source.
6. Perform a leak test to ensure that there are no gas leaks in the system.
7. Determine the compression factor of the ventilator and breathing circuit system by setting the following:
   A. VT—20 ml
   B. Flowrate—100 ml/second

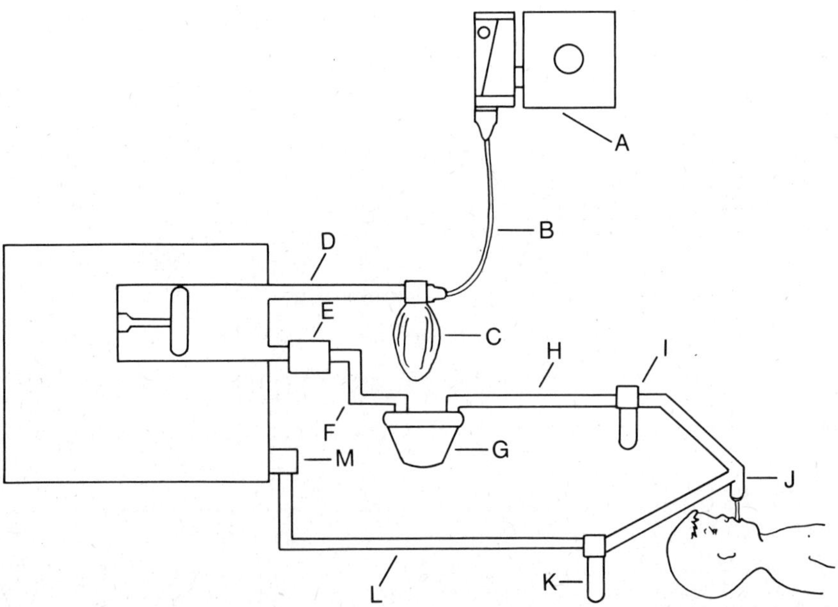

Fig. 44-1. Typical infant breathing circuit used with an infant volume ventilator.

C. Rate—30 bpm
D. Mode—control
E. Sigh interval and inspiratory hold—zero or off
F. Sensitivity—maximum
G. Pressure limit—maximum
H. PEEP—0 cm H_2O

8. Turn the power on.
9. Occlude connection with sterile gauze or sterile gloved hand.
10. Observe peak pressure.
11. Calculate compression factor (CF) by using the following formula:

$$CF = \frac{\text{Set } V_T}{\text{Peak pressure}}, \text{ that is,}$$

$$CF = \frac{20 \text{ ml}}{70 \text{ cm } H_2O}$$

$$CF = 0.29 \text{ ml/cm } H_2O$$

12. Note the CF on your laboratory report.
13. The normal CF for an infant ventilator and breathing circuit system is 0.3 to 0.6 ml/cm H_2O; a larger CF may signify a leak. Check all fittings until you achieve a normal CF
14. Identify the controls found on the Bourns LS 104-150 ventilator (Fig. 44-2).

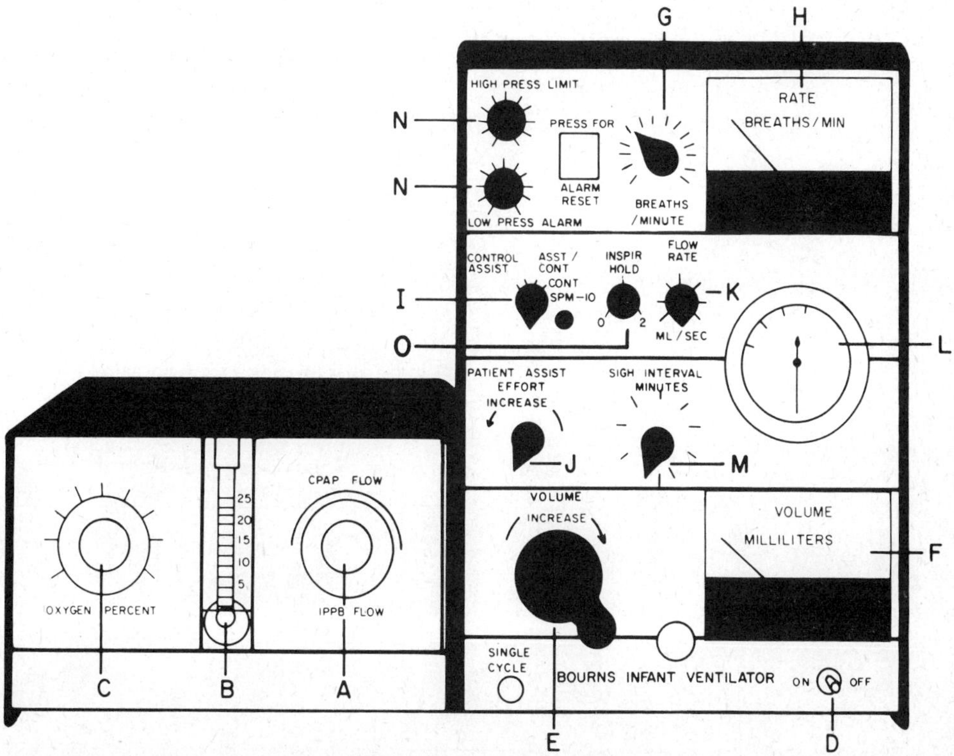

Fig. 44-2. Bourns LS-104-150 ventilator control panel. *(Reproduced with permission from Burton GG, Hodgkin JE: Respiratory Care. A Guide to Clinical Practice, 2nd ed. Philadelphia, JB Lippincott, 1984)*

Exercise B: Activation of Ventilator Settings and Alarms

1. Your patient situation is one of the following:
   A. Baby Boy Eliot—32-week gestation, born by emergency C-section. Baby Eliot was immediately intubated and is being manually ventilated. He is being transferred from the operating room to the intensive care nursery. He weighs 3 kg.
   B. Baby Girl Green—born yesterday at a nearby hospital. She is currently in an oxygen hood, FI_{O_2} 0.8. She has been experiencing episodes of apnea and bradycardia. Baby Green is being transferred to your hospital and you must initiate mechanical ventilation. She weighs 4 kg.
2. Turn the ventilator on and set as follows:
   A. FI_{O_2}—0.9-1.0
   B. Frequency—30/minute
   C. Flowrate—to achieve desired I:E ratio (*i.e.*, 1:2 or 1:3)
   D. Mode—control or IMV
   E. PEEP—2.0 cm H_2O
   F. Humidifier temperature—35°-36°C
   G. VT—7-10 ml/kg
3. Attach patient connection to test lung.
4. Observe for proper function and lung inflation.
5. Observe peak pressure.
6. Calculate compressed volume. Use the following formula:

   Compressed volume (CV) = (Peak pressure − PEEP) × CF

   For example, if the peak pressure was 30 cm H_2O,

   CV = (30 cm H_2O − 0) × 0.29 ml/cm H_2O
   CV = 8.7 ml

7. Readjust volume to compensate for compressed volume. Use the following formula:

   Volume set = desired VT + lost volume, that is,
   Volume set = 14 ml + 8.7 ml
   Volume set = 22.7 ml

8. Note the CV and volume set on your laboratory report.
9. Adjust high pressure limit 10 cm H_2O greater than the average peak pressure.
10. Adjust low pressure limit 5 to 10 cm H_2O less than the average peak pressure.
11. Set alarm time delay 10 seconds greater than the time required for each ventilatory cycle, that is, rate = 30 bpm

    60 seconds ÷ 30 breaths = 2 seconds/breath
    Alarm delay 10 seconds + 2 seconds = 12 seconds

Exercise C: Monitoring the Infant Ventilator

1. Complete the attached ventilator monitoring record. Record the following information:
   A. FI_{O_2} = analyzed value
   B. CPAP/PEEP = cm H_2O of PEEP (if applicable)
   C. Rate = set rate in breaths/minute
   D. IMV/assist/cont = mode selected
   E. Oxygen blender/flowrate = flow in liters/minute from the gas mixing system
   F. Volume set = desired VT + compressed volume

G. Tidal volume = 7 to 10 ml/kg (should equal volume set − compressed volume)
H. Compression factor = factor calculated in Exercise A

2. Complete all other information listed on the ventilator monitoring record.

Exercise D: Determination of "Unknown"

1. Your instructor will establish ventilation using the infant volume ventilator and infant test lung.
2. Determine the following "unknowns":
   A. Compression factor
   B. Volume set
   C. Compressed volume
   D. Delivered tidal volume
   E. Ventilator rate
   F. FI_{O_2}
   G. I:E ratio

RECOMMENDED READING

Blodgett D: Manual of Pediatric Respiratory Care Procedures. Philadelphia, JB Lippincott, 1982

Burgess WR, Chernick V: Respiratory Therapy in Newborn Infants and Children. New York, Thieme-Stratton, 1982

Burton GG, Hodgkin JE: Respiratory Care. A Guide to Clinical Practice, 2nd ed. Philadelphia, JB Lippincott, 1984

Goldsmith JP, Karotkin EH: Assisted Ventilation of the Neonate. Philadelphia, WB Saunders, 1981

Lough MD, Williams TJ, Rawson JE: Newborn Respiratory Care. Chicago, Year Book Medical Publishers, 1979

Thibeault DW, Gregory GA: Neonatal Pulmonary Care. Menlo Park, CA, Addison-Wesley, 1981

Laboratory Performance Evaluation (#44)

Topic: Initiation of Infant Mechanical Ventilation with a Volume-Limited Ventilator

Student ______________________ Course ______________________

Date ______________________ Section ______________________

Performance Elements	Acceptable	Unacceptable	Not Applicable	Comments
1. Obtains necessary equipment and supplies				
2. Washes hands				
3. Prepares infant ventilator for use with test lung or simulated patient A. Assembles and attaches infant breathing circuit B. Performs "leak test" C. Assesses functions of ventilator controls, alarms, monitors				
4. Determines compression factor of infant circuit				
5. Confirms order for CMV				
6. Determines initial ventilator settings for an infant simulation				
7. Activates ventilator alarms and monitors				
8. Attaches activated ventilator to infant test lung or simulated infant				
9. Readjusts infant ventilator controls according to prescription				
10. Rechecks operating alarms and monitors				

Performance Elements	Acceptable	Unacceptable	Not Applicable	Comments
11. Monitors operating infant ventilation system				
12. Records appropriate information in CMV monitoring log				
13. Initials or signs monitoring log				

Knowledge of Procedure

- ☐ Good; student is knowledgeable about rationale and theory related to procedure
- ☐ Fair; student has adequate understanding of rationale and theory related to procedure
- ☐ Poor; student has inadequate understanding of rationale and theory related to procedure

Performance Deficiencies (check those that apply)

- ☐ Excessive time needed to complete procedure
- ☐ Broke aseptic or sterile technique
- ☐ Gross inaccuracy noted
- ☐ Technique may be harmful to patient
- ☐ Incorrect dosage or gas concentration
- ☐ Incorrect equipment assembly/use
- ☐ Unable to answer questions correctly about rationale and/or theory related to procedure
- ☐ Other ____________________

Evaluation Summary

- ☐ Satisfactory performance
- ☐ Unsatisfactory performance

Recommendations of Evaluator
☐ Skills may be applied/observed in clinical setting ☐ Specific evaluation deficiencies require correction ☐ Complete re-evaluation required ☐ Additional laboratory practice required

Signatures:

Evaluator ______________________ Date ______________________

Student ______________________ Date ______________________

Laboratory Report

Student ______________________ Acceptable ______________________

Date ______________________ Unacceptable ______________________

Course ______________________

Topic: Initiation of Infant Mechanical Ventilation with a Volume-Limited Ventilator

Data or Measurements

1. What is the CF of your ventilator and breathing circuit? ______________________

2. What are the calculated values after readjustment:

   Compressed volume ______________________

   Set volume ______________________

3. Infant ventilator monitoring record:

Infant Ventilator Monitoring Record

							Date/time
							Ventilator
							FI_{O_2}
							CPAP/PEEP
							Rate
							Pt. rate
							IMV/assist/cont
							O_2/blender flowrate
							I:E ratio
							Flowrate
							Peak pressure
							Hum. setting
							Insp. gas temp.
							Volume set
							Compressed volume
							Compression factor
							Tidal volume
							Alarm time delay
							High pressure limit
							Low pressure limit
							Set-up changed
							Initials

Scenario: Rounds with the neonatal staff had just begun when the attendant was beeped stat to the delivery room. A few minutes later, you find yourself in the department preparing the volume-limited neonatal ventilator for use on a 1.8 kg infant whose Apgar scores were low and who seems to have both cardiac and pulmonary anomalies. Please respond to the following questions:

1. What is the normal CF for an infant ventilator and breathing circuit?

2. You have just calculated the CF for a ventilator and breathing circuit you are about to use. The value you observe is 0.61 ml/cm H_2O. What would you do?

3. During ventilation of a 6 lb neonate, the set tidal volume is 30 ml, the peak pressure is 35 cm H_2O, and the circuit compression factor is 0.4 ml/cm H_2O. What is the delivered tidal volume? Show your work.

4. What is a volume-limited ventilator?

5. What tidal volume should be delivered to the following infants?
   A. 3.5 kg

   B. 2.8 kg

   C. 800 g

6. What patient cycling modes are available on this ventilator?

chapter 45

Initiation of infant ventilation with a time-cycled ventilator

INTRODUCTION

A time-cycled ventilator terminates inspiration when a preset inspiratory time has elapsed. Because the pressure waveform and subsequently the mean airway pressure may be varied, time-cycled ventilators are commonly used when ventilating infants with poor lung compliance. Currently, several brands of time-cycled infant ventilators are available. The purpose of this chapter is to introduce you to infant ventilation using a time-cycled ventilator.

OBJECTIVES

After completing this chapter, you should be able to do the following:

1. *Assemble a breathing circuit to a time-cycled ventilator and identify the components of the circuit.*
2. *Determine the initial ventilator settings for an apneic infant who requires ventilation.*
3. *Monitor the infant ventilator system during operation.*
4. *Estimate the tidal volume delivered with a time-cycled ventilator.*
5. *Operate a time-cycled ventilator in the pressure-limited and volume-limited modes.*

EQUIPMENT NEEDED

- ☐ Time-cycled infant ventilator (*i.e.*, Bourns BP 200, Baby Bird, Healthdyne Infant Ventilator)
- ☐ Infant breathing circuit
- ☐ Infant test lung
- ☐ 50 psi air and oxygen source(s)
- ☐ Watch with a second hand

☐ Sterile gauze or sterile glove
☐ Oxygen analyzer

ACTIVITIES

Exercise A: Assembly of a Ventilator with a Breathing Circuit and Assessment of Proper Function

1. Your instructor will provide you with a time-cycled ventilator in which the breathing circuit has been fully assembled (Fig. 45-1).
2. Identify the typical components of a breathing circuit used with a time-cycled ventilator:
   A. Inspired gas bacterial filter
   B. Humidifier
   C. Inspiratory line water trap
   D. Patient connection
   E. Proximal airway pressure tubing
   F. Expiratory line water trap
   G. Exhalation valve
3. Disassemble and reassemble the circuit.
4. Fill the humidifier with water and activate the heating element.
5. Connect the high-pressure (50 psi) air and oxygen source (if applicable).

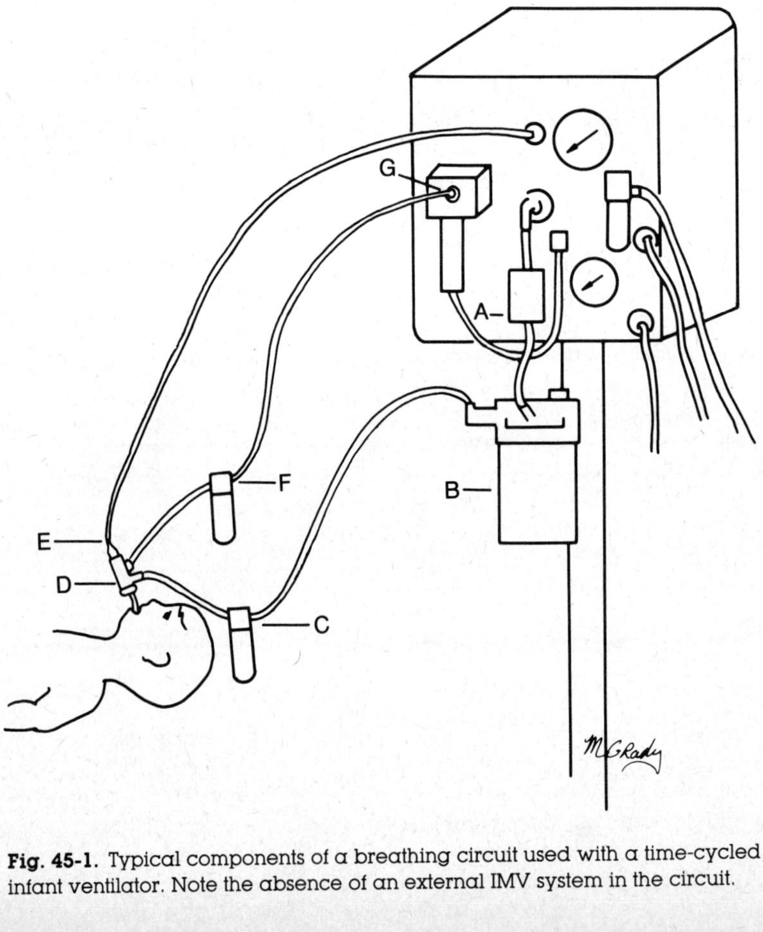

Fig. 45-1. Typical components of a breathing circuit used with a time-cycled infant ventilator. Note the absence of an external IMV system in the circuit.

6. Connect ventilator to electrical source (if applicable).
7. Turn the ventilator power on.
8. Adjust the ventilator controls to provide the following:
   A. Pressure limit—maximum
   B. Flowrate—10 liters/minute.
   C. Rate—15 breaths/minute
   D. FI_{O_2}—0.21
   E. Inspiratory time—1.0 second
   F. I:E ratio—1:2
9. Perform a leak test by allowing the ventilator to cycle and occluding the patient connection with a sterile glove. The proximal airway pressure manometer should indicate a pressure of 80 cm H_2O or greater. If the pressure is less than 80 cm H_2O, check the connections of the breathing circuit and humidifier. A leak may exist in the system. *Note:* The presence of a gas leak in the breathing circuit may be harmful or fatal to an actual infant.
10. Check the high-pressure gas inlet manometers. The manometers should indicate the air and oxygen inlet pressure to the ventilator (usually 35–60 psi).
11. Check the function of all alarms present on the ventilator. Be certain that all alarms are activated before connection to a patient.
12. Locate the diagram of the ventilator control panel assigned by your instructor (Figs. 45-2, 45-3, 45-4, 45-5). Identify the controls, alarms, and monitors found on the ventilator.

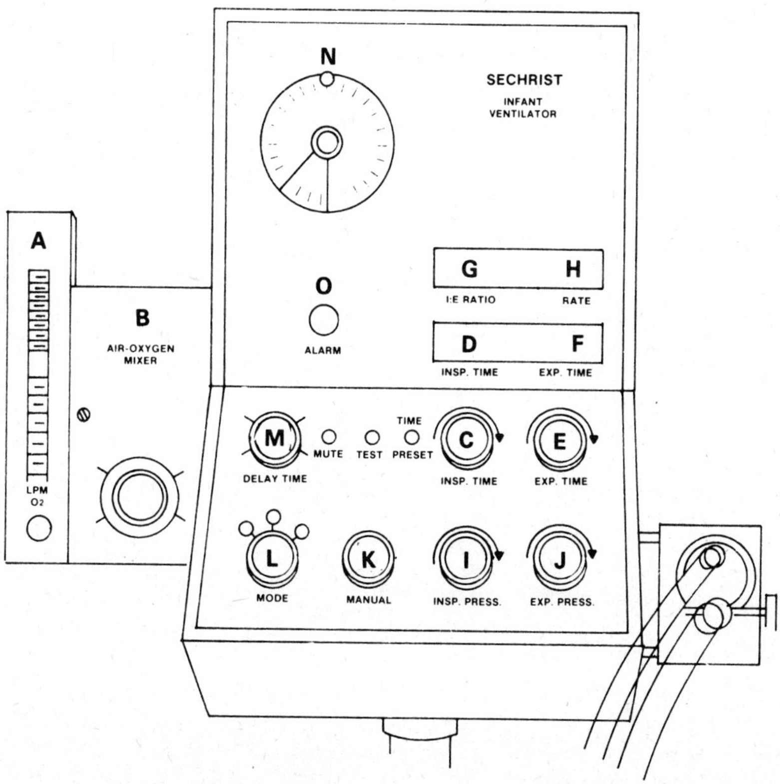

Fig. 45-2. Sechrist IV 100 B ventilator control panel. *(Reproduced with permission from Burton GG, Hodgkin JE: Respiratory Care. A Guide to Clinical Practice, 2nd ed. Philadelphia, JB Lippincott, 1984)*

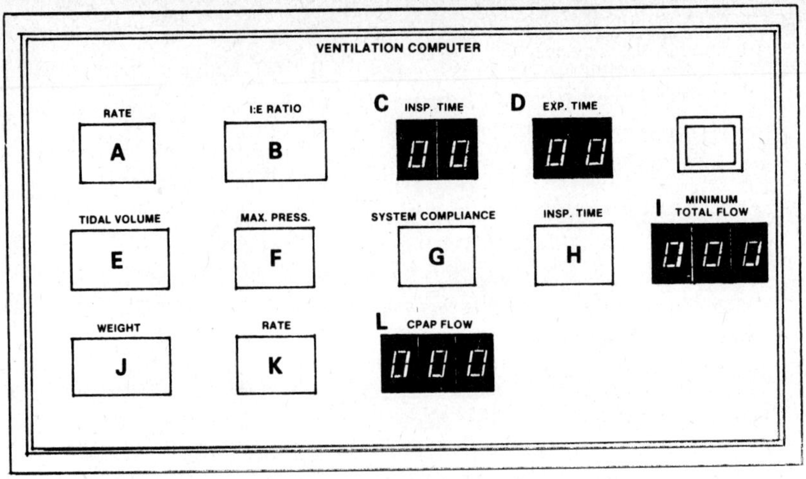

Fig. 45-2. cont.

VENTILATOR BRAND AND MODEL ______________________________

A. ______________________________

B. ______________________________

C. ______________________________

D. ______________________________

E. ______________________________

F. ______________________________

G. ______________________________

H. ______________________________

I. ______________________________

J. ______________________________

K. ______________________________

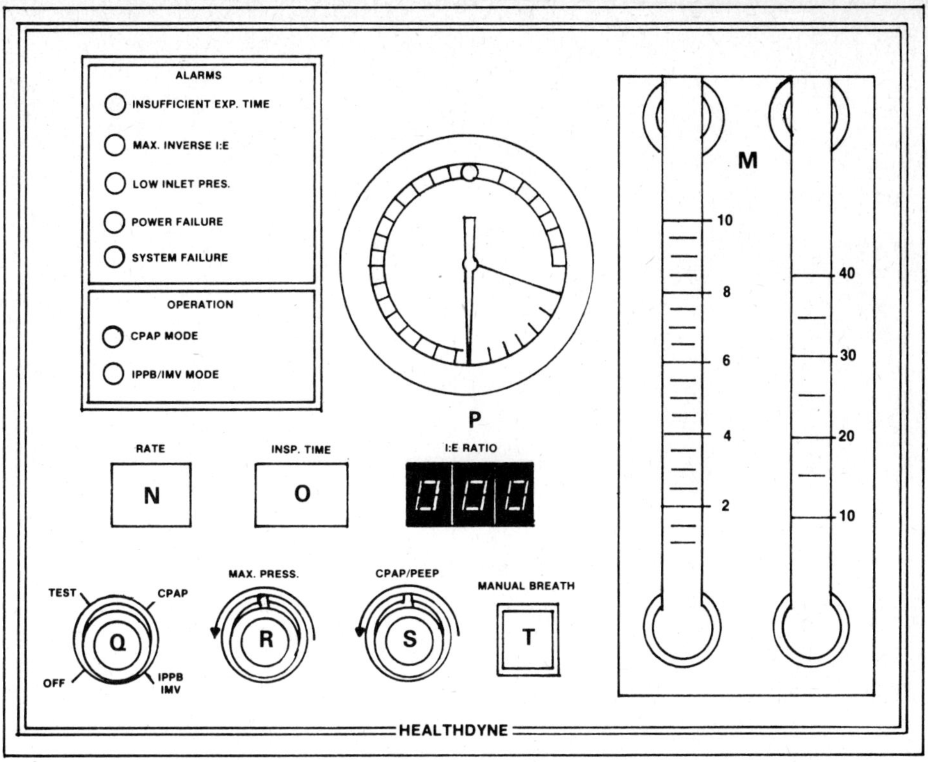

Fig. 45-3. Healthdyne infant ventilator. *(Reproduced with permission from Burton GG, Hodgkin JE: Respiratory Care. A Guide to Clinical Practice, 2nd ed. Philadelphia, JB Lippincott, 1984)*

VENTILATOR BRAND AND MODEL ______________________

A. ______________________ K. ______________________

B. ______________________ L. ______________________

C. ______________________ M. ______________________

D. ______________________ N. ______________________

E. ______________________ O. ______________________

F. ______________________ P. ______________________

G. ______________________ Q. ______________________

H. ______________________ R. ______________________

I. ______________________ S. ______________________

J. ______________________ T. ______________________

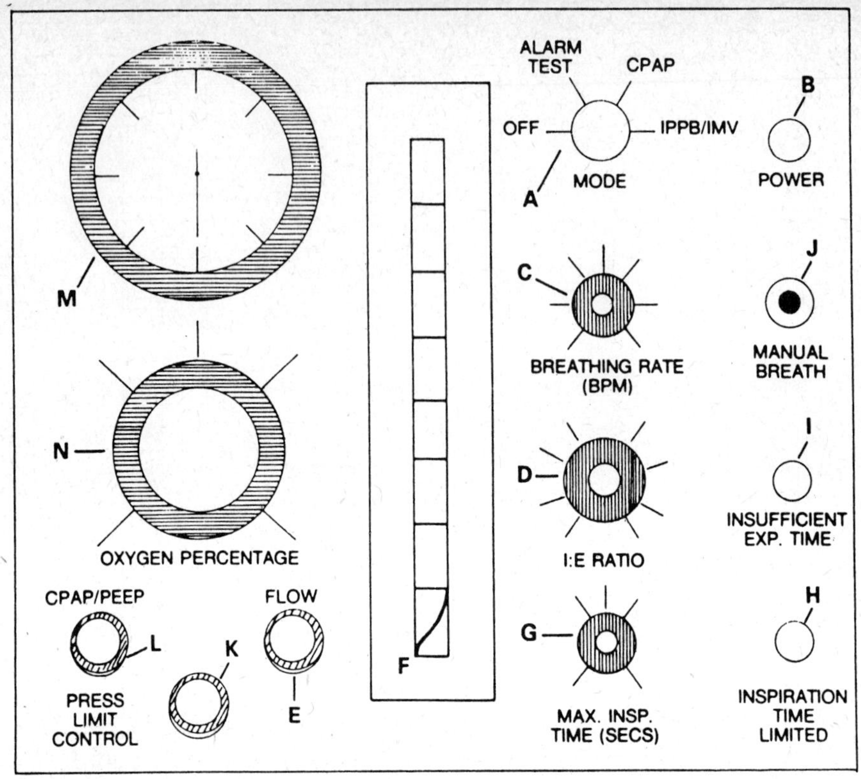

Fig. 45-4. Bourns BP-200 ventilator. *(Reproduced with permission from Burton GG, Hodgkin JJ: Respiratory Care. A Guide to Clinical Practice, 2nd ed. Philadelphia, JB Lippincott, 1984)*

VENTILATOR BRAND AND MODEL ______________________________

A. ______________________________ H. ______________________________

B. ______________________________ I. ______________________________

C. ______________________________ J. ______________________________

D. ______________________________ K. ______________________________

E. ______________________________ L. ______________________________

F. ______________________________ M. ______________________________

G. ______________________________ N. ______________________________

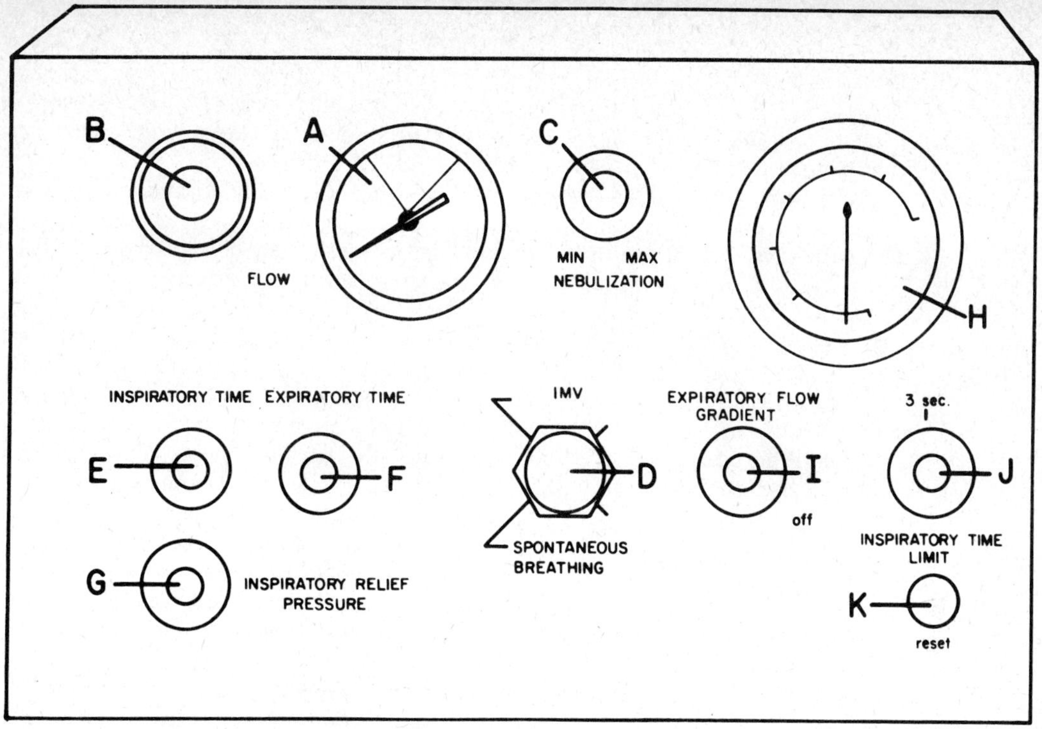

Fig. 45-5. BABYBird ventilator. *(Reproduced with permission from Burton GG, Hodgkin JE: Respiratory Care. A Guide to Clinical Practice, 2nd ed. Philadelphia, JB Lippincott, 1984)*

VENTILATOR BRAND AND MODEL ____________________

A. ____________________

B. ____________________

C. ____________________

D. ____________________

E. ____________________

F. ____________________

G. ____________________

H. ____________________

I. ____________________

J. ____________________

K. ____________________

Exercise B: Selection of Initial Settings

1. Rather than following a ventilation "recipe," the ventilator controls are adjusted according to each infant's condition; however, guidelines may be followed when beginning ventilation with a time-cycled infant ventilator. Review the following guidelines for instituting ventilation for an apneic infant:

   Ventilator Rate: 20–40 breaths per minute. The rate is usually adjusted according to the degree of ventilatory support required.

   Pressure Limit: 18–35 cm H_2O. The pressure limit indirectly controls the tidal volume. *Note:* When the pressure limit is reached, cycling into exhalation may *not* occur. In other words, the pressure limit on infant ventilators functions differently from that on IPPB ventilators. In conjunction with other settings, the pressure limit may determine the pressure waveform.

   Flowrate: 4–10 liters/minute. The flowrate may affect two ventilator functions: The flowrate may affect the proximal pressure waveform and indirectly affect delivered tidal volume; and the flowrate may be the primary source of gas flow in a continuous flow IMV mode. When the flowrate control affects the continuous flow IMV mode, the total flowrate should meet the following requirements:

   a) Flow should exceed two or three times the estimated infant minute volume.
   b) Flow should meet or exceed the infant peak inspiratory flowrate (for a 3.0 kg infant, the peak flowrate approximates 4.0 liters/minute or 66 ml/second)

   Note: Excessive flowrates in infant time-cycled ventilators may cause turbulent flow, increased deadspace ventilation, and high mean airway pressures.

   Inspiratory Time: 0.3–0.7 seconds. Inspiratory time limits may override the I:E ratio control.

   I:E Ratio: Initial ratios of 1 : 1 or 1 : 2 are typically used. The I:E ratio may vary from reverse (2:1) to ratios allowing prolonged exhalation time at low ventilator rates (1 : 10).

   PEEP: 2–10 cm H_2O. PEEP levels rarely exceed 10 cm H_2O in infants.

   Pressure Waveforms: The pressure waveform may be affected by the pressure limit, flowrate, inspiratory time, and lung compliance. In general, low flowrates produce a sine waveform and high flowrates produce a square pressure waveform.

2. Adjust the ventilator controls to typical settings that may be used to ventilate an apneic, 2500 g infant:

   Mode: IMV
   FI_{O_2}: 1.0
   Flow: 5 liters/minute
   Rate: 30 breaths/minute
   I:E ratio: 1:2
   Pressure limit: 25 cm H_2O
   PEEP: 2 cm H_2O

Exercise C: Measurement and Validation of Ventilator Settings

1. Using a sterile glove, completely occlude the breathing circuit patient connection. The proximal airway manometer should indicate the pressure limit; if not, adjust the pressure limit while occluding the patient connection. If you are still unable to achieve the pressure limit, repeat the leak test.
2. Analyze the oxygen concentration.
3. Connect the ventilator breathing circuit to the infant test lung or intubated mannequin.

4. Immediately verify adequate lung inflation. Using a watch with a second hand, time the rate for 60 seconds. *Note:* In a noisy intensive care nursery, it is sometimes helpful to place your hand on the exhalation valve to feel the ventilator cycle when counting the rate.
5. Monitor the inspired gas temperature.
6. Set all alarms.
7. While referring to Table 45-1, determine the inspiratory time and expiratory time when the rate is 30 breaths/minute and the I:E ratio is 1:2.
8. If applicable, verify that the inspiratory time limit control is consistently set with the calculated inspiratory time. *Note:* Because small tidal volumes are difficult to measure accurately and may require the use of special apparatus, the tidal volume is usually adjusted in response to clinical observation of the infant, blood gases, and auscultation.
9. Time-cycled infant ventilators may also be used as volume-limiting devices. Before using as a volume-limiting device, determine the ventilator and breathing circuit compression factor by readjusting the controls to provide the following settings:
   Rate = 30 bpm
   I:E ratio = 1:1
   Flowrate = 3 liters/minute or 50 ml/second
   Pressure limit = maximum
   PEEP = 0 cm H_2O
10. Occlude the patient connection to the breathing circuit while the ventilator cycles. Determine the pressure generated. If the pressure is 80 cm H_2O, the compression factor may be calculated by the following:

$$\text{Compression factor} = \frac{\text{Volume set}}{\text{Pressure}}$$
$$= \frac{50 \text{ ml}}{80 \text{ cm}} H_2O$$
$$= 0.63 \text{ ml/cm } H_2O$$

11. Determine the desired tidal volume. The tidal volume may be determined by multiplying the infant's body weight (kg) by 7 to 10 ml/kg.
   Example: What is the desired tidal volume for a 2.0 kg infant?

$$2.0 \text{ kg} \times 10 \text{ ml/kg} = 20 \text{ ml}$$

12. Determine the inspiratory time required to deliver a volume of 20 ml if the flowrate is 3.5 liters/minute from Table 45-2.
13. The tidal volume may be calculated with the following formula:

$$V_T = \text{Inspiratory time (seconds)} \times \text{flowrate (ml/second)}$$
$$V_T = 0.34 \text{ seconds} \times 58 \text{ ml/second}$$
$$V_T = 19.7 \text{ ml}$$

14. Connect the breathing circuit to the test lung or infant mannequin. Allow the ventilator to cycle and determine the peak pressure. (Be sure the pressure limit is set about 10 cm H_2O higher than the peak pressure.)
15. Determine the volume of gas captured by the gas compression and tubing compliance. Determine the "lost" volume by multiplying the peak pressure by the compression factor. For example, if the peak pressure equals 25 cm H_2O and the compression factor is 0.63 ml/cm H_2O, the lost volume may be determined by the following:

$$\text{Volume lost} = \text{Peak pressure} \times \text{Compression factor}$$
$$= 25 \text{ cm } H_2O \times 0.63 \text{ ml/cm } H_2O$$
$$= 16 \text{ ml}$$

Table 45-1. Inspiratory and Expiratory Time Resulting from Intersection of Ventilator Rate (Horizontal Column) and I:E Ratio (Vertical Column)

Ventilator Rate / One Cycle Time

I:E Ratio	22	21	20	19	18	17	16	15	14	13	12	10	9	8	7	6	5	4	3	2
	2.7	2.9	3.0	3.2	3.3	3.5	3.8	4.0	4.3	4.6	5.0	6.0	6.7	7.5	8.6	10	12	15	20	30
4/1	2.16/0.54	2.32/0.58	2.4/0.6	2.56/0.64	2.64/0.66	2.8/0.7	3.04/0.76	3.2/0.8	3.44/0.86	3.68/0.92	4.0/1.0	4.8/1.2	5.36/0.34	6.0/1.5	6.88/1.72	8.0/2.0	9.6/2.4	12.0/3.0	16.0/4.0	24.0/6.0
3/1	2.02/0.67	2.12/0.73	2.25/0.75	2.4/0.8	2.47/0.82	2.63/0.88	2.85/0.95	3.0/1.0	3.23/1.07	3.45/1.15	3.75/1.25	4.50/1.50	5.02/1.67	5.62/1.87	6.45/2.15	7.5/2.5	9.0/3.0	11.3/3.7	15.0/5.0	22.5/7.5
2/1	1.8/0.9	1.93/0.96	2.0/1.0	2.1/1.06	2.2/1.1	2.33/1.16	2.53/1.26	2.66/1.33	2.86/1.43	3.06/1.53	3.33/1.66	4.0/2.0	4.46/2.24	5.0/2.5	5.73/2.86	6.66/3.33	8.0/4.0	10.0/5.0	13.3/6.6	20.0/10.0
1.5/1	1.62/0.8	1.74/1.16	1.8/1.2	1.92/1.28	1.98/1.32	2.1/1.4	2.28/1.52	2.4/1.6	2.58/1.72	2.76/1.84	3.0/2.0	3.6/2.4	4.02/2.68	4.5/3.0	5.16/3.48	6.0/4.0	7.2/4.8	9.0/6.0	12.0/8.0	18.0/12.0
1/1	1.35/1.35	1.45/1.45	1.5/1.5	1.6/1.6	1.65/1.65	1.75/1.75	1.9/1.9	2.0/2.0	2.15/2.15	2.3/2.3	2.5/2.5	3.0/3.0	3.35/3.35	3.75/3.75	4.3/4.3	5.0/5.0	6.0/6.0	7.5/7.5	10.0/10.0	15.0/15.0
1/1.5	1.08/1.62	1.16/1.74	1.2/1.8	1.28/1.92	1.32/1.98	1.4/2.1	1.52/2.28	1.6/2.4	1.72/2.58	1.84/2.76	2.0/3.0	2.4/3.6	2.68/4.02	3.0/4.5	3.48/5.16	4.0/6.0	4.8/7.2	6.0/9.0	8.0/12.0	12.0/18.0
1/2	0.9/1.8	0.96/1.93	1.0/2.0	1.06/2.1	1.1/2.2	1.16/2.33	1.26/2.53	1.33/2.66	1.43/2.86	1.53/3.00	1.66/3.33	2.0/4.0	2.2/4.46	2.5/5.0	2.86/5.73	3.3/6.6	4.0/8.0	5.0/10.0	6.6/13.3	10.0/20.0
1/3	0.67/2.02	0.73/2.12	0.75/2.25	0.8/2.4	0.82/2.47	0.88/2.63	0.95/2.85	1.0/3.0	1.07/3.23	1.15/3.45	1.25/3.75	1.50/4.50	1.67/5.0	1.87/5.62	2.15/6.45	2.5/7.5	3.0/9.0	3.75/11.25	5.0/15.0	7.5/22.5
1/4	0.54/2.16	0.58/2.32	0.6/2.4	0.64/2.56	0.66/2.64	0.7/2.8	0.76/3.04	0.8/3.2	0.86/3.44	0.92/3.68	1.0/4.0	1.2/4.8	1.34/5.36	1.5/6.0	1.72/6.88	2.0/8.0	2.4/9.6	3.0/12.0	4.0/16.0	6.0/24.0
1/6	0.38/2.31	0.41/2.48	0.43/2.57	0.45/2.74	0.47/2.83	0.5/3.0	0.54/3.26	0.57/3.42	0.61/3.64	0.65/3.94	0.71/4.29	0.86/5.14	0.96/5.74	1.07/6.43	1.23/7.37	1.43/8.57	1.71/10.2	2.14/12.9	2.80/17.1	4.29/25.7
1/10	0.24/2.45	0.26/2.63	0.27/2.72	0.29/2.90	0.30/3.0	0.31/3.18	0.34/3.45	0.36/3.63	0.39/3.90	0.41/4.18	0.45/4.54	0.54/5.45	0.61/6.09	0.68/6.81	0.78/7.81	0.90/9.09	1.09/1.09	1.30/13.6	1.81/18.1	2.72/27.2

(continued)

Table 45-2. Inspiratory Time Required to Produce a Given Tidal Volume (Horizontal Column) at a Given Flowrate (Vertical Column) Using a Time-Cycled Ventilator

Tidal Volume (ml)

Flow Rate (liters/minute)	Flowrate (ml/second)	3.0	4.0	5.0	6.0	7.0	8.0	9.0	10.0	11.0	12.0	13.0	14.0	15.0	16.0	17.0	18.0	19.0	20.0
0.5	8.3	0.36	0.48	0.60	0.72	0.84	0.96	1.08	1.20	1.30	1.40	1.60	1.68	1.80	1.92	2.04	2.16	2.28	2.40
1.0	16.6	0.18	0.24	0.30	0.36	0.42	0.48	0.54	0.60	0.66	0.72	0.78	0.84	0.90	0.96	1.02	1.08	1.14	1.20
1.5	25.0	0.12	0.16	0.20	0.24	0.28	0.32	0.36	0.40	0.44	0.48	0.52	0.56	0.60	0.64	0.68	0.72	0.76	0.80
2.0	33.3	0.09	0.12	0.15	0.18	0.21	0.24	0.27	0.30	0.33	0.36	0.39	0.42	0.45	0.48	0.51	0.54	0.57	0.60
2.5	41.6	0.07	0.09	0.12	0.14	0.16	0.19	0.21	0.24	0.26	0.28	0.31	0.33	0.36	0.38	0.40	0.43	0.45	0.48
3.0	50.0	0.06	0.08	0.10	0.12	0.14	0.16	0.18	0.20	0.22	0.24	0.26	0.28	0.30	0.32	0.34	0.34	0.36	0.40
3.5	58.3	0.05	0.06	0.08	0.10	0.12	0.13	0.15	0.17	0.18	0.20	0.22	0.24	0.25	0.27	0.29	0.30	0.32	0.34
4.0	66.7	0.04	0.05	0.07	0.08	0.10	0.11	0.13	0.14	0.16	0.17	0.19	0.20	0.22	0.23	0.25	0.26	0.28	0.29
4.5	75.0	0.04	0.05	0.06	0.08	0.09	0.10	0.12	0.13	0.14	0.16	0.17	0.18	0.20	0.21	0.22	0.24	0.25	0.26
5.0	83.3	0.03	0.04	0.06	0.07	0.08	0.09	0.10	0.12	0.13	0.14	0.15	0.16	0.18	0.19	0.20	0.21	0.22	0.24
5.5	91.6	0.03	0.04	0.05	0.06	0.07	0.08	0.09	0.10	0.12	0.13	0.14	0.15	0.16	0.17	0.18	0.19	0.20	0.21
6.0	100.0	0.03	0.04	0.05	0.06	0.07	0.08	0.09	0.10	0.11	0.12	0.13	0.14	0.15	0.16	0.17	0.18	0.19	0.20
6.5	108.3	0.02	0.03	0.04	0.05	0.06	0.07	0.08	0.09	0.10	0.11	0.12	0.129	0.13	0.14	0.14	0.166	0.17	0.18
7.0	116.6	0.02	0.03	0.04	0.04	0.05	0.06	0.07	0.08	0.09	0.10	0.11	0.12	0.12	0.13	0.14	0.15	0.16	0.17
7.5	125.0	0.02	0.03	0.04	0.04	0.05	0.06	0.07	0.08	0.08	0.09	0.10	0.11	0.12	0.128	0.13	0.14	0.15	0.16
8.0	133.3	0.02	0.03	0.03	0.04	0.05	0.06	0.06	0.07	0.08	0.09	0.09	0.11	0.11	0.12	0.12	0.13	0.14	0.15

(continued)

Table 45-1. *(Continued)*

I:E Ratio	Ventilator Rate 60	50	40	38	36	35	34	33	32	31	30	29	28	27	26	25	24	23
One Cycle Time	1.0	1.2	1.5	1.6	1.7	1.7	1.8	1.81	1.9	1.93	2.0	2.1	2.1	2.2	2.3	2.4	2.5	2.6
4/1	0.8/0.2	0.96/0.24	1.2/0.3	1.28/0.32	1.36/0.34	1.36/0.34	1.44/0.36	1.44/0.36	1.52/0.38	1.54/0.38	1.6/0.4	1.64/0.41	1.68/0.42	1.76/0.44	1.84/0.46	1.92/0.48	2.0/0.5	2.08/0.52
3/1	0.75/0.25	0.9/0.3	1.12/0.37	1.2/0.4	1.27/0.42	1.27/0.42	1.35/0.45	1.35/0.45	1.42/0.47	1.42/0.47	1.5/0.5	1.57/0.52	1.57/0.52	1.65/0.55	1.72/0.57	1.80/0.60	1.87/0.62	1.95/0.65
2/1	0.66/0.33	0.8/0.4	1.0/0.5	1.06/0.53	1.13/0.56	1.13/0.56	1.20/0.60	1.20/0.60	1.26/0.63	1.26/0.63	1.33/0.66	1.33/0.66	1.4/0.7	1.46/0.73	1.53/0.76	1.6/0.8	1.66/0.83	1.73/0.86
1.5/1	0.6/0.4	0.72/0.48	0.9/0.6	0.96/0.64	1.02/0.68	1.02/0.68	1.08/0.72	1.08/0.72	1.14/0.76	1.14/0.76	1.2/0.8	1.26/0.84	1.26/0.84	1.32/0.88	1.38/0.92	1.44/0.96	1.5/1.0	1.56/1.04
1/1	0.5/0.5	0.6/0.6	0.75/0.75	0.8/0.8	0.85/0.85	0.85/0.85	0.9/0.9	0.9/0.9	0.95/0.95	0.95/0.95	1.0/1.0	1.05/1.05	1.05/1.05	1.1/1.1	1.15/1.15	1.2/1.2	1.25/1.25	1.3/1.3
1/1.5	0.4/0.6	0.48/0.72	0.6/0.9	0.64/0.96	0.68/1.02	0.68/1.02	0.72/1.08	0.72/1.08	0.76/1.14	0.76/1.14	0.8/1.2	0.84/1.26	0.84/1.26	0.88/1.32	1.92/1.38	0.96/1.44	1.0/1.5	1.04/1.56
1/2	0.33/0.66	0.4/0.8	0.5/1.0	0.53/1.06	0.56/1.13	0.56/1.13	0.60/1.20	0.60/1.20	0.63/1.26	0.63/1.26	0.66/1.33	0.7/1.4	0.7/1.4	0.73/1.46	0.76/1.53	0.8/1.6	0.83/1.66	0.86/1.73
1/3	0.25/0.75	0.3/0.9	0.37/1.12	0.4/1.2	0.42/1.27	0.42/1.27	0.45/1.35	0.45/1.35	0.47/1.42	0.47/1.42	0.5/1.5	0.52/1.57	0.52/1.57	0.55/1.65	0.57/1.72	0.60/1.80	0.62/1.87	0.65/1.95
1/4	0.2/0.8	0.24/0.96	0.3/1.2	0.32/1.28	0.34/1.36	0.34/1.36	0.36/1.44	0.36/1.44	0.38/1.52	0.38/1.52	0.4/1.6	0.41/1.64	0.42/1.68	0.44/1.76	0.46/1.84	0.48/1.92	0.5/2.0	0.52/2.08
1/6	0.14/0.86	0.17/1.03	0.21/1.24	0.23/1.37	0.24/1.46	0.24/1.46	0.26/1.54	0.26/1.54	0.27/1.62	0.27/1.62	0.28/1.71	0.3/1.8	0.3/1.8	0.31/1.89	0.32/1.92	0.34/2.05	0.36/2.14	0.37/2.22
1/10	0.09/0.90	0.10/1.09	0.14/1.36	0.15/1.45	0.15/1.54	0.15/1.54	0.16/1.63	0.16/1.63	0.17/1.72	0.17/1.72	0.18/1.80	0.19/1.90	0.19/1.90	0.20/2.09	0.20/2.09	0.21/2.18	0.22/2.27	0.23/2.36

Table 45-2. *(Continued)*

Flow Rate (liters/minute)	Flowrate (ml/second)	Tidal Volume (ml) 21.0	22.0	23.0	24.0	25.0	26.0	27.0	28.0	29.0	30.0	31.0	32.0	33.0	34.0	35.0	36.0	37.0	38.0
0.5	8.3	2.50	2.65	2.77	2.89	3.01	3.13	3.25	3.37	3.49	3.61	3.73	3.85	3.97	4.09	4.21	4.33	4.45	4.57
1.0	16.6	1.26	1.32	1.38	1.44	1.50	1.56	1.62	1.68	1.74	1.80	1.86	1.92	1.98	2.04	2.10	2.16	2.22	2.28
1.5	25.0	0.84	0.88	0.92	0.96	1.00	1.04	1.08	1.12	1.16	1.20	1.24	1.28	1.32	1.36	1.40	1.44	1.48	1.52
2.0	33.3	0.63	0.66	0.64	0.72	0.75	0.78	0.81	0.84	0.87	0.90	0.93	0.96	0.99	1.02	1.05	1.08	1.11	1.14
2.5	41.6	0.50	0.52	0.55	0.57	0.60	0.62	0.64	0.66	0.69	0.72	0.74	0.76	0.79	0.81	0.84	0.86	0.88	0.91
3.0	50.0	0.42	0.44	0.46	0.48	0.50	0.52	0.54	0.56	0.58	0.60	0.62	0.64	0.66	0.68	0.70	0.72	0.74	0.76
3.5	58.3	0.36	0.37	0.39	0.41	0.42	0.44	0.46	0.48	0.49	0.51	0.53	0.54	0.56	0.58	0.60	0.61	0.63	0.65
4.0	66.7	0.31	0.32	0.34	0.35	0.37	0.38	0.40	0.41	0.43	0.44	0.46	0.47	0.49	0.50	0.52	0.53	0.55	0.56
4.5	75.0	0.28	0.29	0.30	0.32	0.33	0.34	0.36	0.37	0.38	0.40	0.41	0.42	0.44	0.45	0.46	0.48	0.49	0.50
5.0	83.3	0.25	0.26	0.27	0.28	0.30	0.31	0.32	0.33	0.34	0.36	0.37	0.38	0.39	0.40	0.42	0.43	0.44	0.45
5.5	91.6	0.22	0.24	0.25	0.26	0.27	0.28	0.29	0.30	0.31	0.32	0.33	0.34	0.36	0.37	0.38	0.39	0.40	0.41
6.0	100.0	0.21	0.22	0.23	0.24	0.25	0.26	0.27	0.28	0.29	0.30	0.31	0.32	0.33	0.34	0.35	0.36	0.37	0.38
6.5	108.3	0.19	0.20	0.21	0.22	0.23	0.23	0.24	0.25	0.26	0.27	0.28	0.29	0.30	0.31	0.32	0.33	0.34	0.35
7.0	116.6	0.18	0.18	0.19	0.20	0.21	0.22	0.23	0.24	0.24	0.25	0.26	0.27	0.28	0.29	0.30	0.30	0.31	0.32
7.5	125.0	0.16	0.17	0.18	0.19	0.20	0.21	0.22	0.22	0.23	0.24	0.24	0.25	0.26	0.27	0.28	0.28	0.29	0.30
8.0	133.3	0.15	0.16	0.17	0.18	0.18	0.19	0.20	0.21	0.21	0.22	0.23	0.24	0.24	0.25	0.26	0.27	0.27	0.28

16. The volume lost must be compensated for by increasing the flowrate and recalculation of the lost volume.
17. Adjust the ventilator to provide volume ventilation to a 3200 g infant, given the following information:
    Flowrate = 6 liters/minute
    Compression factor = 0.5 ml/cm H_2O
    Peak pressure = 24 cm H_2O
    Rate = 25 breaths/minute
    I:E ratio = 1:3
18. Record the following information on the laboratory report:
    Compression factor
    Desired tidal volume
    Delivered tidal volume
    Volume lost
    Inspiratory time
    Expiratory time
    Pressure limit

Exercise D: Monitoring the Infant Ventilator System

1. Adjust the ventilator to provide pressure-limited ventilation to a simulated 2.0 kg neonate. Adjust the controls to provide the following settings:
    FI_{O_2}—0.85
    Mode—IMV
    Rate—35 breaths/minute
    Pressure limit—23 cm H_2O
    PEEP—+6 cm H_2O
    I:E ratio = 1:2
2. Using the monitoring record, monitor and record the ventilator settings. Be sure to time the rate for a full minute, analyze the oxygen concentration, and determine the inspiratory and expiratory time.

Exercise E: Determination of "Unknown"

1. Your instructor will provide you with a fully assembled and functional time-cycled infant ventilator. Monitor and record all of the ventilator settings, time the rate, analyze the FI_{O_2}, and check the function of all alarms. Record the data on the monitoring record.

RECOMMENDED READING

Blodgett D: Manual of Pediatric Respiratory Care Procedures. Philadelphia, JB Lippincott, 1982

Burgess WR, Chernick V: Respiratory Therapy in Newborn Infants and Children. New York, Thieme-Stratton, 1982

Burton GG, Hodgkin JE: Respiratory Care. A Guide to Clinical Practice, 2nd ed. Philadelphia, JB Lippincott, 1984

Goldsmith JP, Karotkin EH: Assisted Ventilation of the Neonate. Philadelphia, WB Saunders, 1981

Lough MD, Williams TJ, Rawson JE: Newborn Respiratory Care. Chicago, Year Book Medical Publishers, 1979

Thibeault DW, Gregory GA: Neonatal Pulmonary Care. Menlo Park, CA, Addison-Wesley, 1981

Laboratory Performance Evaluation (#45)

Topic: Initiation of Infant Mechanical Ventilation with a Time-Cycled Infant Ventilator

Student ______________________ Course ______________________

Date ______________________ Section ______________________

Performance Elements	Acceptable	Unacceptable	Not Applicable	Comments
1. Obtains appropriate equipment and supplies				
2. Washes hands				
3. Prepares infant ventilator for use with test lung or simulated patient A. Assembles and attaches infant breathing circuit B. Performs "leak test" C. Assesses function of ventilator controls, alarms, monitors				
4. Determines compression factor of the infant circuit				
5. Repeats "leak test"				
6. Confirms CMV order				
7. Determines initial ventilator settings for an infant simulation				
8. Activates ventilator alarms and monitors				
9. Attaches activated ventilator to infant test lung or simulated patient				
10. Readjusts infant ventilator controls according to prescription				

Performance Elements	Acceptable	Unacceptable	Not Applicable	Comments
11. Rechecks alarms and monitors				
12. Monitors infant ventilator system				
13. Records appropriate information in CMV monitoring log				
14. Initials or signs monitoring log				

Knowledge of Procedure

☐ Good; student is knowledgeable about rationale and theory related to procedure

☐ Fair; student has adequate understanding of rationale and theory related to procedure

☐ Poor; student has inadequate understanding of rationale and theory related to procedure

Performance Deficiencies (check those that apply)

☐ Excessive time needed to complete procedure

☐ Broke aseptic or sterile technique

☐ Gross inaccuracy noted

☐ Technique may be harmful to patient

☐ Incorrect dosage or gas concentration

☐ Incorrect equipment assembly/use

☐ Unable to answer questions correctly about rationale and/or theory related to procedure

☐ Other ____________________

Evaluation Summary

☐ Satisfactory performance

☐ Unsatisfactory performance

Recommendations of Evaluator

☐ Skills may be applied/observed in clinical setting

☐ Specific evaluation deficiencies require correction

☐ Complete re-evaluation required

☐ Additional laboratory practice required

Signatures:

Evaluator ______________________ Date ______________________

Student ______________________ Date ______________________

Laboratory Report

Student ______________________ Acceptable ______________________

Date ______________________ Unacceptable ______________________

Course ______________________

Topic: Initiation of Infant Ventilation with a Time-Cycled Ventilator

Data or Measurements

1. What is the name of the ventilator you are using for this laboratory exercise? ________

   From Exercise D:

   Compression factor ______________________

   Desired tidal volume ______________________

   Delivered tidal volume ______________________

   Volume lost ______________________

   Inspiratory time ______________________

   Expiratory time ______________________

   Pressure limit ______________________

Scenario: Responding to a call from the delivery room, you are confronted with the following scene: The neonatologist and delivery room nurse are applying resuscitative efforts to a newborn while obstetricians have begun closing the wound caused by the cesarean section. "Let's go ahead and intubate him," the neonatologist said, "and transport him to the nursery. Everything's set up and waiting."

Aside from a brief and transient episode of bradycardia, the transport to the intensive care nursery was uneventful. A time-cycled ventilator is at the bedside. The baby's weight is 3.4 kg. Initially, you have decided to use the ventilator in the pressure-limiting mode and an FI_{O_2} of 0.40.

Please answer the following questions:

1. What initial settings would you recommend to provide full ventilatory support?

   Ventilation rate ______________________

   I:E ratio ______________________

   Pressure limit ______________________

   Patient cycling mode ______________________

   Flowrate ______________________

2. In infant time-cycled ventilators, what causes the termination of the inspiratory phase?

3. As applied to infant time-cycled ventilators, compare and contrast pressure limiting with pressure cycling.

4. What are two possible hazards of excessive flowrates used with an infant time-cycled ventilators?

5. Classify the ventilator used to complete these laboratory exercises:

A. Name of ventilator ______________________

Powered ______________________

Cycled ______________________

Circuits ______________________

Modes ______________________

6. When providing volume-limited ventilation to an infant, what tidal volume is desirable for an infant weighing

A. 2.2 kg?

B. 3.8 kg?

C. 900 gm?

D. 5 lb?

7. If the ventilator rate is 35 breaths/minute and the I : E ratio is 1 : 2, what are the inspiratory and expiratory times?

Infant Ventilator Monitoring Record

							Date/time
							Ventilator
							FI_{O_2}
							CPAP/PEEP
							Rate
							Pt. rate
							IMV/assist/cont
							O_2/blender flowrate
							I:E ratio
							Flowrate
							Peak pressure
							Hum. setting
							Insp. gas temp.
							Volume set
							Compressed volume
							Compression factor
							Tidal volume
							Alarm time delay
							High pressure limit
							Low pressure limit
							Set-up changed
							Initials

chapter 46

Intermittent mandatory ventilation

INTRODUCTION

Intermittent mandatory ventilation (IMV) is a mode of ventilation that combines a patient's spontaneous breathing with positive pressure (mandatory) breaths from a ventilator. IMV can provide a transition from ventilation that is controlled by the ventilator to spontaneous ventilation by the patient. IMV is most commonly used as a weaning technique but can also be used as a maintenance technique to help promote respiratory muscle activity. Many ventilators offer an IMV mode, or it can be added externally. The purpose of this chapter is to introduce you to internal and external IMV.

OBJECTIVES

At the completion of this chapter, you should be able to do the following:

1. *Assemble an IMV setup and attach it externally to a ventilator.*
2. *Assess proper function of a ventilator when IMV is incorporated.*
3. *Determine when a ventilator has continuous flow IMV or demand flow IMV.*
4. *Use a ventilator that provides IMV.*
5. *Discuss the indications for the use of IMV.*

EQUIPMENT NEEDED

- ☐ Ventilator with IMV mode
- ☐ Small-bore oxygen tubing
- ☐ 12 inch large-bore tubing
- ☐ IMV manifold or two "T"-adapters and a one-way valve
- ☐ Oxygen inlet adapter
- ☐ 3 liter reservoir bag
- ☐ 22 mm adapter
- ☐ Adult breathing circuit
- ☐ Gas mixing system (blender or air and oxygen flowmeter)

- ☐ 50 psi gas source(s)
- ☐ Test lung or lung analog
- ☐ Oxygen analyzer

ACTIVITIES

Exercise A: Assembly and Attachment of External IMV to a Ventilator

1. Your instructor will provide an adult ventilator with a breathing circuit attached.
2. Remove the tubing from the ventilator gas outlet to the humidifier inlet (Fig. 46-1)
3. Consult Figure 46-1 and identify the following components of the IMV setup:
   - **A.** 22 mm adapter
   - **B.** "T" adapter
   - **C.** One-way valve
   - **D.** "T"-adapter
   - **E.** Oxygen inlet adapter
   - **F.** Small-bore oxygen tubing
   - **G.** 3 liter reservoir bag
   - **H.** Oxygen blender and flowmeter
4. Assemble the IMV setup as shown in Figure 46-1. Attach it to the humidifier inlet of the breathing circuit. After attachment of the setup, perform a leak test.
5. If you do not have a gas mixing system as shown in Figure 46-1, use one air and one oxygen flowmeter and blend the gases manually.

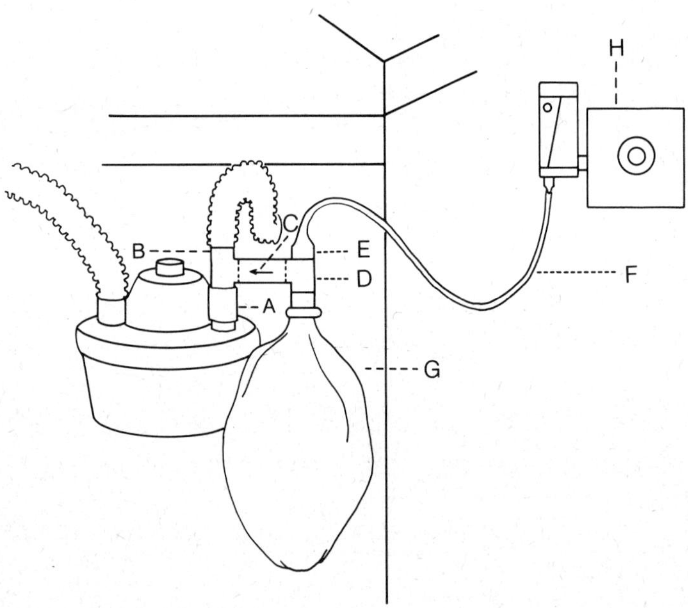

Fig. 46-1. External IMV circuit with gas blender.

Exercise B: Initiation of IMV Using an External Setup and Assessment of Function

1. After attempting the IMV setup, adjust standard ventilator setings. Use an FI_{O_2} between 0.21 and 1.0. Have your instructor check these settings.
2. Adjust the supplemental gas flow to the IMV setup at 10 to 15 liters/minute. Excessive supplemental gas flows may result in resistance to flow through the tubing cir-

cuit, causing "inadvertent PEEP." Inadequate flows may increase the work of breathing.

3. Attach the patient wye to the test lung.
4. Observe the 3 liter reservoir bag during mandatory inspirations and during expiration. Observe the one-way valve at these times also. Note your observation on the laboratory report.
5. Turn the IMV rate to 2 breaths/minute. Disconnect the patient wye from the test lung and feel for continuous air flow between mandatory breaths. If properly functioning, flow should be felt. This is referred to as a continuous flow IMV.
6. Analyze the oxygen concentration with a continuous readout analyzer. The oxygen concentration should remain stable during mandatory breaths and during continuous flow (Fig. 46-2).

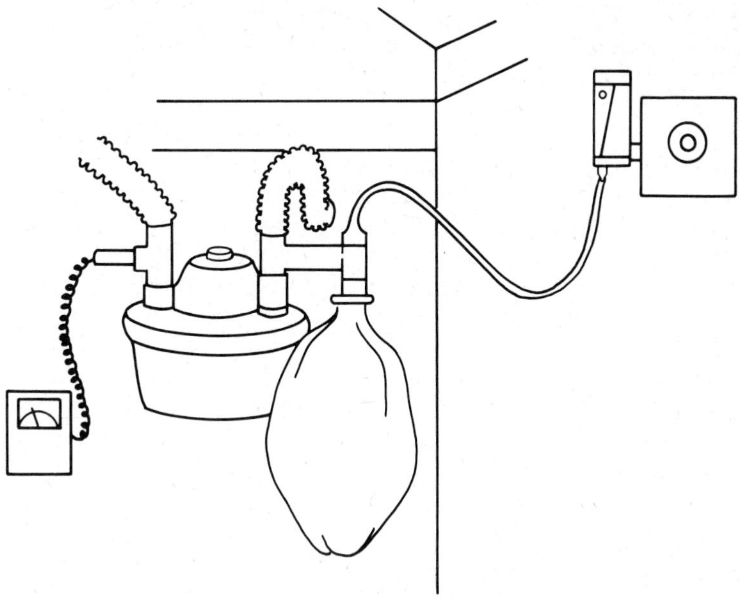

Fig. 46-2. Analysis of oxygen concentration delivered in an IMV system. Note that the analysis is made downstream from gas mixing.

Exercise C: Initiation of IMV Using a Ventilator That Provides IMV and Assessment of Function

1. Obtain a ventilator that provides an IMV mode (i.e., Bear II, MA-II, Servo 900B).
2. Set the ventilator in the IMV mode.
3. Render the ventilator operational by selecting standard ventilator settings. Select a frequency of 2 breaths/minute.
4. Feel for air flow at the patient wye between mandatory breaths. If air flow is present, you have a continuous flow IMV. If no air flow is felt, you have a demand flow IMV. Indicate which type you have on your laboratory report.

Exercise D: Determination of "Unknown"

1. Your instructor will provide you with an adult ventilator with an operational external IMV setup.

2. Determine the total IMV flow, the F_{IO_2}, and whether the system is functioning properly.
3. Note these observations on your laboratory report.

RECOMMENDED READING

Burgess WR, Chernick V: Respiratory Therapy in Newborn Infants and Children. New York, Thieme-Stratton, 1982

Burton GG, Hodgkin JE: Respiratory Care: A Guide to Clinical Practice, 2nd ed. Philadelphia, JB Lippincott, 1984

Goldsmith JP, Karotkin EH: Assisted Ventilation of the Neonate. Philadelphia, WB Saunders, 1981

Lough MD, Williams TJ, Rawson JE: Newborn Respiratory Care. Chicago, Year Book Medical Publishers, 1979

McPherson S: Respiratory Therapy Equipment, 3rd ed. St Louis, CV Mosby, 1985

Thibeault DW, Gregory GA: Neonatal Pulmonary Care. Menlo Park, CA, Addison–Wesley, 1981

Laboratory Performance Evaluation (#46)

Topic: Intermittent Mandatory Ventilation

Student ____________________ Course ____________________

Date ____________________ Section ____________________

Performance Elements	Acceptable	Unacceptable	Not Applicable	Comments
1. Obtains appropriate equipment and supplies				
2. Identifies components of an external IMV system: A. Power/gas source B. Gas reservoir/mixing system C. One-way valves D. Safety relief mechanisms E. Pressure manometers F. Gas humidification source				
3. Washes hands				
4. Assembles external IMV system				
5. Attaches external IMV system to mechanical ventilator				
6. Makes appropriate adjustments of ventilator to accommodate the external IMV				
7. Assesses function of external IMV: A. Adequate flow B. Safety relief C. Prescribed FI_{O_2} D. One-way valves E. Gas temperature F. Gas humidification				
8. Records appropriate information in CMV monitoring log				

Performance Elements	Acceptable	Unacceptable	Not Applicable	Comments
9. Initials or signs monitoring log				
10. Initiates IMV of ventilator incorporated system				

Knowledge of Procedure

☐ Good; student is knowledgeable about rationale and theory related to procedure

☐ Fair; student has adequate understanding of rationale and theory related to procedure

☐ Poor; student has inadequate understanding of rationale and theory related to procedure

Performance Deficiencies (check those that apply)

☐ Excessive time needed to complete procedure

☐ Broke aseptic or sterile technique

☐ Gross inaccuracy noted

☐ Technique may be harmful to patient

☐ Incorrect dosage or gas concentration

☐ Incorrect equipment assembly/use

☐ Unable to answer questions correctly about rationale and/or theory related to procedure

☐ Other ____________________

Evaluation Summary

☐ Satisfactory performance

☐ Unsatisfactory performance

Recommendations of Evaluator

- ☐ Skills may be applied/observed in clinical setting
- ☐ Specific evaluation deficiencies require correction
- ☐ Complete re-evaluation required
- ☐ Additional laboratory practice required

Signatures:

Evaluator ______________________ Date ______________________

Student ______________________ Date ______________________

Laboratory Report

Student ______________________ Acceptable ______________________

Date ______________________ Unacceptable ______________________

Course ______________________

Topic: Intermittent Mandatory Ventilation

Data or Measurements

1. What is the action of the IMV reservoir bag and one-way valve during mandatory inspiration and expiration?

2. What ventilator are you using that provides IMV?

   Is the IMV continuous or demand flow?

3. What are your observations from the determination of unknown exercise?

   A. Flowrate ______________________

   B. FI_{O_2} ______________________

   C. Assessment of function:

Scenario: You have been asked to consult on a difficult weaning case (Mr. Williams) in the medical intensive care unit. After consulting with the medical resident and your supervisor, you have been given permission to review Mr. Williams' case and to assume personal responsibility for his weaning. As you review the case, you discover that every Friday night, usually between 9:00 p.m. and 12:00 a.m., someone switches Mr. Williams from the IMV mode (internal) to assist/control with a control rate of 10 breaths/minute. You have changed Mr. Williams' ventilator from one with internal IMV to one with external IMV. Please answer the following questions:

1. What is one indication for the use of IMV?

2. What would occur if the supplemental gas flow to the external IMV setup:
   A. exceeded 15 liters/minute?
   B. was inadvertently decreased to 5 liters/minute?

3. Draw a simple schematic of an external IMV setup. Be sure to indicate gas flow through the diagram. Clearly label one-way valves.

4. What would occur if the IMV setup was assembled with the one-way valve in the wrong direction?

5. In Mr. Williams' case, why would changing from IMV to assist/control make weaning more difficult?

6. When using external IMV, how is the oxygen concentration to the IMV controlled?

7. Can PEEP and IMV be administered simultaneously?

8. What differentiates CPAP from IMV?

9. What hazards, if any, are associated with IMV?

chapter 47

Ventilator weaning and pressure support ventilation

INTRODUCTION

There is no absolute technique used to wean patients from mechanical ventilation. Each patient has a unique medical history associated with the reason(s) that he needed mechanical ventilation in the first place. Therefore, each patient must be considered separately when the weaning process begins.

There are some standardized guidelines used before every weaning attempt. First, the patient's general condition must be improved or stable. Some general factors must be optimized before weaning, such as the following:

1. Normal acid-base status
2. Stable cardiac status (no arrhythmias)
3. Adequate nutritional intake
4. Normal electrolyte status
5. No fever or infection

Pulmonary mechanics test a patient's ability to perform the muscular work of breathing. Pulmonary mechanics (see previous laboratory exercise) should be completed at least twice each day during the patient's ventilator course. In this way, trends can be detected. The pulmonary mechanics test values acceptable for weaning are as follows:

1. Vital capacity: $\geq$ 15 ml/kg
2. Minute ventilation: 6-10 liters
3. Respiratory frequency: $<$25-30 breaths/minute
4. Tidal volume: $\geq$ 7 ml/kg
5. Negative inspiratory force: ≤ -25 cm H_2O

The patient's ability to oxygenate must also be assessed before weaning. The physiologic measurements that may indicate acceptable oxygenation are as follows:

1. Alveolar-arterial oxygen difference: $PA\text{-}aO_2 < 300\text{-}350$ mm Hg (FI_{O_2} 1.0)
2. Partial pressure of arterial oxygen $>$ 60 mm Hg ($FI_{O_2} \leq 0.40$)
3. Shunt fraction $<$ 15%

Three methods are commonly used to wean patients from mechanical ventilation: T-piece trials of spontaneous breathing, intermittent mandatory ventilation (IMV), and synchronized intermittent mandatory ventilation (SIMV) and pressure support ventilation (PSV). There are advantages and disadvantages to each method. You must choose the method that will work best for each patient. In general, T-piece trial is used for patients who have been ventilated for short periods, and IMV may be used for patients who have been ventilated for a moderate amount of time. PSV can be used for patients who may not meet the pulmonary mechanics criteria and have been difficult to wean.

Pressure support ventilation (PSV) is a novel form of mechanical ventilation. Because of its relative newness, a definite protocol still needs to be established; however, there are guidelines that can be implemented to assure patient safety.

PSV augments spontaneous breaths with a set amount of pressure. During a spontaneous inspiration, a set amount of pressure is supplied while the patient controls the inspiratory flow, time, and volume. The airway flow, volume, and pressure curves during PSV are shown in Figure 47-1. PSV appears to optimize respiratory muscle function in patients with respiratory failure. The advantages of PSV are a reduction in patient ventilatory work that results in a more efficient and comfortable spontaneous breathing pattern and a shift in the character of the patient's work of breathing to optimize respiratory muscle reconditioning.

PSV can be applied during SIMV, IMV, or CPAP modes. Many newer mechanical ventilators offer the option of PSV. Some examples of ventilators that offer the PSV mode include the Puritan Bennett 7200, Siemens Servo 900C, and Bourns Bear 5.

PSV may be used to wean patients from mechanical ventilation. The initial pressure support level is determined by the exhaled pressure support volume. The amount of pressure support should result in a spontaneous tidal volume (VT) of 10 to 12 ml/kg of body weight. The frequency of mandatory breaths given in addition to the pressure supported breaths is determined by the Pa_{CO_2}. When patients are on pressure support

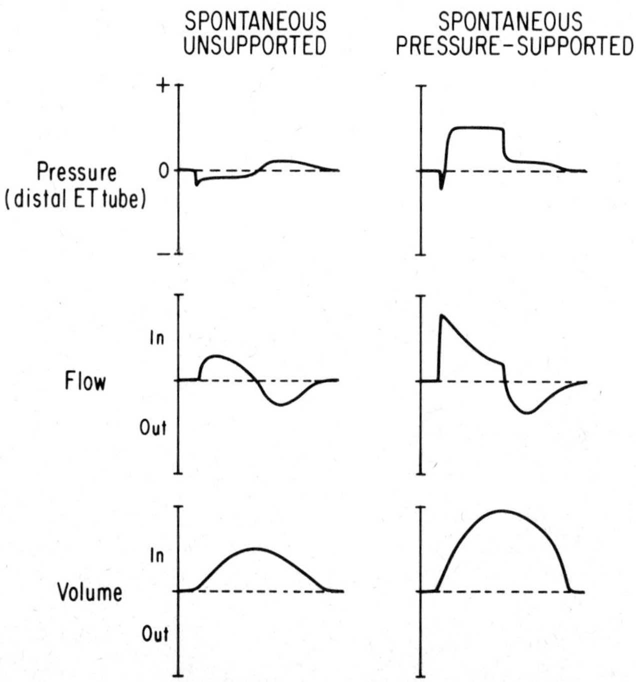

Fig. 47-1. Airway flow, volume, and pressure curves during pressure support ventilation. *(Courtesy of Neil R. MacIntyre, M.D.)*

and SIMV or IMV, the mandatory breath rate should be gradually decreased as tolerated before reducing the pressure support level.

PSV can also be used to overcome the airway resistance of flow through an endotracheal tube. Subjective evidence indicates that low level PSV provides for increased patient comfort. The purpose of this chapter is to introduce you to the techniques of ventilator weaning and pressure support ventilation.

OBJECTIVES

After completing this chapter, you should be able to do the following:

1. *Identify three methods of ventilator weaning.*
2. *Demonstrate the use of IMV and "T"-piece trials as used for weaning.*
3. *Identify two methods of PSV.*
4. *Demonstrate the use of PSV as indicated for weaning a patient from mechanical ventilation.*
5. *Demonstrate the use of low level PSV as indicated to overcome airflow resistance.*

EQUIPMENT NEEDED

- ☐ Ventilator with a pressure support option (i.e., Siemens-Servo 900C, Puritan Bennett 7200, Bear 5)
- ☐ Mechanical lung or lung analog
- ☐ Ventilator with IMV mode
- ☐ Heated nebulizer
- ☐ Ventilator breathing circuit
- ☐ Briggs "T"-piece adapter
- ☐ Oxygen and air flowmeter or oxygen blender

ACTIVITIES

Exercise A: Initiation of Weaning Using IMV

Patient Situation: Mr. Stevens is a 53 kg man who has been ventilated for 3 days. His initial diagnosis was ventilatory failure caused by pneumonia. He is being treated with antibiotics and is now afebrile. His chest x-ray film shows clearing of previous consolidation. His present ventilator settings are as follows:

- ☐ Frequency: 15 breaths/minute
- ☐ FI_{O_2}: 0.40
- ☐ Tidal volume: 800 ml
- ☐ Flowrate: 50 liters/minute
- ☐ PEEP: 0

Mr. Stevens' arterial blood gas values and pulmonary mechanics results suggest that ventilator weaning is indicated. The physician in charge wants to use IMV. Mr. Stevens' vital signs are BP 110/70, pulse 70/minute, and spontaneous frequency 15/minute.

1. Set up a ventilator according to the above settings using a mechanical lung or lung analog.
2. On your laboratory report, note the measurements that would indicate Mr. Stevens is ready for weaning.
3. Explain the procedure to Mr. Stevens.
4. Switch the ventilator mode to IMV.

5. Decrease the IMV rate to 13 breaths/minute.
6. In the clinical setting, arterial blood gases (ABGs) would be obtained in 15 to 30 minutes.
7. Assuming the ABGs are acceptable and the other psysiologic variables remain stable, continue weaning. The IMV rate should be decreased in increments of 2 breaths per adjustment.
8. The ventilator can be discontinued when the patient tolerates an IMV rate of zero for 20 minutes.

Exercise B: Initiation of Weaning Using "T"-Piece Trials

1. Reconsider the previous patient situation. In this case, Mr. Stevens' physician wants him weaned using "T"-piece trials.
2. Set up a Briggs "T"-piece with corregated tubing, reservoir tubing, and heated nebulizer. Set the FI_{O_2} at 0.45 at a flow of 10 to 15 liters/minute. Nebulization should be delivered at 37°C. Analyze the FI_{O_2}.
3. Explain the procedure to the patient.
4. Attach the Briggs "T"-piece to an intubated mannequin.
5. Simulate monitoring of vital signs by using your laboratory partner. Vital signs should be monitored every 5 minutes and the "T"-piece trial discontinued if the vital signs change in the following manner:
   - A. Blood pressure: increase or decrease 10 mm Hg
   - B. Pulse increase > 20/minute
   - C. Respiratory frequency: increase > 10 breaths/minute

   In a real clinical situation, the trial would also be terminated if the patient experienced severe anxiety or instability in the physiologic measurements mentioned previously.
6. Return the mannequin to the ventilator on the original settings.
7. In a clinical situation, if ABGs were acceptable, another "T"-piece trial would be attempted in the next hour. Trial durations would increase in increments of 5 to 15 minutes per hour as tolerated. When the patient tolerates 45 to 60 minutes of spontaneous breathing, weaning can progress more rapidly.

Exercise C: Demonstration of Use of PSV in Weaning a Simulated Patient from Mechanical Ventilation

Patient Situation: Ms. Baker is a 45 kg postcardiac surgery patient. She has received ventilation for 24 hours. Ms. Baker has been heavily sedated, but now the sedation level has decreased.

1. Assemble a ventilator for patient use.
2. Adjust the ventilator controls for full ventilatory support in the IMV or SIMV mode. Have your instructor check these initial settings.
3. Attach the ventilator to the mechanical lung.
4. Add pressure support. The level of PSV should result in a spontaneous V_T of 10 to 12 ml/kg. You will need to simulate spontaneous breathing by manually compressing the mechanical lung. Adjust the level of pressure support by adjusting the pressure support control or selecting the value on the numerical key pad.
5. Observe the pressure manometer at peak pressure support (spontaneous) inspiration. The peak pressure should be ≤ the "peak pressure" during a mandatory breath.
6. On your laboratory report, chart the arterial blood gas results that would indicate Ms. Baker is ready for weaning.
7. Proceed to wean Ms. Baker. You would do this by decreasing the IMV rate by 2

breaths every 15 to 30 minutes, obtaining arterial blood gases with each increment decrease. For laboratory purposes, these decreases can be done very rapidly.

8. When you have decreased the IMV rate to zero, begin to decrease the pressure support level by increments of 3 to 5 cm H_2O.
9. Discontinue the ventilator when the pressure support level is 3 to 5 cm H_2O. In a clinical setting, oxygenation must also be considered before the ventilator can be discontinued.

Exercise D: Demonstration of Use of Low-Level PSV When Used with PEEP

1. Adjust the ventilator controls as you did in Exercise C for Ms. Baker. If you did not use PEEP, please add 5 cm H_2O at this time.
2. Add 5 cm H_2O pressure support.
3. Simulate spontaneous respirations by manually compressing the mechanical test lung. Be certain that your compression creates adequate pressure.
4. At peak pressure support inspiration, the manometer should read 5 cm H_2O pressure support plus 5 cm H_2O PEEP.

RECOMMENDED READING

Blodgett DJ: Manual of Respiratory Care Procedures. Philadelphia, JB Lippincott, 1980

Burton GG, Hodgkin JE: Respiratory Care. A Guide to Clinical Practice, 2nd ed. Philadelphia, JB Lippincott, 1984

MacIntyre NR: Respiratory function during pressure support ventilation. Chest 89:677–683, 1986

McPherson SP, Spearman CB: Respiratory Therapy Equipment, 3rd ed. St Louis, CV Mosby, 1985

Prakash O, Meij S: Cardiopulmonary response to inspiratory pressure support during spontaneous ventilation vs. conventional ventilation. Chest 88: 403–408, 1985

Shapiro BA, Harrison RA, Kacmarek RM, Cane RD: Clinical Application of Respiratory Care, 3rd ed. Chicago, Year Book Medical Publishers, 1985

Laboratory Performance Evaluation (#47)

Topic: Ventilator Weaning and Pressure Support Ventilation

Student ______________________ Course ______________________

Date ______________________ Section ______________________

Performance Elements	Acceptable	Unacceptable	Not Applicable	Comments
1. Thoroughly reviews CMV log of simulated weaning situation				
2. Evaluates cardiovascular and oxygenation status				
3. Obtains necessary equipment for performing bedside pulmonary mechanics				
4. Washes hands				
5. Performs bedside pulmonary mechanics				
6. Suggests appropriate weaning technique				
7. Obtains order for initiating weaning procedures.				
8. Initiates prescribed weaning procedure A. IMV B. T-tube C. Pressure support ventilation				
9. Monitors status of simulated patient immediately after initiation of weaning.				
10. Logs obtained results in CMV monitoring log				
11. Signs or initials monitoring log				

Knowledge of Procedure

- ☐ Good; student is knowledgeable about rationale and theory related to procedure
- ☐ Fair; student has adequate understanding of rationale and theory related to procedure
- ☐ Poor; student has inadequate understanding of rationale and theory related to procedure

Performance Deficiencies (check those that apply)

- ☐ Excessive time needed to complete procedure
- ☐ Broke aseptic or sterile technique
- ☐ Gross inaccuracy noted
- ☐ Technique may be harmful to patient
- ☐ Incorrect dosage or gas concentration
- ☐ Incorrect equipment assembly/use
- ☐ Unable to answer questions correctly about rationale and/or theory related to procedure
- ☐ Other ______________________________

Evaluation Summary

- ☐ Satisfactory performance
- ☐ Unsatisfactory performance

Recommendations of Evaluator

- ☐ Skills may be applied/observed in clinical setting
- ☐ Specific evaluation deficiencies require correction
- ☐ Complete re-evaluation required
- ☐ Additional laboratory practice required

Signatures:

Evaluator ______________________ Date ______________________

Student ______________________ Date ______________________

Laboratory Report

Student ______________________ Acceptable ______________________

Date ______________________ Unacceptable ______________________

Course ______________________

Topic: Ventilator Weaning and Pressure Support Ventilation

Review Questions

1. Fill in the following values that indicate Mr. Stevens (from Exercise A) is ready for weaning.

   Vital capacity (VC) ______________________

   Minute ventilation (VE) ______________________

   Frequency (f) ______________________

   Tidal volume (VT) ______________________

   Negative inspiratory force (NIF) ______________________

2. Fill in the following values that indicate that Mr. Stevens' "T"-piece trial can be continued.

   BP ______________________

   Pulse ______________________

   Frequency ______________________

3. Fill in the ABG values that indicate that Ms. Baker is ready for weaning.

   pH ______________________

   Pa_{CO_2} ______________________

   Pa_{O_2} ______________________

   HCO_3 ______________________

   O_2 Sat. ______________________

4. What will the pressure manometer read at peak pressure support (spontaneous) inspiration in the following example:

   PIP = 30 cmH_2O
   f = 10 breaths/minute
   Mode = IVM
   PEEP = 5 cm H_2O
   Pressure support = 20 cm H_2O

5. Explain two methods of pressure support and when it is appropriate to use each method.

6. Ms. Carter has been mechanically ventilated for 2 weeks. She is on assist/control. Briggs "T"-piece trials have been attempted several times but were unsuccessful. Ms. Carter's original diagnosis was respiratory failure secondary to COPD. Explain why Ms. Carter might benefit from pressure support ventilation.

Mr. White has been on the Bear 5 ventilator for 8 days. His ventilator settings are as follows:

f = 12 breaths/minute
VT = 800 ml
FI_{O_2} = 0.35
Flowrate = 45 liters/minute
PEEP = 0

7. A physician wants pressure support added to the ventilator settings in an attempt to begin weaning.

   A. How can you determine what level of pressure support will be appropriate for Mr. White?

   B. After pressure support is initiated, explain the step-by-step procedure you would use to wean Mr. White.

chapter 48

Oximetry and capnography

INTRODUCTION

Oximetry and capnography are both noninvasive techniques used in monitoring and analyzing respiratory gases. Oximetry is used to measure oxygen saturation of hemoglobin and is indicated whenever a noninvasive measurement of oxygen saturation is desired. Some examples in which oximetry may be used include weaning during continuous mechanical ventilation, exercise testing, pulmonary rehabilitation, fiberoptic bronchoscopy, anesthesia, and sleep apnea studies.

Capnography is used to monitor the concentration of carbon dioxide (PE_{CO_2}) in exhaled gas. Changes in metabolism (CO_2 production), circulation, and ventilation will alter PE_{CO_2}. The graphic recording of CO_2 in exhaled gas is referred to as a capnogram.

Capnography can be used to detect any of the following conditions: hyperventilation, CO_2 retention, and apnea. It is also useful when changes in exhaled CO_2 should be closely monitored in conditions such as weaning from mechanical ventilation and during surgery. The purpose of this chapter is to introduce you to the noninvasive monitoring techniques of capnography and oximetry.

OBJECTIVES

After completing this chapter, you should be able to do the following:

1. *Perform noninvasive gas measurements using an oximeter and a capnograph.*
2. *Prepare an oximeter and capnograph for patient use.*
3. *Obtain a capnogram tracing.*
4. *Obtain arterial oxygen saturation (Sa_{O_2}) using an oximeter and exhaled carbon dioxide (PE_{CO_2}) measurements using a capnograph.*
5. *Observe and measure the effects of exercise on Sa_{O_2} and PE_{CO_2}.*
6. *State indications for use of oximetry and capnography.*

ACTIVITIES

Exercise A: Preparation of an Oximeter for Patient Use

1. Consult your instructor or the technical manual for calibration instructions. Calibrate the oximeter before use to ensure accuracy.
2. Turn oximeter on and allow it to warm up.

Exercise B: Preparation of the Patient and Obtainment of Baseline Sa_{O_2} Measurement

1. Explain the procedure to your laboratory partner.
2. If using the ear lobe probe, promote vascularization of the ear lobe.
   - **A.** Massage ear lobe with an isopropyl alcohol pad for 10 to 20 seconds.
   - **B.** A mild redness signifies sufficient vascularization.
   - **C.** Apply the ear probe on the ear lobe.
   - **D.** Center the ear probe on the fleshy part of the lobe.
3. If using the finger probe, attach to the fingertip (Fig. 48-1).
4. Wait the appropriate length of time for the oximeter to stabilize. (Consult your instructor or technical manual.)
5. Obtain an Sa_{O_2} measurement as displayed on the front panel readout. This is your baseline value. Note this value on your laboratory report.
6. Set high and low alarms (2% above and below value obtained), if desired.

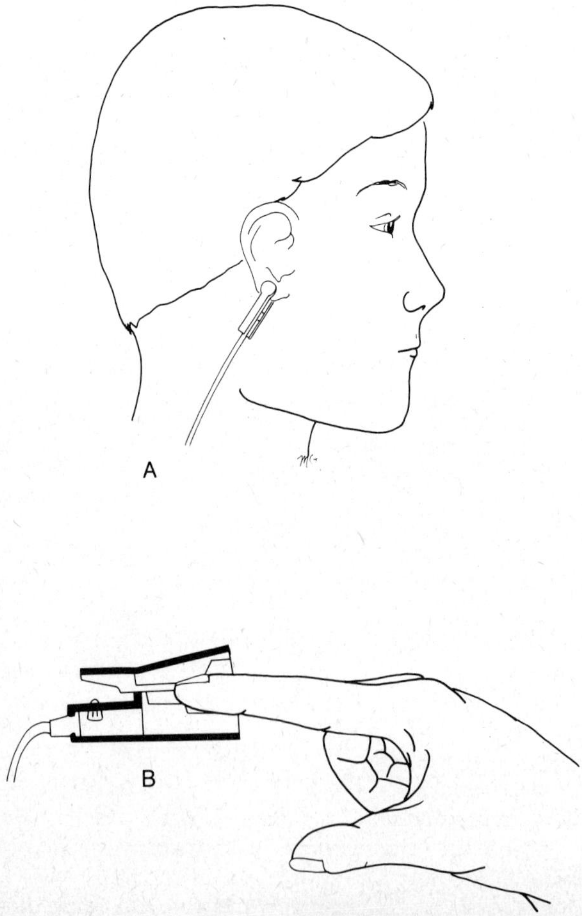

Fig. 48-1. A. Ear lobe oximetry probe. **B.** Fingertip oximetry probe.

Exercise C: Obtainment of Sa_{O_2} Measurement During Exercise

1. Leave ear or finger probe attached to your laboratory partner as described in Exercise B.
2. Have your laboratory partner jog in place for 5 minutes.
3. Obtain an Sa_{O_2} measurement after 4½ minutes while jogging is still taking place. Note this reading on your laboratory report.
4. Disconnect the ear probe and turn oximeter power off.

Exercise D: Preparation of a Capnograph for Patient Use

1. Consult your instructor or the technical manual for calibrating instructions. Calibrate the capnograph before use to ensure accuracy. A calibration gas of approximately 5% CO_2 and 95% air is often used to calibrate a capnograph.
2. Explain the procedure to your laboratory partner.
3. Turn power on and allow sufficient time for warmup.
4. Attach sampling tube to capnograph.
5. Connect sampling tube that is supplied with the capnograph to your laboratory partner by taping it to the skin at the nose. The tube should go into the nostril about ½ to ¾ of an inch. If you were using this with an intubated patient, the sample gas would be taken through an adapter connected between the wye and the tracheal tube (Fig. 48-2).

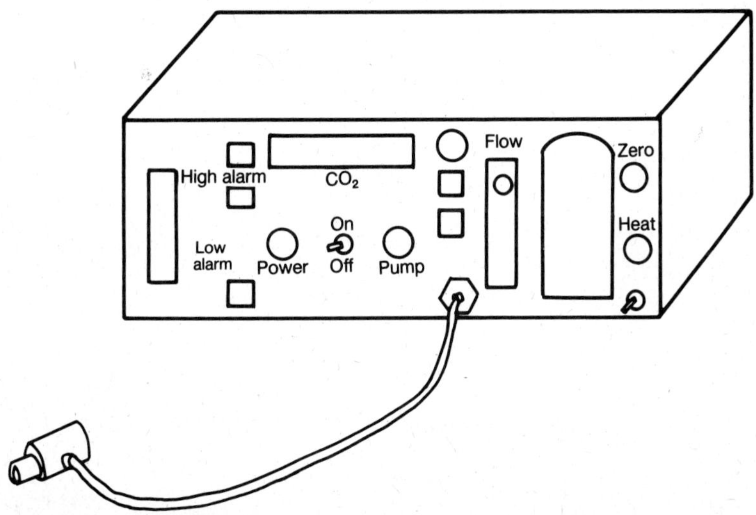

Fig. 48-2. Capnograph and adapter for mechanical ventilator wye connector.

Exercise E: Obtainment of a Baseline PE_{CO_2} Measurement

1. Have your laboratory partner breathe normally for 3 minutes.
2. Record the highest PE_{CO_2} reading obtained on your laboratory report. This will be your baseline value.
3. Set high and low alarms 5% above and below the baseline value desired.

Exercise F: Obtainment of a Capnogram Tracing

1. While your laboratory partner continues to breathe normally, turn the recorder at a fast speed so that phases of exhalation can be distinguished (Fig. 48-3).
2. Remove capnogram and attach it to your laboratory report.

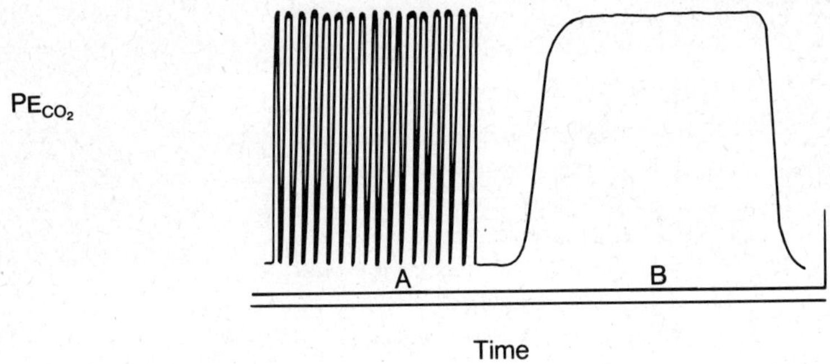

Fig. 48-3. Sample capnogram at (A) slow speed and (B) high speed. *(Courtesy of IL Laboratories, Lexington, MA)*

Exercise G: Observation and Measurement of the Effects of Exercise on PE_{CO_2}

1. Have your laboratory partner jog in place for 5 minutes while still connected to the capnograph.
2. Obtain PE_{CO_2} measurement after 4½ minutes. Record this value on your laboratory report.

RECOMMENDED READING

Kinasewitz G: Use of end-trial capnography during mechanical ventilation. Respir J 27:2, February 1982

Kochansky M: Ear oximetry as a method of determining home oxygen prescriptions. Respir Care, 29:12, December 1984

Rebuck A, D'uzzo A: The accuracy and response characteristics of a simplified ear oximeter. Chest 83(6), June 1983

Laboratory Performance Evaluation (#48)

Topic: Capnography and Oximetry

Student ______________________ Course ______________________

Date ______________________ Section ______________________

Performance Elements	Acceptable	Unacceptable	Not Applicable	Comments
1. Obtains necessary equipment and supplies				
2. Identifies components of oximeter				
3. Identifies components of capnograph				
4. Prepares (calibrates) device				
5. Washes hands				
6. Prepares sample site (simulated patient)				
7. Attaches sensor to prepared sampling site				
8. Uses proper technique to obtain baseline measurement				
9. Obtains correct reading from device				
10. Obtains correct oximetry results: A. Resting B. Exercise				
11. Obtains correct capnography results: A. Resting B. Exercise				
12. Documents obtained results				

Knowledge of Procedure

☐ Good; student is knowledgeable about rationale and theory related to procedure

☐ Fair; student has adequate understanding of rationale and theory related to procedure

☐ Poor; student has inadequate understanding of rationale and theory related to procedure

Performance Deficiencies (check those that apply)

☐ Excessive time needed to complete procedure

☐ Broke aseptic or sterile technique

☐ Gross inaccuracy noted

☐ Technique may be harmful to patient

☐ Incorrect dosage or gas concentration

☐ Incorrect equipment assembly/use

☐ Unable to answer questions correctly about rationale and/or theory related to procedure

☐ Other ______________________________

Evaluation Summary

☐ Satisfactory performance

☐ Unsatisfactory performance

Recommendations of Evaluator

☐ Skills may be applied/observed in clinical setting

☐ Specific evaluation deficiencies require correction

☐ Complete re-evaluation required

☐ Additional laboratory practice required

Signatures:

Evaluator ____________________ Date ____________________

Student ____________________ Date ____________________

Laboratory Report

Student ______________________ Acceptable ______________________

Date ______________________ Unacceptable ______________________

Course ______________________

Topic: Oximetry and Capnography

Data or Measurements

1. Values obtained from the ear or finger oximetry:

   A. Baseline Sa_{O_2} ______________________

   B. Exercise Sa_{O_2} ______________________

2. What values were obtained from ear oximetry?

   A. Baseline exhaled CO_2 ______________________

   B. Exercise exhaled CO_2 ______________________

3. Attach the CO_2 tracing obtained below.

Scenario: You have assumed responsibility for weaning Mr. Jones from his mechanical ventilator. Currently, he is using a combination of pressure support and intermittent mandatory ventilation (IMV). If his progress continues, he will be gradually placed on IMV only and then the ultimate test, T-tube trials. In an attempt to find your approach to weaning Mr. Jones, you are continuously monitoring his oxygen and carbon dioxide levels using capnography and oximetry. The use of capnography and oximetry has also alleviated any fears among the night nursing staff that they may not notice if he becomes fatigued and suffers a respiratory arrest. Please answer the following questions:

1. Specifically, how may oximetry and capnography be useful in determining the exercise tolerance of Mr. Jones?

2. Could capnography be used to assess Mr. Jones' deadspace to tidal volume ratios?

3. Specifically, how would you use oximetry to determine the BEST FI_{O_2} for Mr. Jones?

4. Could oximetry be used as a guide for changing the FI_{O_2} during situational changes (for example, increased FI_{O_2} during eating)?

5. How might capnography be useful in the intensive care nursery?

6. Compare and contrast oximetry and transcutaneous gas analysis?

7. What hazards, if any, are associated with oximetry and capnography?

8. State two indications for monitoring Sa_{O_2}.

9. Name three situations in which the exhaled PE_{CO_2} values would be abnormal?

10. What was the effect of exercise on Sa_{O_2}, and what is a possible explanation for the change, if any?

